withdrawn
12/6/23

MRI Handbook

MRI Handbook

MR Physics, Patient Positioning, and Protocols

Muhammed Elmaoğlu
Department of Medical Imaging Technologies
Yeni Yüzyıl University, Yılanlı Ayazma Caddesi 26,
Cevizlibağ Topkapı, Istanbul, Turkey

Azim Çelik, PhD
General Electric Medical Systems
Siteler Mah. 1313 Sokak, Tuncaylar Sitesi A Blok Kat: 9 No: 20
Antalya, Turkey

Foreword by
Muzaffer Basak

Springer

Azim Çelik, PhD
General Electric Medical Systems
Siteler Mah. 1313 Sokak
Tuncaylar Sitesi A Blok Kat: 9
No: 20, Antalya, Turkey
azim.celik@yahoo.com

Muhammed Elmaoğlu
Department of Medical
Imaging Technologies
Yeni Yüzyil University
Yilanli Ayazma Caddesi 26
Cevizlibağ Topkapi
Istanbul, Turkey
Muhammed.Elmaoglu@ge.com

ISBN 978-1-4614-1095-9 e-ISBN 978-1-4614-1096-6
DOI 10.1007/978-1-4614-1096-6
Springer New York Dordrecht Heidelberg London

Library of Congress Control Number: 2011938684

Printed on acid-free paper

Springer is part of Springer Science+Business Media (www.springer.com)

This book is dedicated to my late father, late mother, my dear wife and my two beautiful children.

Azim Çelik

Preface

After the first MR image was acquired in experimental phantom tubes almost 40 years ago, magnetic resonance imaging (MRI) has developed significantly and become one of today's most interesting and irreplaceable imaging modalities. MRI is used to find answers to medical questions by utilizing various contrast mechanisms independently or in combination, which is different from other imaging modalities. However, using an MRI system effectively depends mainly on a good understanding of underlying physical principles, correct use of the MR protocols, correct patient positioning, and graphical prescription. These main sections form the basis of a good MR scanning routine in clinical practice.

In this book, MRI principles, patient positioning, and protocols are explained in a very easy to understand manner and supported with hundreds of pictures for everyday routine clinical scanning. The book itself is based on the 25 years of combined, unique experience of the authors on teaching MRI principles, creating protocols, teaching routines, and advanced MRI in many different countries. We have witnessed again and again that MRI scanning and applications may differ significantly depending on countries and institutes. Therefore, we organized this book in an easy to follow manner with intuitive sections, so that anyone can look up a specific topic or entire section very easily as described below.

Basic MRI Principles: From Chaps. 1–5, basic MRI principles that anybody who works or plans to work with an MRI should know are explained in a clear and concise manner. For cross-reference among different MR manufacturers, pulse sequence naming tables are created to include the old and new pulse sequences.

MR safety, patient positioning, graphical prescription, and protocol examples: From Chaps. 6–11 the practical scanning information for MR users are given in easy to follow sections, supported by pictures and protocol tables. Based on patient safety, these chapters are designed to explain tips and tricks for best MR image quality with coil positioning, patient positioning, graphical prescriptions, and sample protocols. This book is a product of a diligent and intensive work and we believe that it will guide you to understand how to get excellent MRI images. We truly hope that this book will be a great resource for all MR technicians, radiology specialists, assistants, research associates, and everyone who wants to learn MRI.

Azim Çelik, PhD
Muhammed Elmaoğlu, RT

Foreword

Dear Reader,

Magnetic resonance imaging has almost always been one of the most difficult imaging modalities to learn due to its somewhat complicated physical principles and difficulties of "fine tuning" the protocols for patients. However, it has always been the center of attention due to its noninvasive and safer nature for clinical routine.

There have been a number of books published recently on MRI by respectable colleagues explaining MRI, its principles, and clinical applications. These books brought tremendous wealth of knowledge to the MRI community and are well appreciated by many radiologists all over the world. However, the book you are holding is completely different than what I have seen so far. It explains the MRI physics in a very easy to understand manner and more importantly provides much needed information on patient positioning, graphical prescriptions, and protocols in pictures. The saying "A picture is worth a thousand words" is the best way to describe this book I believe. Even though I am aware that each institute has their own techniques and protocols they use for everyday routine, based on American College of Radiology (ACR) recommendations, this book can be a reference book for MR radiographers who want a new way of scanning or additional ways of scanning to improve their work practices.

I would like to congratulate the authors for taking their time to write this very valuable book and hope that it will contribute significantly to the MRI community.

Istanbul, Turkey — Muzaffer Basak

Contents

Part I

Basic MRI Principles

Chapter 1

A Brief History of Magnetic Resonance Imaging

Magnetic resonance imaging is one of the most important imaging modalities in our modern world. We strongly believe that it is very important to remember and honor the many outstanding people who contributed to magnetic resonance. The next few pages are devoted to introduce the readers a brief history of magnetic resonance imaging and hope that you enjoy it as much as we do.

The Beginning

It is somewhat difficult to exactly define the beginning of magnetic resonance imaging. However, we would like to honor the famous mathematician *Jean Baptiste-Joseph Fourier* as one of the early contributors due to his Fourier Transform theory. The Fourier Transform is one of the most essential foundations of magnetic resonance imaging.

Felix Bloch and *Edward Purcell* can be surely named as the inventors of nuclear magnetic resonance (NMR) in real terms. However, other scientists working on proton spins starting from 1920s had also quite important findings. Specifically, in 1924, *Wolfgang Pauli* started talking about the nuclear spin concept. Following year, *George Eugene Uhlenbeck* and *Samuel A. Goudsmit* drew attention to the electron's rotation around the nucleus. In 1926, *Pauli* and *Charles Alton Darvin* adapted the electron spin concept to quantum mechanics theory developed by *Edwin Schrödinger* and *Werner Heisenberg*. The theoretical basis of NMR continued to be formed with smaller steps during 1930s. In 1933, *Otto Stern* and *Walther Gerlach* were first to show the magnetic

M. Elmaoğlu and A. Çelik, *MRI Handbook: MR Physics, Patient Positioning, and Protocols*, DOI 10.1007/978-1-4614-1096-6_1,

moments of protons' hydrogen atoms by diffracting beams of these atoms. Their experiments have also been the experimental proof of the most important physical basis of magnetic resonance, low- and high-energy proton levels.

I.I. Rabi, at Columbia University (New York) laboratories, worked intensively on these topics. Although the early studies of *Rabi* were considered to be successful, his experiments failed to prove the fundamental concept of magnetic resonance and magnetic moments. However, his visit to *Cornelis Jacobus Gorter* laboratories in Holland made a big difference. *Gorter* was working on the same subject and he made some suggestions to *Rabi*. Afterwards, *Rabi* succeeded to show magnetic moments and published his well-known article titled "*A New Method of Measuring Nuclear Magnetic Moment.*"

In 1946, two scientists (*Felix Bloch* and *Edward Purcell*) working independently described a physicochemical phenomenon of the certain nuclei in the periodic table. Their invention is considered to be the start of NMR by many people, and *Bloch* and *Purcell* were awarded the *Nobel Prize* in 1952.

Purcell was born in Illinois, USA. After working at Massachusetts Institute of Technology (MIT), he joined Harvard University. *Bloch* was born in 1905 in Zurich. He lectured at Leipzig University until 1933 and, in 1934, he joined Stanford University. Later on, he returned back to Zurich and died there in 1983.

Following *Bloch* and *Purcel's* seminal work, scientists continued to work on NMR concept. Until 1970s, the studies made a significant progress on NMR and became the cornerstone of modern magnetic resonance imaging. These key studies were:

- In 1955/1956, Erik Odeblad and Gunnar from Stockholm published the results of their studies on the properties of living cells and the relaxation times.
- Between 1956 and 1970, a great deal of studies were done on the T1 and T2 relaxation times of the blood and muscle T1 and T2 relaxation times, diffusion concept, and intracellular and extracellular water exchange.
- Between 1960 and 1970, NMR signals were acquired from animal models.

Design of the First MR Scanner

In 1972, *Raymond Damadian* (Downstate Medical Centre, Brooklyn) measured the T1 and T2 relaxation times of the normal tissue and tumor in rats and showed that tumors had longer relaxation times using an NMR apparatus. These studies can be considered as the first clinically relevant studies of NMR.

Damadian filed for a patent for an NMR apparatus without going into details on this subject.

Studies on Blood Flow Volume Measurement with MRI

Flow measurements with MRI started in 1980s in true sense. However, in 1959, *Jay Singer* studied the relaxation properties of blood. Later in 1967, *Alexander Ganssen*, invented an NMR scanner consisting of a number of small coils to measure the blood flow in whole body. At this point of the time, all the efforts were still on NMR scanners and they were significantly different than MRI scanners, as they did not have any imaging capabilities.

Development of Spatial Encoding Concept in MRI

In 1973, late *Paul Lauterbur* from University of Illinois – Urbana – Champaign came up with a bright idea of using gradients in three planes (Gx, Gy, and Gz) to excite the selected slice location (spatial encoding). Later on, Lauterbur used a back projection technique used for computed tomography and reconstructed the first ever MR image. Even though, *Erwin Hahn* used the gradients for developing spin echo concept earlier, Lauterbur's discovery made a revolution for MR imaging and paved the way for other researchers such as *Hinshaw, Andrew*, and *Moore*. The first ever reconstructed MR images of test tubes look quite simple but they marked the beginning of today's MRI.

Richard Ernst, thought about using Fourier Transformation instead of back projection technique after he attended a lecture of *Lauterbur* in North Carolina. In 1975, he successfully applied Fourier Transformation to image reconstruction.

Peter Mansfield from Nottigham improved the MRI technique with studies he did in 1973, 1975, and 1977. He further developed the utilization of gradients in magnetic field and created mathematical models in 1977 with *Andrew A. Maudsey*. He achieved to image a human finger and in 1978 they imaged an abdomen. *Mansfield* was the first to use the fundamental technique that today we call echo planar imaging (EPI).

The First MRI System

In 1974, Jim Hutchison, Bill Edelstein, and their colleagues from the University of Aberdeen, England, developed the first prototype MR equipment. These scientists imaged a rat by using spin echo technique and in 1980 they started to receive images by Ernst technique.

Development of Fast Imaging Techniques

By the end of 1970s, commercial companies saw the potential in MR and started commercial investments. Hence, studies on MR equipment accelerated. In 1986, *Hennig, A. Nauerth* and *Hartmut Friedburg* together developed quick imaging techniques today known as fast spin echo or turbo spin echo. In 1986, at the same time with *Hennig, Haase* and *Frahm* developed and started using the fast gradient echo technique, which is even faster than fast spin echo.

Clinical Applications

Early MR images were based on proton weighting. Later on T1-weighted imaging was also used clinically. In 1982–1983, when researchers realized that T2-weighted spin echo imaging shows pathologies better, T2-weighted imaging became an irreplaceable part of clinical MR imaging.

Contrast media that has a great effect on angiographic studies attracted attention in 1980s and Schering became the first company to apply for patent in 1981 for Gd-DTPA.

In 1987, EPI technique was used to scan a total phase of heart in real time, and in the same year, *Charles Dumoulin* succeeded to scan the blood vessels without contrast media by developing the magnetic resonance angiography.

In 1993, functional magnetic resonance imaging (fMRI) technique was developed by using EPI technique. Therefore, a technique developed for cardiac imaging became the main technique to investigate the unknowns of human brain. Since then, fMRI is still one of the most important research areas of MR imaging.

In 1994, researchers succeeded to scan lung by inhaling the hyperpolarized xenon gas (129Xe) at New York State Hospital in Stony Brook and in Princeton University.

In 1998, FDA (Food and Drug Administration) allowed the marketing of equipments up to 4 T. In 2002, again the same administration allowed the use of 3 T equipments on brain or body.

Equipments with higher magnetic field got attention of the clinicians as they improved the image quality while decreasing the scan time. These equipments are believed to contribute a great deal in spectroscopy, fMRI, diffusion tensor imaging, and MRA techniques.

In 2003, late Paul Lauterbur and Sir Peter Mansfield became the recipient of the Nobel Prize to acknowledge their outstanding contributions to the field of magnetic resonance imaging.

Chapter 2

Fundamentals of Magnetic Resonance Imaging

Concept of Magnetization

All the materials and living objects around us are composed of atoms. Atoms consist of three main particles that are positively charged protons, negatively charged electrons, and neutrons without any charge. The protons and neutrons are located within the nucleus of the atoms and electrons are located outside the nucleus as shown in Fig. 2.1a. The elements in the nature have additional properties called atomic weight and atomic number. Atomic number is simply the number of protons in the nucleus. Atomic weight is the sum of protons and neutrons in the nucleus. The most abundant atom in the human body is the hydrogen atom and it has the same atomic number and atomic weight, which is equal to one. All atoms can have the same atomic number. However, they can have different atomic weights (different number of neutrons) and those are called isotopes.

Positively charged protons in the nucleus continuously rotate around an axis and create their own magnetic field as shown in Fig. 2.1b. The magnetic field created by this proton will be oriented in the axis of rotation. Therefore, we can imagine this rotation and magnetization like a magnet bar with poles as shown in Fig. 2.2.

The magnetic field or magnetization is created with rotational motion of positively charged protons. As we have shown in Fig. 2.1b., this magnetization can be represented by a vector called magnetic vector. When this proton is placed within a magnetic field B_0, they start rotation or precessing around the

M. Elmaoğlu and A. Çelik, *MRI Handbook: MR Physics, Patient Positioning, and Protocols*, DOI 10.1007/978-1-4614-1096-6_2,

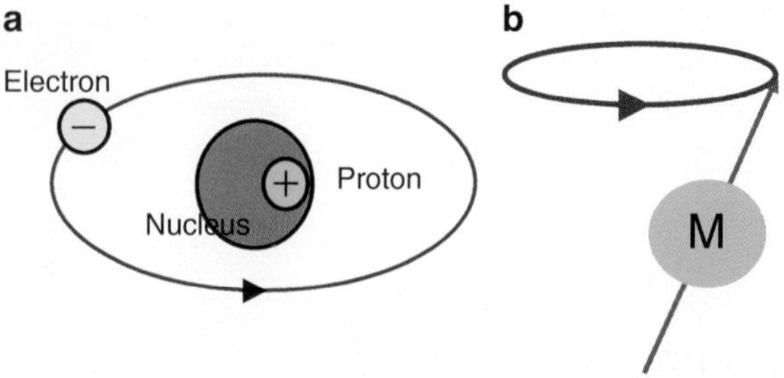

Figure 2.1 Composition of an atom (a) and postively charged protons' rotational motion (b).

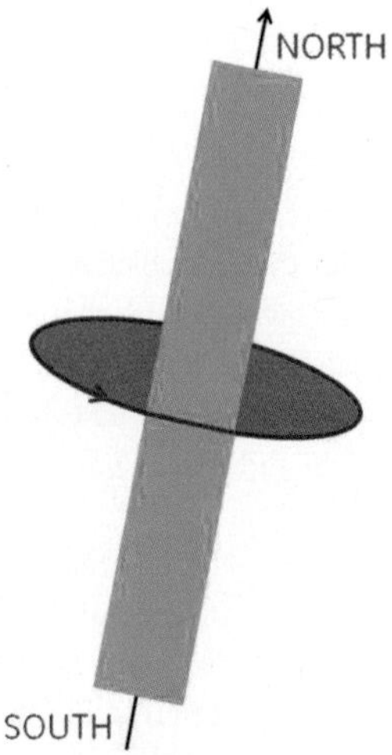

Figure 2.2 A magnet bar closely resembles the rotation and directional motion of positively charged proton.

axis (just like a gyroscope) of magnetic field direction. This interaction with the proton's magnetic vector and magnetic field B_0 creates magnetic resonance. Later in the book and also in many other MR physics-related books, you will read the term spin a lot and it is the right place to explain what it means. Spin is an important property of the nucleus and directly related to magnetic resonance. If a nucleus has an even atomic number and atomic weight, then, we can say that this nucleus has *no spin* and it is invisible to MR. In other words, those elements cannot be imaged with MRI. Luckily, all the elements in the nature with the exception of argon and cerium have at least one isotope that has a spin. A nucleus would have a fractional spin (such as 1/2, 3/2, or 5/2) if it has an odd atomic weight and an integer spin (such as 1, 2, or 3) if it has an even atomic weight and odd atomic number. Among all the nucleus in human body, ^{1}H nucleus has a ½ spin and it is the most abundant atom (present in 99.98% of the tissues) in the body. Therefore, it is the choice of nucleus in the majority of MRI scanning applications today. However, phosphorus (^{31}P), sodium (^{23}Na), and carbon (^{13}C) are also imaged with MRI for a number of applications and research as of today.

Magnetic Resonance and Static Magnetic Field Concepts

Now, we know that in human body, each atom with a spin behaves like a mini magnet bar with its own magnetization or magnetic vector. If we place those billions and billions of mini magnets within a large magnetic field (placing the patient on MR table into the magnet bore), these tiny magnetic vectors start interacting with the strong magnetic field (e.g., 1.5 T) and start rotating at a certain speed as we will define below. For a hydrogen proton, those magnetic vectors can be either parallel or antiparallel to the main magnetic field direction. Energy levels of protons determine whether they are parallel or antiparallel to the main magnetic field. We can say that protons parallel to static field have low energy levels and protons antiparallel to static field have high energy levels. To better understand this concept, we can consider swimmers in a river. A strong swimmer with high energy would be able to swim against the current in the river. However, a rather weak swimmer with low energy level would swim with the current in the river. From this simple analogy, we can remember that protons with low energy are like weaker swimmers: they cannot be aligned against the main static field.

A very interesting fact about protons is that the number of protons parallel to main magnetic field is slightly larger than the number of protons antiparallel to main static field. To be more specific, the difference between the number of protons parallel and antiparallel to main magnetic field is only *about* 45 out of 10 million protons at 1.5 T. Isn't it amazing ? Luckily, we have so many protons in the body that we approximately have 2×10^{15} more protons in a $1 \times 1 \times 5$-mm voxel producing the total magnetization (M_0), which is a vectoral summation of all the tiny magnetic vectors of each proton. Just to be clear, the above number (2×10^{15}) is not the total number of protons in the voxel but the difference between parallel and antiparallel protons in that small voxel.

The protons placed in a strong magnetic field start rotating around their axis at a frequency (number of loops per second) determined by a constant number and magnetic field strength. This rotational motion is called magnetic resonance and is defined by Larmor equation, the most essential equation of magnetic resonance:

$$w_o = \gamma * B_o, \tag{2.1}$$

where

γ = A proton-specific constant called GyroMagnetic Ratio. It is 42.57 MHz/T for hydrogen proton.

B_o = Applied main static field in the unit of Tesla (e.g., 3.0 T).

w_o = The rotational speed or frequency of the protons placed in the magnetic field in the unit of MHz (megahertz).

From this equation, we can simply calculate the Larmor frequency of hydrogen protons as 63.8 MHz at 1.5 T and 21.28 MHz at 0.5 T magnetic field (Fig. 2.3).

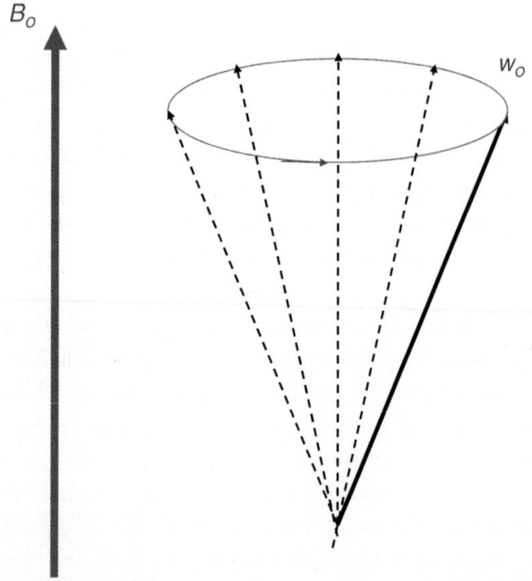

Figure 2.3 **The protons placed in static field B_0 immediately start rotating (resonating) with w_0 at counterclockwise direction.**

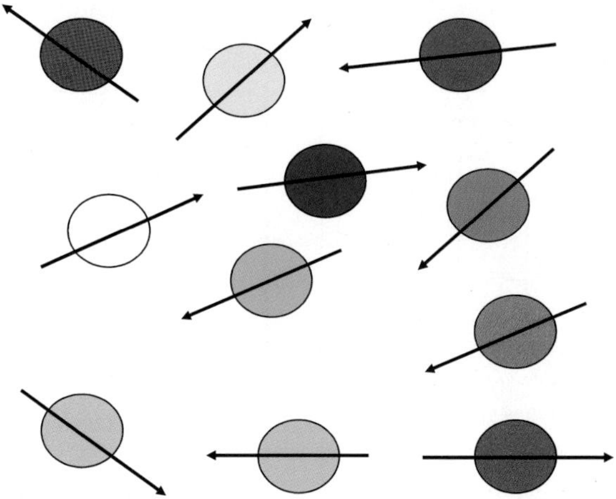

Figure 2.4 Magnetic vectors of the protons are randomly oriented when there is no external static field present.

When the protons are not exposed to an external strong magnetic field, they would still have a magnetization vector due to the earth's small magnetic field. However, in this case, they do align almost randomly in any direction as shown in Fig. 2.4. If we sum up all these individual magnetic vectors, we practically get zero total magnetization.

When we place all these randomly oriented protons in a strong magnetic field in the bore of an MRI scanner, these independent vectors becomes either parallel or antiparallel to main magnetic field. If we consider an unrealistic voxel with only 10 protons, let us assume that 6 orange-colored protons become parallel and 4 white-colored protons become antiparallel to 1.5 T main static field B_o as shown in, Fig. 2.5a. Then we end up having a net 2 protons creating, total magnetization in this voxel. If we double the main static field from 1.5 to 3.0 T, then 9 orange-colored protons would be parallel to the stronger magnetic field and only 1 white colored protons would be antiparallel to magnetic field as shown in Fig. 2.5b. Then, we end up having 8 protons creating the total magnetization. Therefore, we can increase the MR signal fourfold by doubling the main static field from 1.5 to 3.0 T. However, in this case, the noise in the voxel is doubled and we can claim only a twofold real MR signal increase.

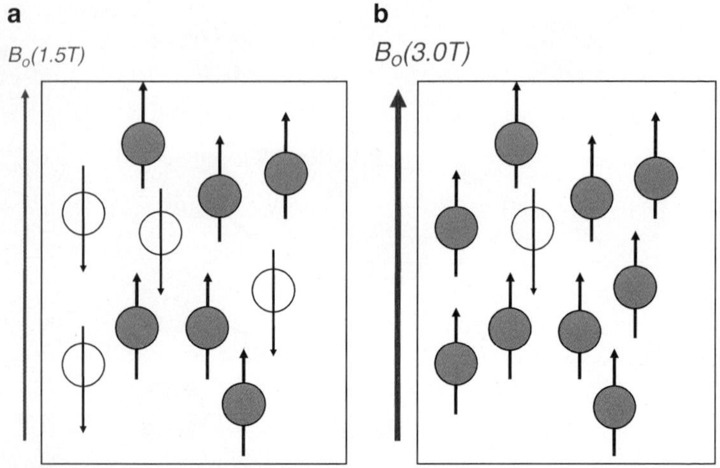

Figure 2.5 Protons' magnetic vectors become parallel (*orange* colored) or antiparallel (*white* colored) to main magnetic field. The difference of parallel and antiparallel protons becomes smaller at lower magnetic field (a) and larger at a larger magnetic field (b).

MR Signal Formation and *B*1 Field

In the previous section, we described the concepts of magnetic resonance and main static field B_0. The sum of all individual magnetic vectors of the protons produces a combined magnetic vector, which we call as total magnetization M_0. The next step is producing an MR signal, but how?

When we look at Fig. 2.3, we see that the rotational motion of the protons resembles the rotation of a gyroscope. The longitudinal (M_z) projection vector of this magnetization is pretty much unchanged. As we can remember from early school science experiments, we cannot measure a signal if we do not have a dynamic magnetic vector. Therefore, this M_0 magnetization is not very useful for us as such. We somehow have to manipulate this magnetization, so that we can produce a dynamic magnetic vector to be able to measure some type of *MR signal*. This is the place where a new dynamic and short duration magnetic field B_1 come into the picture.

The B_1 pulse or simply the *rf-pulse* is the first thing we apply in a routine MR scan to tilt the magnetization M_0 to transverse plane. To be able to tilt the continuously rotating spins at w_0 frequency, we need to apply a force (B_1 pulse) rotating at the same speed. Under this condition, the rotating (precessing) spins can be pushed from the longitudinal plane (*Z*-axis) to transverse plane (XY-plane) with a relatively small force. Since the applied small force (*B*1 pulse) has the same exact w_0 frequency, the precessing protons will be stationary for the B_1 force as shown in Fig. 2.6. To understand this concept, let's consider a child on a merry-go-round. If we stand up on the ground next to a rotating (precessing) merry-go-round, we cannot touch the child on the merry-go-round because of its rotation. However, if start running around merry-go-round with the same speed, the child on merry-go-round will look like as if he is standing next to us. In this condition, we can touch him, hold his hand, and even can apply a *small force*. The precessing protons in the body can be considered as the child on merry-go-round and the B_1 pulse can be considered as the running person around merry-go-round at the same speed.

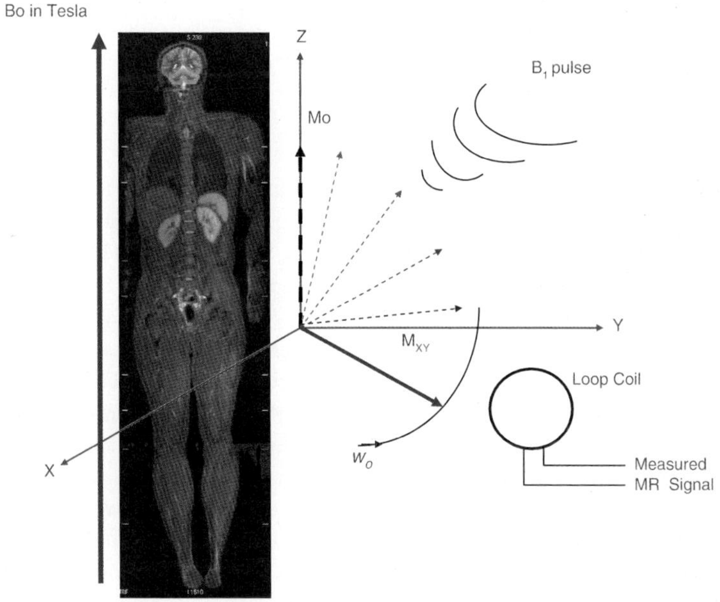

Figure 2.6 When the B_1 rf-pulse is applied, total magnetization M_0 is tilted from *Z*-axis to XY-axis and it continues to precess in XY-plane at Larmor frequency (w_0). When a coil is positioned perpendicular to magnetization MXY, a current (MR signal) is inducted based on Faraday's principle on the coil.

There are three conditions we need to maintain to efficiently tilt the magnetization from *Z*-axis to XY-plane. These are:

- The frequency of B_1 rf-pulse should be the same as the precession or resonance frequency of w_o.
- B_1 rf-pulse should be applied long enough to create the desired tilt (flip angle) of the magnetization.
- B_1 rf-pulse should be perpendicular to main static field.

Once we tilt the M_o magnetization to XY-plane, we can call it M_{XY} as shown in Fig. 2.6. M_{XY} magnetization continues to rotate on XY-plane at w_o frequency. Under this condition, if we place a coil perpendicular to M_{XY} magnetization, a current is inducted in the coil based on well-known Faraday's principle. The current resulting from precessing magnetization is called MR signal. As you can imagine, we need to apply a B_1 rf-pulse just long enough to tilt M_o to 90° exactly on to XY-plane. However, we can create a tilt angle or *flip angles* of 90°, 180°, 45°, or 112° by simply adjusting the duration and strength of B_1 rf-pulse. Please note that the B_1 rf-pulse here is also an external magnetic field somewhat similar to B_0 main static field but much smaller.

MR Signal Spatial Encoding and Gradients

In the previous section, we made a great progress and learned how to create and measure an MR signal at the coil. Now, we can manipulate the total magnetization in a region of interest and produce a signal, but we still do not know where this combined signal comes from or how to separate them. This is due to the fact that all the protons in this large region of interest are making almost the same precessional motion no matter where they are located within the region. It is also important that the measured total MR signal in this case has a certain frequency (same as w_o). To understand this problem better, let us think about a big room with 100 people in it. If we want to locate Jane and James in the room, we can create a simple manipulation and ask them to speak in a tone significantly different than the other people in the room. This way, by tuning to the tone in their voice, we can know where they are located. Similar to this analogy, we can manipulate precessing protons within a region of interest by means of *gradients* and locate their *spatial* location.

Even though this concept may sound complicated, it is quite simple. We know that all the protons in the region are precessing at the same Larmor frequency w_o, which is determined by the main static field. If we somehow label those protons with small frequency change with respect to their location (spatial encoding), then each proton will start precessing with a frequency slightly less or more than the Larmor frequency w_0. Therefore, by just looking at the measured MR signal frequency components, we can easily locate the spatial coordinates of our protons. This frequency labeling is called *spatial encoding* and done using a spatially changing magnetic field called *gradients*. The gradients are typically within 1–3% of the main static field and have a unit of milli Tesla per meter (mT/m). To locate a proton in a plane, we need at least two coordinates. Therefore, MR imaging has to have spatial encoding in two directions at least.

Frequency Encoding Gradients

MR signal frequency labeling (spatial encoding) in frequency direction can be done with a spatially changing gradient as shown in Fig. 2.7. Frequency encoding direction can be any direction and is used to refer to frequency direction or readout direction in MR pulse sequence diagram. In Fig. 2.7, frequency encoding gradient is applied only in one direction to spatially encode the precession

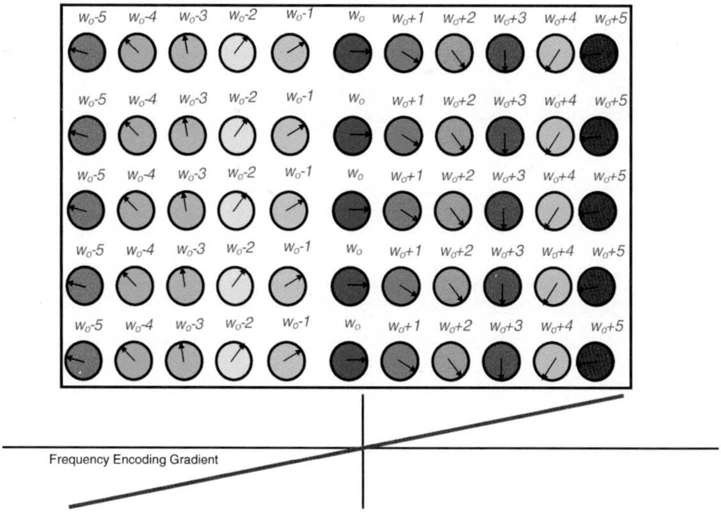

Figure 2.7 Frequency encoding gradient is applied only in one direction here to encode all the protons in the same column with the same frequency as shown with the color-coded figure above.

frequencies of the protons from $w_0 - 5$ to $w_0 + 5$. Since we know exactly this spatial encoding scheme, we can easily tell that we measured signal from protons in the first column if we have $w_0 - 5$ frequency component in the MR signal. As you may have already noticed, there are protons in the center, and the precession frequency of those protons becomes w_0 at the zero crossing of the gradient. In the case of a one dimensional (1D) gradient encoding, all the protons in the same column do have the same precession frequency (coded with the same color) while the protons in each row do have a slightly different precession frequency.

The frequency encoding gradient as shown in Fig. 2.7 is a simple and efficient way of assigning a frequency label to protons' spatial location. However, we obviously need at least one more gradient to spatially encode protons accurately.

Phase Encoding Gradients

Let us consider another 1D gradient commonly called phase encoding gradient as shown in Fig. 2.8. Phase encoding gradient application is almost identical to frequency encoding gradient other than the gradient application direction.

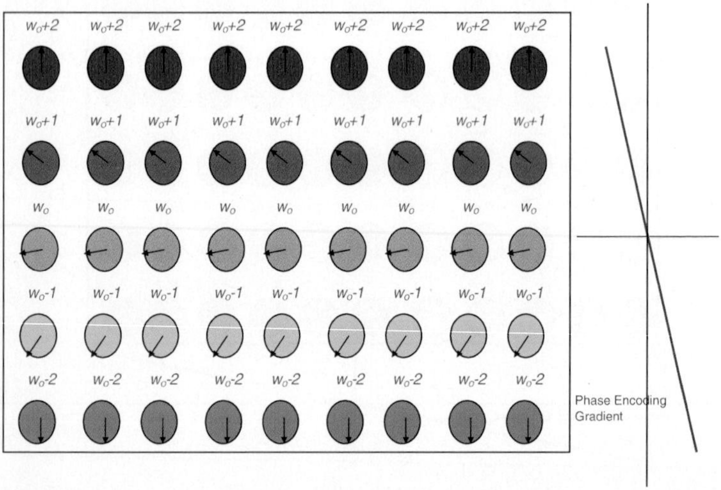

Figure 2.8 Phase encoding gradient is applied only in one direction here to encode all the protons in the same row with the same frequency as shown with the color-coded figure above.

In Fig. 2.8, phase encoding gradient is applied only in one direction to spatially encode the precession frequencies of the protons from $w_0 - 2$ to $w_0 + 2$. Since we know exactly this spatial encoding scheme, we can easily tell that we measured signal from protons in the first row if we have $w_0 + 2$ frequency component in the MR signal. As you may have already noticed, there are protons in the center, and the precession frequency of those protons becomes w_0 at the zero crossing of the gradient. In case of a one dimensional (1D) gradient encoding, all the protons in the same row do have the same precession frequency (coded with the same color) while the protons in each column do have a slightly different precession frequency.

For a better understanding, we looked at frequency encoding and phase encoding gradients independently in these two sections. As we mentioned before, we do combine at least two gradient encoding axes to spatially encode the gradient in a 2D plane (e.g., a single slice of MR image). When frequency and phase encoding gradients are applied in a certain order, we label (spatially encode) all the protons in each row and column very accurately. Therefore, we can know their location by looking at the frequency component of the MR signal using a mathematical transformation called *Fourier Transform*.

Slice Select Encoding Gradients

Frequency and phase encoding gradients are vital to spatially label the protons in a given 2D slice of the anatomy, but how can we choose the desired 2D slice location? Somewhat similar to above gradient, we apply a third spatial encoding gradient called slice select gradient to be able to choose a 2D slice of interest in the body. If we do not apply this gradient correctly, then we can end up having a liver image instead of a desired pelvic image.

The slice select gradient is applied for any MR imaging acquisition during the application of the B_1 rf-pulse. The slice select gradient in combination with the rf-pulse properties and gradient strength is used to choose the thickness and location of the 2D slice. For a 3D imaging, an additional slice select gradient is applied to encode the protons in the third slice encoding dimension.

K-Space or Raw Data

The MR signal recorded at the coil is the raw data or k-space data as we call it. The k-space data are complex data as the engineers call and do have two main components: *real* and *imaginary*. The magnitude raw data (k-space) can be calculated by taking the square root of the sum of real and imaginary k-space components squared. The resulting magnitude k-space image is shown in Fig. 2.9. Similar to magnitude k-space, phase k-space data can be calculated from the real and imaginary raw data. However, in practice magnitude MR image and/or phase MR image can be created only after Fourier Transformation is applied to the raw data or k-space data.

How can we make sense out of these bright spots shown below in the so-called k-space data. Well, you cannot make any sense of it because the k-space data are like an encrypted message. It shows the frequency components

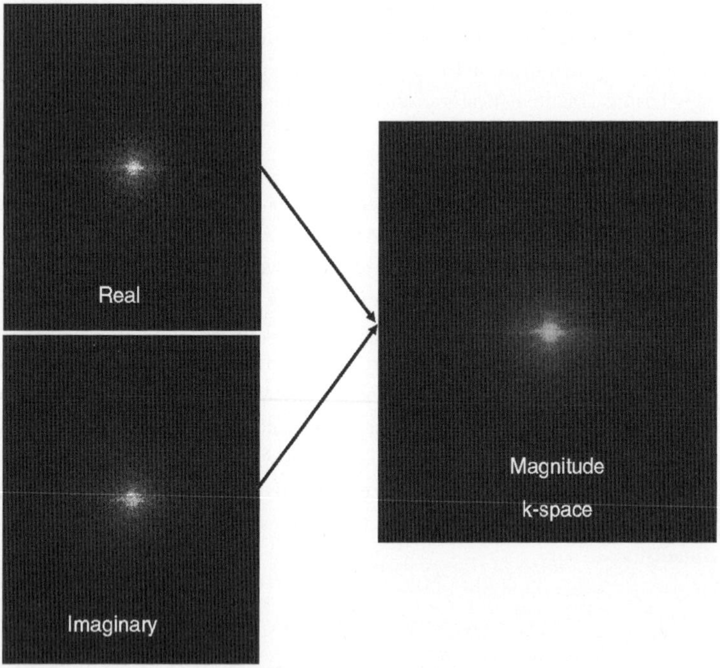

Figure 2.9 The k-space data can be acquired as real and imaginary components and then be combined to create a magnitude k-space data.

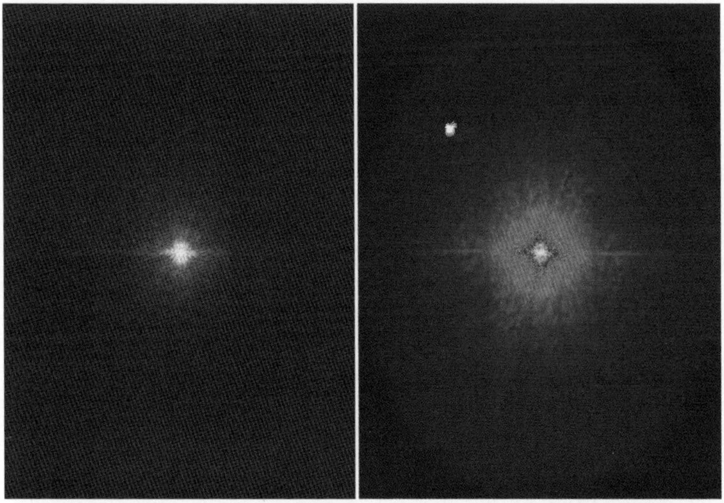

Figure 2.10 A typical gray-scale k-space and a simple color-coded k-space that is identical to the gray scale image are shown to visualize the extension of k-space information.

of the data but the users cannot really make any use of it, even though it carries a huge amount of information. There are multiple ways of looking at the k-space image, for example in color as shown in Fig. 2.10. The color image does not really change anything. However, it makes it easier to human eye to see the extension of k-space information due to the addition of a simple color coding.

The k-space data have dense center region or the bright spot as we can see in Fig. 2.10. The central part of k-space data has in fact carries most of the information. For example, the red circle in Fig. 2.11 has almost 90% of the whole data. We will see in the later section what happens if we remove it.

Fourier Transform and MR Image Reconstruction

In the previous sections, we learned that a strong stationary magnetic field B_0 is used to create a net magnetization. Having learned that B_1 rf-pulse is applied to tip the net magnetization in transverse plane, so that we can measure an MR signal from the protons in the region. Finally, spatially changing low-level magnetic fields, called gradients, are applied to spatially encode or tag the protons with small frequency variation per location, so that we can later on decode this labeling and successfully create an MR image.

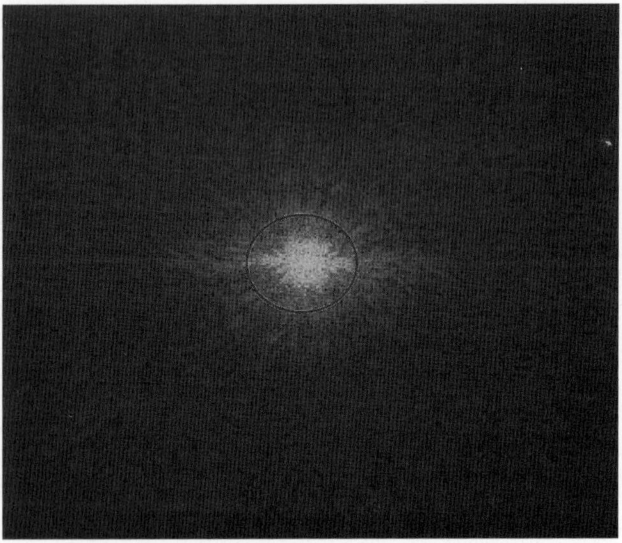

Figure 2.11 A zoomed version of k-space data is shown. Almost 90% of all data is included in the dense central portion (encircled in *red*) of k-space.

Transforming the frequency-encoded raw MR data recorded at the system can be done with Fourier Transformation. Fourier Transformation is a mathematical model transforming the frequency-encoded data from raw data domain or k-space to time domain or MR image domain. A typical Fourier Transformation converts the encrypted MR data to a beautiful, high resolution T2-weighted image as shown in Fig. 2.12.

The Fourier Transformation in your MR scanner is all done in the background without any user intervention or manipulation. As you can imagine, applying a mathematical transformation to a data requires a certain time and computational power of electronics. If you have an older MR scanner, you notice that the MR images come some time later after the acquisition is finished, especially with the relatively large data volume acquisitions such as 3D data acquisitions or functional MRI acquisition with multiple repetitions. This reconstruction delay simply occurs due to the time required to *process* all these raw MR data to create MR images. With the very fast progress on the computer and computing power within the last few years, you will see that MR images

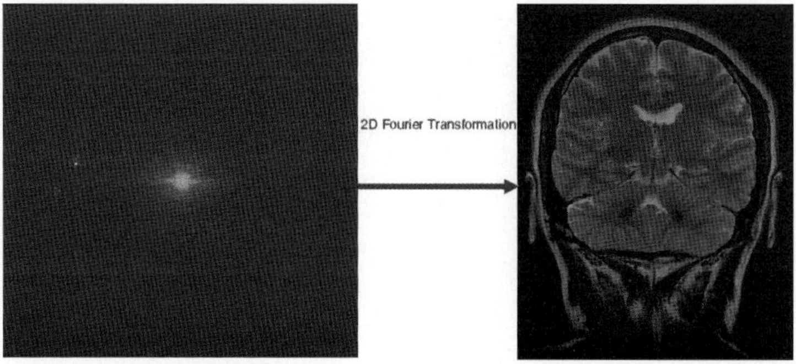

Figure 2.12 A high resolution image is created by means of a 2D Fourier Transformation as shown.

reconstructed almost instantly at the end of MR acquisition. The ability to transform images is commonly related to your scanner's *recon engine* or image reconstruction hardware and software. Despite the incredible recon speeds of the new MR scanners today, the recon speed may still be a limiting factor in certain MR acquisition. Why is it so? Fortunately or unfortunately, the typical MR data acquisition volumes have been increasing tremendously with the introduction of multichannel coil systems and introduction of parallel imaging to many clinical applications.

It might be important to note that other reconstruction techniques such as projection reconstruction can also be used for MR image reconstruction. However, Fourier Transformation is still the main image transformation method in commercial MR sequences and systems.

K-Space or Raw Data Manipulations

The raw or k-space MR data carry a great deal of information as we had mentioned before. In the modern MRI, we manipulate the raw data to create faster imaging sequences. We would like to expose you briefly how the k-space relates to reconstructed image in this section and we will elaborate on this at the later chapters for some of the new imaging techniques.

In the first case, let's remove 90% of whole k-space by cutting it off, filling this space with zeros and then applying a Fourier Transformation as shown in Fig. 2.13. Even if we cut most of the original k-space data, the reconstructed image still makes it possible to identify all the main structure in the brain but is

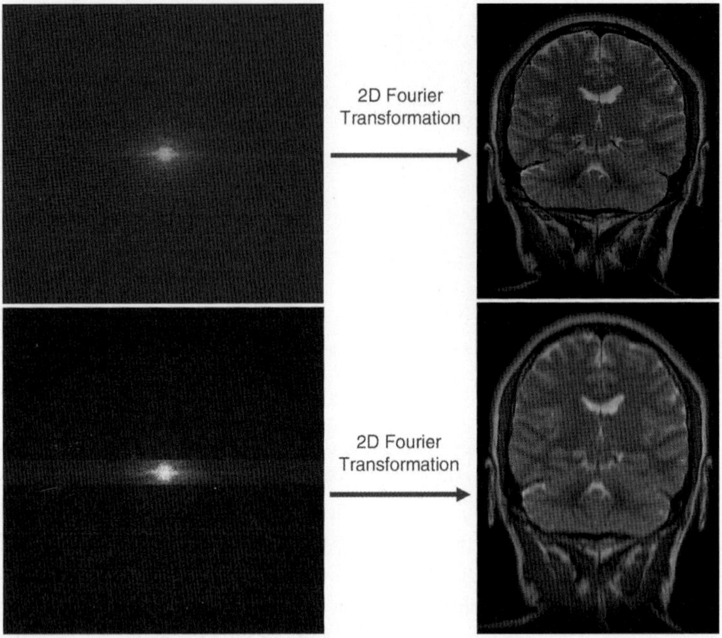

Figure 2.13 The effects of removing the outer portions of k-space data on the reconstructed image are shown in lower part.

visibly much more blurry. The removed sections of the k-space in this case will remove the high frequent components or edge details of the image and we will get a blurry image as shown in Fig. 2.13 compared to original image.

In the second case, let's remove 10% of whole k-space by cutting off only the central portion of raw data in circular fashion and apply a Fourier Transformation as shown in Fig. 2.14. Even if we cut very little of the original k-space data in this case, the reconstructed image is almost useless. A careful look at the image reveals that we can only see the edges of ventricles and sulcus but nothing else. The removed sections of the k-space in this case will remove the low frequency components or morphological details of the image and we will get an edgy image as shown in Fig. 2.14 compared to original image.

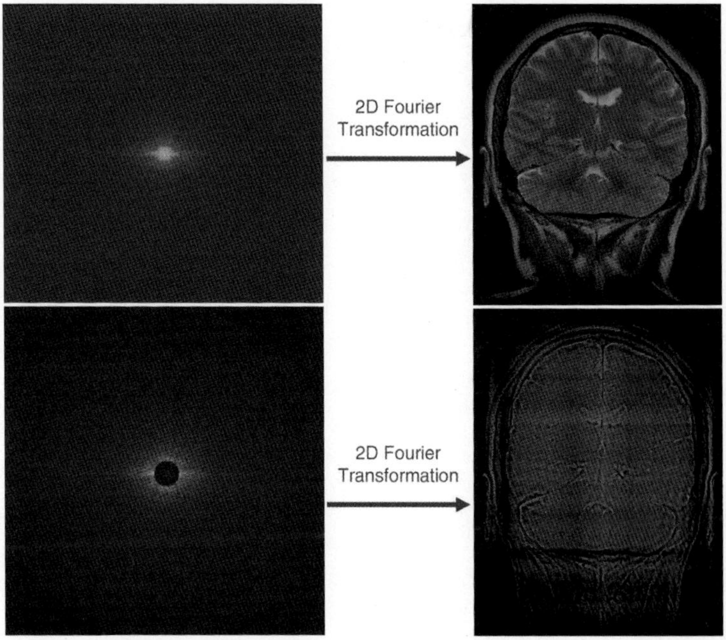

Figure 2.14 The effects of removing the central portion of k-space data on the reconstructed image are shown in the lower part.

Congratulations! This chapter was the most difficult part of magnetic resonance imaging. If you think that you have a pretty good understanding of the concepts here, then you are very much ready to tackle the remaining chapters with a great confidence.

Chapter 3

The Relaxation Concept in MRI

Relaxation Concept and Its Relevance to MR Imaging

In Chap. 2, we learned that MR signal is created by rf pulses and spatial encoding with the gradients. However, there is still a major question. What happens to MR signal when we tilt it to transverse plane? This is a very valid question and can be answered only with the relaxation concept. Therefore, we will be looking at the relaxation concept in this chapter and will see how T1 and T2 contrast is related to tissue relaxation.

T1 and T2 relaxation are the two main concepts we have to know about. T1 relaxation can be defined in simple terms as the time needed for the water protons to return to their initial state after the application of a 90° rf pulse. The T1 relaxation is very much dependent on interaction of protons with their environment (spin and lattice interaction). T2 relaxation can be described as the time for spins to lose their teamwork (coherence) due to their interactions among them (spin and spin interaction). Let's take a closer look at them for a better understanding.

T1 Relaxation

Let's revisit Fig. 2.6 and think about application of a typical 90° rf pulse. The 90° rf pulse will tilt the magnetization vector M_z from *Z*-axis all the way to transverse plane or XY-axis. At this moment, we turn off rf pulse, otherwise we end up with a higher *flip angle* greater than 90°. Then, what happens? Let's remember the swimmer in the strong current example from Chap. 2. If we have swimmers (spins in this case) swimming along with the current in the river (B_0), they will move smoothly. If we throw a rope and start pulling them to the river bank, they will be coming close to river bank (transverse plane)

M. Elmaoğlu and A. Çelik, *MRI Handbook: MR Physics, Patient Positioning, and Protocols*, DOI 10.1007/978-1-4614-1096-6_3,

because of the rope (rf pulse). However, when we release the rope, they will start moving away from the river bank back to the strong current of the river. How long it takes for them to go back to their initial swimming stage (before the rf pulse) is very much dependent on the river bank structure, water depth, their strength, and the river current (swimmer and their environment). Very similar to this example, all the spins tilted to XY-plane with the application of the rf pulse will return to their initial state in a certain time dependent on their interaction with their environment. For example, spins in a fat return back to their original state very fast. However, spins in a fluid such as cerebro spinal fluid (CSF) takes much longer (almost 10 times longer) than fat spins to return back to their original state. The time required for spins to *relax* back to their original state is explained with the energy exchange between the spins and their environment (lattice). Therefore, T1 relaxation is defined as the time needed for protons to return back to their initial state in *Z*-axis (Fig. 3.1).

T1 Relaxation Curve

When a 90° rf pulse applied to our spins aligned with B_o in *Z*-axis, $M_{z,\ Total}$ becomes zero. However, it returns back to its original value in a relatively short time as we call *T1 relaxation time*. The T1 time will be different for each tissue type in our body due to different structures of the tissues. As an MR physicist or reader, you can easily create a T1 relaxation graph if you have few key parameters. A sample T1 relaxation curve is plotted in Fig. 3.2a and b for different tissue types. In the brain, the two most common tissue types, gray matter (GM) and white matter (WM), have some similarities and their T1 relaxation curves also look somewhat similar as shown in Fig. 3.2a. On the other hand, WM and CSF are completely different tissues and the T1 relaxation curve also shows a significant difference as shown in Fig. 3.2b. From these plots, we can also get a feeling that which TR choice can give the biggest difference between different tissue types. I almost hear that now you are asking the question: *How do we plot those curves and what do they mean*?

In MR, we can measure some key tissue parameters such as T1 and T2 relaxation time. We can also model or *formulate* MR signal in relatively simple equations. Equation (3.1) shows a MR signal formula for a spin echo sequence. In this sequence, we see the inherent tissue parameters such as proton density, T1 relaxation time, and T2 relaxation time. We also see the user-defined parameters such as TR and TE.

$$\text{MR signal} \propto \text{PD} * \underbrace{[1 - e^{-TR/T1}]}_{\text{T1 Component}} * \underbrace{e^{-TE/T2}}_{\text{T2 Component}}, \tag{3.1}$$

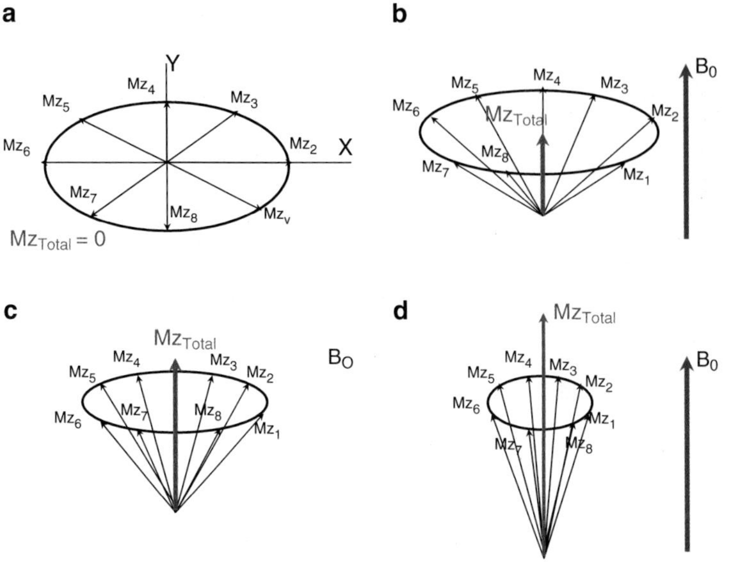

Figure 3.1 Magnetization vector (Mz, total) tilted completely to transverse plane 90° rf pulse is turned off (a) and it starts relaxing back to the initial state in time as shown in (b–d).

where

- PD: Tissue proton density
- T1: Tissue T1 value
- T2: Tissue T2 value
- TR: User-defined parameter called repetition time
- TE: User-defined parameter called echo time

In this equation, we can almost separate the T1 effect and T2 effect as shown above. If we somehow can eliminate the T2 effect of MR signal, we can measure an MR signal only dependent on T1 effect or weighting. On the other hand, if we can eliminate the T1 effect of MR signal, we can measure an MR signal only dependent on T2 effect or weighting. If we can somehow eliminate both T1 and T2 effects, we can measure an MR signal only dependent on the PD effect. This should give us some clues on how do we obtain T1 weighted, T2 weighted, or PD weighted MR images. Let me elaborate more on what I mean.

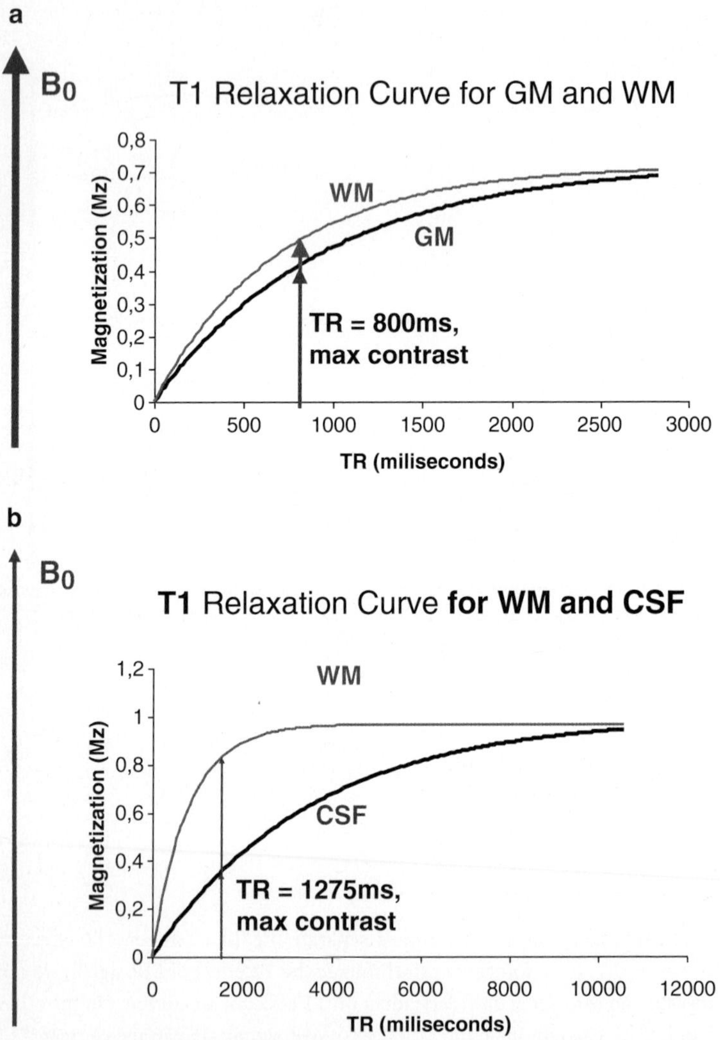

Figure 3.2 When excitation rf pulse is turned off, tissue magnetization returns back to original state at tissue-specific times. This magnetization change can be calculated and plotted for different tissue types as shown above for GM and WM (a) and WM and CSF (b).

In this equation, the T2 component of the MR signal is given by a simple exponential function, $e^{-TE/T2}$. If you choose a very short echo time TE (much shorter than the T2 of the tissue of interest) such as 10 ms, then you can make $e^{-TE/T2}$ very close to 1 and practically eliminate this component or T2 effect of MR signal.

Then, you can write the same formula as T1 weighted equation as shown in (3.2).

$$\text{MR signal}_{\text{T1 weighted}} \propto \text{PD} * [1 - e^{-TR/T1}], \tag{3.2}$$

where

- PD: Tissue proton density
- T1: Tissue T1 value
- TR: User-defined parameter called repetition time

As you can see, this equation is not dependent on T2 value and therefore has no T2 effect. From this simple equation, we can calculate and plot the T1 behavior of the tissues as shown below. The T1 curves shown in Fig. 3.2 can be plotted from (3.2) using simple softwares such as excel and we can even calculate the optimal TR time, which can produce the maximum T1 contrast between tissue types.

Definition and Measurement of T1 Time

In the previous sections, we learned that T1 value is related to the time for the z-magnetization to return back to its original state. In MR physics, T1 time is described as the time needed for the Mz magnetization (z-magnetization) to return back to 63% of its initial or original value. The z-magnetization recovery occurs when the spins start transferring their energy back to the surroundings (lattice). Therefore, T1 relaxation is also called *spin-lattice relaxation* and also *longitudinal* (*Z*-axis) *relaxation*. Please note that the return of the magnetization to the original value is going to be an exponential graph simply because its physical basis is the exponential function given in (3.2). We now defined T1 time for a tissue but how do we measure it?

As shown in Fig. 3.3, the sample tissue in this example reached its original value of 1.0 (Mz) in 3,100 ms. To measure T1 time, we need to look at how much time passed for the z-magnetization to reach 63% of its original value. From the *Y*-axis, we look 0.63 (63% of 1.0) and find out 750 ms has passed to

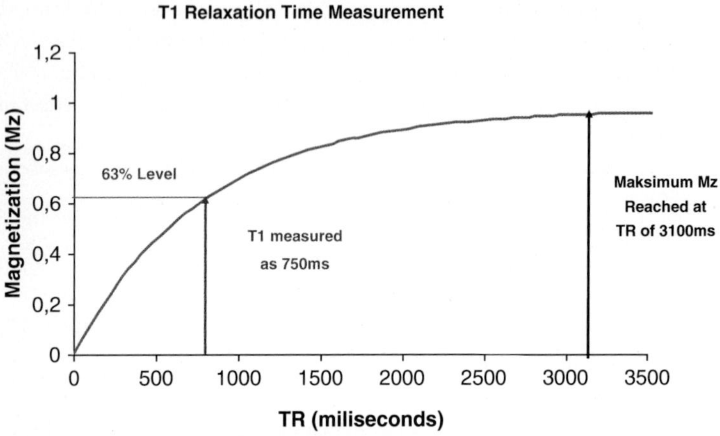

Figure 3.3 The T1 relaxation time is defined as the time required for z-magnetization to reach 63% of its original value. The times required for z-magnetization to reach its original value and 63% values are shown in the plot above.

reach 0.63 after the rf excitation pulse. BINGO then our T1 time for this sample tissue is 750 ms.

In theory, you can easily set up a simple experiment on a phantom by repeatedly measuring MR signal at different TR times and plot an MR signal very similar to what we have shown in Fig. 3.3. Then, you can experimentally measure the T1 value of the phantom or any tissue in fact. However, in practice, we use an inversion pulse sequence with a fixed TR time. We plot the graph by changing the inversion time (TI) and then measure the T1 value or T1 relaxation time of the tissue. Remember that each tissue has a different T1 time and this enables us to see different tissue types in a T1 weighted image.

T1 Weighted Imaging or T1 Contrast

When we look at Fig. 3.2 carefully, we can easily realize that if we want to see a difference between different tissue types, we have to choose a relatively shorter TR time. For example, if we want a good contrast between GM and WM, we should choose TR somewhere around 800 ms not 3,000 ms. Because at 3,000 ms TR time, the signal from GM and WM practically becomes identical and we cannot see any difference. Please note that the 800 ms optimal TR time is calculated from (3.2) by using the 1.5 T T1 relaxation time given in literature. If we ever want to see a great contrast between WM and CSF though for some unknown reasons, then TR time should be around 1,275 ms. Therefore, the TR time is a very critical parameter to create a good T1 weighted imaging in a simple spin echo sequence. In more complicated fast and ultrafast sequences, flip angle also becomes an additional parameter affecting the T1 weighting in the image. As we have given in Table 3.1, we have quite many different tissue types and also a number of pathologies with different T1 relaxation times. Considering that in the brain T1 values range from 100 to 1,000 ms for most tissues, we recommend using a TR time somewhere between 400 and 800 ms in 1.5 T. In the later chapters of the book, the exact TR time choice is also given in each protocol, so that readers can have a reference TR value optimizing the T1 weighting with an excellent contrast and acceptable scan times.

A typical T1 weighted image is shown in Fig. 3.4 acquired with a turbo spin echo sequence. In a T1 weighted imaging, there is a simple rule we should remember: *The tissue signal in a T1 weighted imaging is inversely proportional to its T1 relaxation time.* This simple statement comes from the fact that $1-e^{-TR/T1}$ value of (3.2) will be small for a tissue with a long T1 value (CSF) and quite large for a tissue with short T1 value (fat). We can easily confirm this fact from the T1 weighted imaging by looking at hyperintense fat signal and hypointense CSF signal.

T2 Relaxation

I am hoping that you learned what the T1 relaxation is and how to measure it. Now, it is time to take a look at T2 relaxation and its great importance for MR imaging. Let's again assume that we applied the 90° rf excitation pulse and tilted M_z-magnetization to XY-plane as shown in Fig. 2.6. The excitation pulse will be turned off exactly when the spin tilted to XY-plane. As we remember from the T1 relaxation, the spins will start returning back to their original state in *Z*-axis as soon as we turn off rf pulse. At this point, all spins rotate or move at the same speed (Larmor frequency) in XY-plane like a huge group of people (coherence). However, in time, spins start moving at slightly different speed and the coherence will be disappeared. To understand this spin behavior, we can consider marathon runners. All the runners will start running at the start signal all together and will look like the coherent group. After a short while, some of the runners will slow down because they will bump into the other runners (spins) nearby, get exhausted, or run slower than others. After 1 h or so, you will see

Table 3.1 The MR signal intensities, parameters range for T1, T2, and PD weighted imaging for select tissues in the brain.

For spin echo pulse sequences	TR range	TE range	MR signal intensity
T2 weighted imaging	Longer than 2,000 ms	80–150 ms	CSF: very bright GM: bright WM: darker Fat: darkest (bright in FSE sequences)
T1 weighted imaging	450–900 ms at 3 T 400–800 ms at 1.5 T 375–600 ms at 1.0 T 300–350 ms at 0.2 T	Minimum	CSF: darkest GM: darker WM: bright Fat: brightest
PD weighted imaging	Longer than 2,000 ms	Minimum	CSF: very bright GM: bright WM: darker Fat: darkest

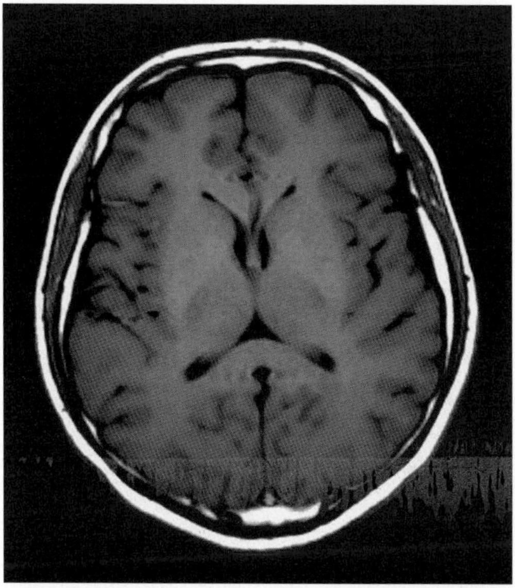

Figure 3.4 A typical fast spin echo–based T1 weighted imaging is shown.

marathon runners with almost no coherence. Similar to this example, the spins in the XY-plane start losing coherence because of the fact that they rotate at slightly different speed depending on which type of tissue they are located and the slightly different magnetic field they experience. The disappearance of the coherence is shown in Fig. 3.5 from time zero (a) to 100 ms (d). At time zero, we will have the maximum MR signal. Later on, we will start getting less and less signal due to both T1 and T2 relaxation effects.

T2 Relaxation Curve

If we place the coil and measure signal with the application of excitation RF pulse (90°), we will see an exponentially decaying signal, which is called free induction decay (FID). This FID signal will look like the exponential decay signal shown in Fig. 3.6. When we want to get a T2 weighted image, we somehow have to eliminate the T1 component of MR signal given in (3.1). A simple way of doing this is to choose a long TR. With the longer TR (greater than 2,000 ms), the T1 component of the MR signal $(1-e^{-TR/T1})$ will be very close

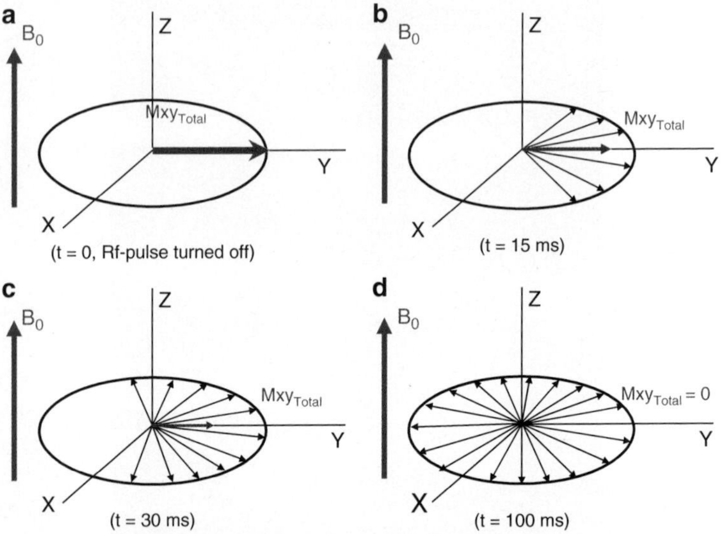

Figure 3.5 With the application of excitation rf pulse, z-magnetization is pushed to XY-plane (a) and produces a coherent signal. In time, the coherence disappears as shown in (b–d).

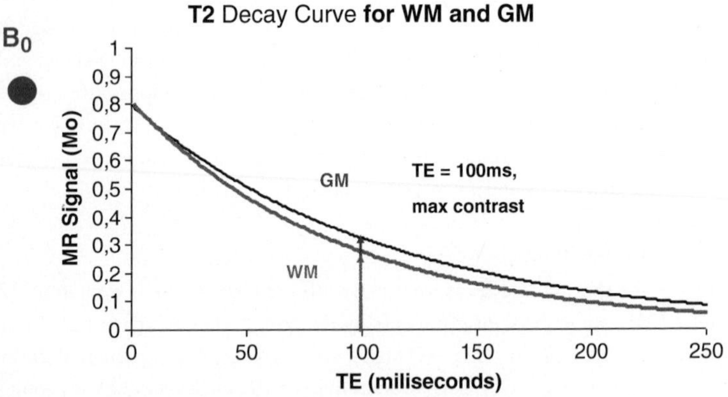

Figure 3.6 The T2 relaxation curve is shown for GM and WM using (3.3).

to 1.0. Therefore, it will have almost no effect in the resulting MR signal. The longer the TR used, the less the T1 effect will be. Assuming a longer TR, we can rewrite the MR signal for a simple spin echo sequence as shown in (3.3), and it will be only a function of user-defined echo time TE as shown below.

$$\text{MR signal}_{\text{T2 weighted}} \propto \text{PD}^* \underbrace{e^{-\text{TE/T2}}}_{\text{T2 Component}}, \tag{3.3}$$

where:

- PD: Tissue proton density
- T2: Tissue T2 value
- TE: User-defined parameter called echo time

From this simple formula, we can calculate and plot a T2 relaxation curve as shown in Fig. 3.6 (for GM and WM) and Fig. 3.7 (for CSF and WM). From this curve, we can even calculate the optimum TE value to give the maximum contrast between different tissues. For example, using a TR value of 5,000 ms and PD, T1, and T2 values reported in literature at 1.5 T for GM and WM, we can calculate the MR signal using (3.3) for TE times ranging from 1 to 500 ms with an ordinary software. Then, by simply looking at the MR signal difference at each TE times, we can calculate the optimal TE times resulting

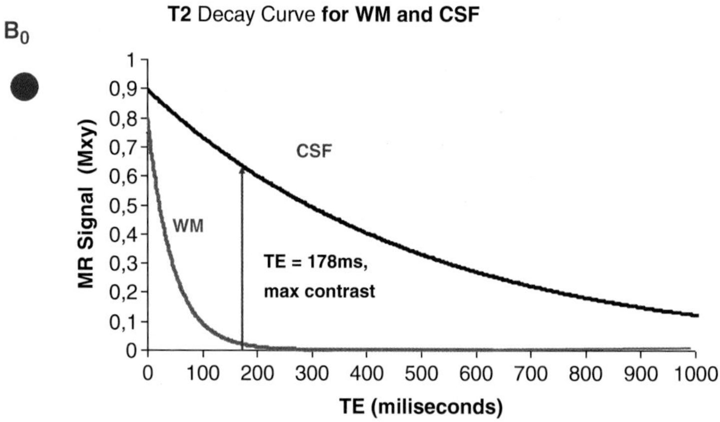

Figure 3.7 **The T2 relaxation curve is shown for CSF and WM using (3.3).**

in the maximum contrast between GM and WM. When I did this calculation using the reference T1 and T2 values given in Table 3.1, I found 100 ms as the optimum TE value maximizing the contrast between these two tissue types. However, in literature, there is a somewhat wide range of the measured T1 and T2 values; therefore, this calculation should be treated as theoretical and can be valid only for spin echo type pulse sequences. The gradient echo or ultrafast pulse sequences have different MR signal models and this formula does not apply to them in the same exact form. However, the basic discussion above is intended for exposing our readers to underlying principles of contrast weighting mechanisms and MR signal optimization of different tissue types.

Definition and Measurement of T2 Time

T2 time is defined as the time required for transverse MR magnetization (MR signal), Mxy, to reach 37% of its initial value. Since the transverse magnetization decay or T2 decay occurs due to the interaction of spins with each other, it is also spin-spin relaxation time. Unlike the T1 relaxation curve, T2 relaxation curve will be an exponentially decaying function as shown in Fig. 3.8.

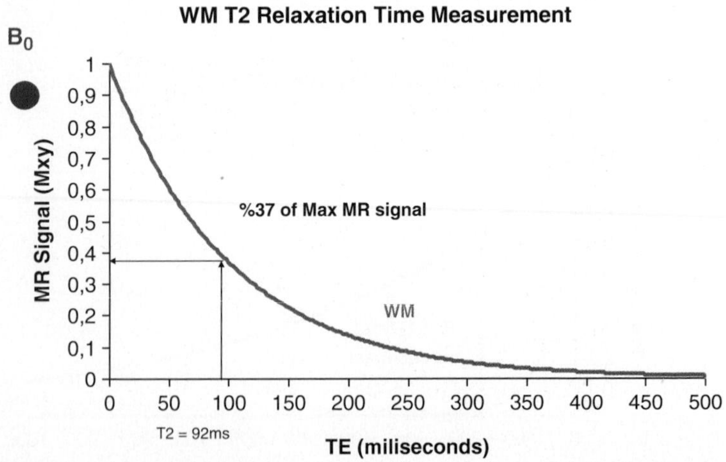

Figure 3.8 Exponentially decaying curve and 37% of initial transverse plane magnetization are shown for T2 measurement.

Using (3.3), we can easily vary TE time from zero to several 1,000 ms and exactly find the TE time resulting 37% of the initial signal as shown in Fig. 3.8. In this example, we calculate the T2 value of WM in the brain as 92 ms. In practice, we can also measure T2 value of any tissue by choosing a minimum of three or four different TE times and fitting the resulting signal intensities to an exponential function. However, the TE times should be chosen smartly for the tissue type and higher number of echo times should be used for better accuracy.

T2 Weighted Imaging or T2 Contrast

When we look at Fig. 3.9 carefully, we can easily realize that if we want to see a difference between different tissue types, we have to choose a long TR time (longer than 2,000 ms) and appropriate TE time. Here, the *appropriate* TE time would be longer than 85 ms to get an acceptable T2 contrast. As you remember, we had a simple discussion on the calculation of optimum TE time providing the best contrast between GM and WM using (3.3). We found that 100 ms TE

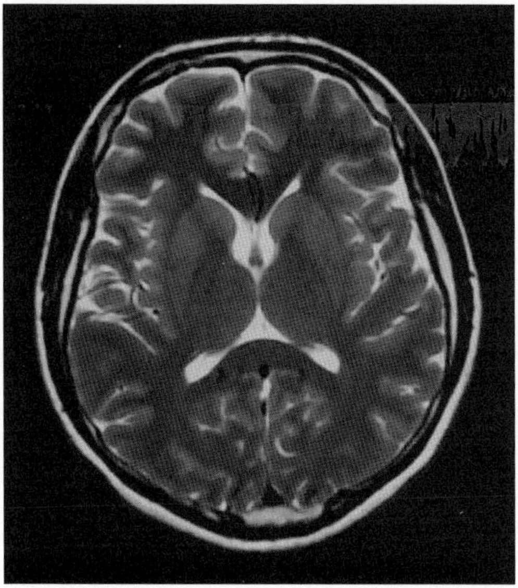

Figure 3.9 A typical T2 weighted imaging of the brain.

Table 3.2 Selected T1 and T2 relaxation times of various tissues at 0.2 and 1.5 T.

	T1 in ms (0.2 T)	T1 in ms (1.5 T)	T2 in ms
Brain			
Gray matter (GM)	525	921	101
White matter (WM)	420	787	92
Tumor	660	1,073	121
Meningioma	580	979	103
Glioma	835	959	111
Edema	660	1,090	113
Bone			
Bone marrow	600	732	106
Osteosarcoma	730	973	85
Breast			
Fibrotic tissue	405	868	49
Adipose tissue	185	259	84
Tumors	480	976	80
Carcinoma	451	923	94
Adenocarcinoma	485	1,167	81
Kidney			
Normal tissue	412	652	58
Tumors	730	907	83
Liver			
Normal tissue	245	493	43
Tumors	710	905	84
Hepatoma	615	1,077	84
Chirrosis	322	438	45
Muscle			
Normal tissue	405	868	47
Tumors	590	1,083	87
Carcinoma	603	1,046	82
Fibrosarcoma	825	1,011	65
Pancreas			
Normal tissue	300	513	60

time provides the optimum contrast between GM and WM based on the TR choice and T1 and T2 relaxation times given in Table 3.2. For some reason, if we want to obtain the maximum T2 contrast between WM and CSF, a similar calculation tells us that 178 ms TE time would be the optimal choice at 1.5 T again. Obviously, we cannot and should not try to calculate the optimal TE for each scan. However, we need to keep in mind that the optimal TE selection would vary for anatomy of interest and we need to use the recommended range of TE times for clinical scanning. As a simple example, TE time for a routine brain imaging can vary from 85 to 130 ms while it can vary from 500 to 1,000 ms for an MRCP examination.

In a T2 weighted image, there is a simple rule we should remember: *The tissue signal in a T2 weighted image is proportional to its T2 relaxation time.* This simple statement comes from the fact that $e^{-TE/T2}$ value of (3.3) will be large for a tissue with a long T2 value (e.g., CSF) and quite small for a tissue with short T2 value (e.g., fat). We can easily confirm this fact from the T2 weighted imaging by looking at hyperintense CSF signal and hypointense fat signal. Please note that T2 imaging with FSE or TSE type sequences results in a hyperintense fat signal because of what we call J-coupling effect. Multiple echoes in those sequences recover the fat signal and fat looks much brighter than it should for a routine T2 imaging as shown in Fig. 3.9.

A Simple Experimental Method for T2 Contrast

It is rather simple to visualize the T2 relaxation time effect and T2 contrast changes in routine clinical scanners. You basically need to choose a T2 protocol from your database and vary TE time within a certain range. In the example shown below, the TE times are varied from 12.6 to 100 ms with approximately 13 ms increase in each image (Fig. 3.10).

The varying TE times with a long TR sequence can be used to measure the T2 relaxation times of the tissues in the body. This can be done quite easily in a clinical setting using simple T2 weighted sequences. However, most of the new scanners can combine parallel imaging with multiple echo sequences to reduce the scan time of such an acquisition from 20 to 3–4 min as shown in this example.

From the individual set of images, you can create T2 relaxation curves very similar to the Fig. 3.6 for GM and WM as shown below at Fig. 3.11.

As some or hopefully most of you can guess, we can experimentally measure the true T2 relaxation time of the tissues from Fig. 3.11 by fitting the T2 curves to an exponential function. If we do it for the whole image, we can

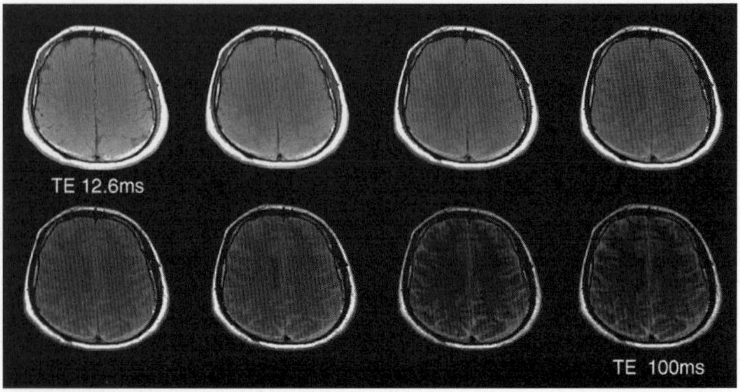

Figure 3.10 A long TR FSE images with echo times ranging from 12.6 to 100 ms are shown. Please note the transition from PD contrast to T2 contrast with increasing TE times.

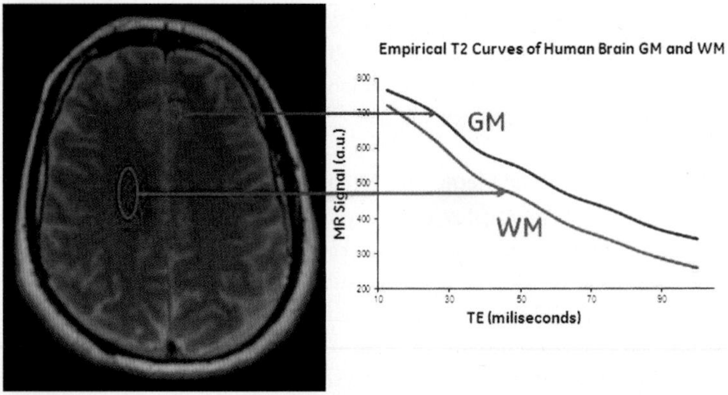

Figure 3.11 The T2 relaxation curves are shown for GM and WM from a simple experimental protocol on the scanners.

create a T2 map of the brain. The T2 map image below simply shows the true T2 relaxation times of the tissues. For example, for the WM and GM regions of interest highlighted on Fig. 3.11, we can measure the T2 relaxation times as 85 and 106 ms for WM and GM, respectively (Fig. 3.12).

The T2 map looks quite interesting and similar to the T2 weighted image as expected. Since the T2 weighting is directly proportional to the tissue T2

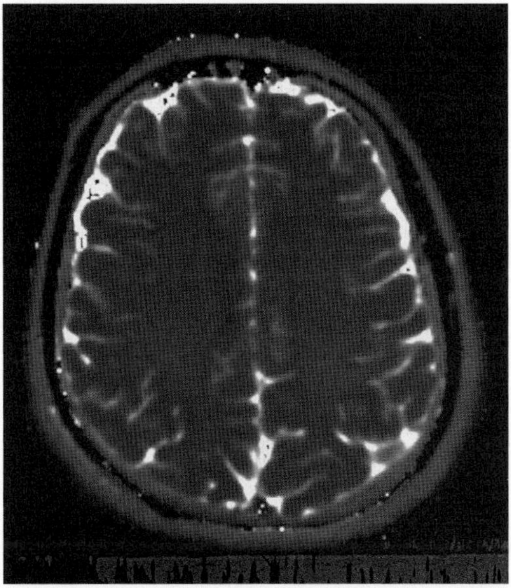

Figure 3.12 The empirically (experimentally) calculated T2 map of the brain is shown.

relaxation times, the WM T2 values look hypointense compared to both GM and CSF. This is a perfect example of applying the theoretical basis of what we have learned so far to the simple practical cases to have a better feel and understanding of fundamental MR concepts.

T2* Relaxation

T2* relaxation time is essentially same as T2 relaxation time. However, there are some differences that need more emphasize. The T2* relaxation does include a relaxation time called T2′ in addition to T2 relaxation time. T2′ relaxation time is a relaxation time resulting from the field inhomogeneties. Any spin echo–based sequences would produce only T2 contrast excluding some special acquisition techniques. On the other hand, gradient echo–based sequences would produce only T2* contrast. T2* is always smaller than T2 relaxation time of a tissue. T2* relaxation time is defined as

$$1/T2^* = 1/T2 + 1/T2' \quad \text{or}$$
$$R2^* = R2 + R2'. \tag{3.4}$$

Unlike T2 relaxation time, the T2* relaxation time is machine and patient dependent. Therefore, T2* relaxation times can be measured on need basis for each patient or different type of tissues. For example, the diseases manifesting themselves with iron overload or iron deficiency can be detected or monitored with T2* relaxation time measurements. You basically need to choose a T2* protocol from your protocol database and vary TE time within a certain range. In the example shown below, the TE times are varied from 1.4 to 41.6 ms with approximately 2.7 ms increase in each image (Fig. 3.13).

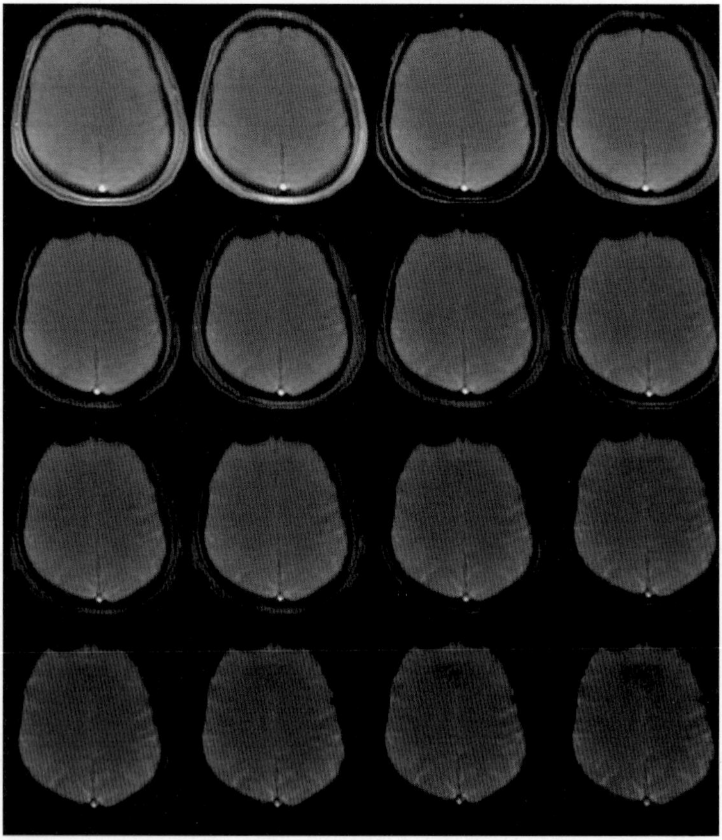

Figure 3.13 **T2* weighted images with echo times ranging from 1.4 to 41.6 ms are shown.**

The varying TE times can be used to measure the T2* relaxation times of the tissues in the body. This can be done quite easily in a clinical setting using simple T2* weighted sequences. However, most of the new scanners can combine parallel imaging with multiple echo sequences to reduce the scan time of such an acquisition from 5 min to 15 to 20 sec as shown in this example.

From the individual set of images, you can create T2* relaxation curves very similar to the T2 relaxation times for GM and WM as shown below at Fig. 3.14.

As you already know from the previous section on T2 measurement, we can experimentally measure the true T2* relaxation time of the tissues from Fig. 3.14 by fitting the T2* curves to an exponential function. If we do it for the whole image, we can create a T2* Map of the brain. The T2* map image below simply shows the true T2* relaxation times of the tissues. For example, for the WM and GM regions of interest highlighted on Fig. 3.14, we can measure the T2* relaxation times as 65 and 75 ms for WM and GM, respectively. Please note the changes on T2* relaxation times. The *T2* and T2* relaxation times from the same WM and GM regions are measured as 85 vs. 65 and 106 vs. 75 ms for these tissue types.

The T2* map looks quite interesting and similar to the T2 map as expected. Since the T2* weighting is also directly proportional to the tissue T2* relaxation times, the WM T2* values look hypointense than both GM and CSF. You can also notice some signal loss on the anterior part of the T2* map compared

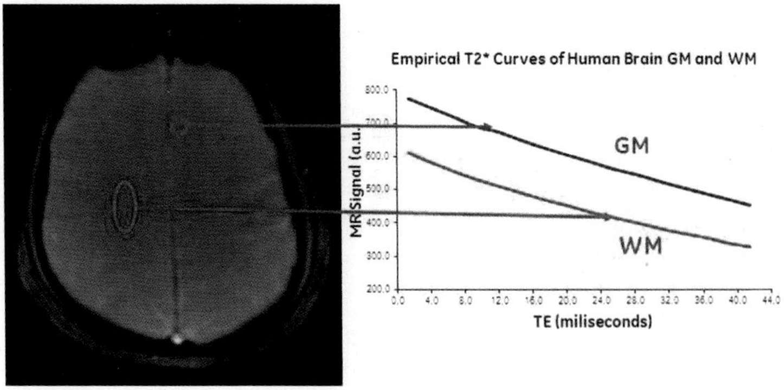

Figure 3.14 The T2* relaxation curves are shown for GM and WM from a simple experimental protocol on the scanners.

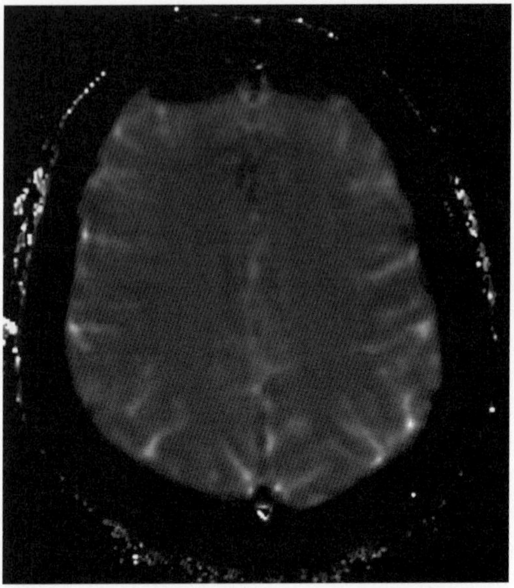

Figure 3.15 The empirically (experimentally) calculated T2* map of the brain is shown.

to T2 map of the brain. This is a typical visual confirmation of increased susceptibility effects seen with gradient echo–based images. This is a perfect example of applying the theoretical basis of what we have learned so far to the simple practical cases to have a better feel and understanding of fundamental MR concepts (Fig. 3.15).

Proton Density Weighted (PD) Imaging

Proton density (PD) or spin density of a tissue is directly proportional to number of hydrogen protons or water content of the tissue. The number of protons or the proton density in the tissue will be low in firm tissues (e.g., fat) and high in fluids (e.g., CSF). When we had the T1 and T2 relaxation discussions above, we had proton density (PD) factor in all cases as shown in (3.1), (3.2), and (3.3). This is because of the fact that PD cannot be eliminated from the MR signal. However, we can almost eliminate the T1 and T2 effects from MR signal given in (3.1) by choosing a long TR (greater than 2,000 ms) and very short T2

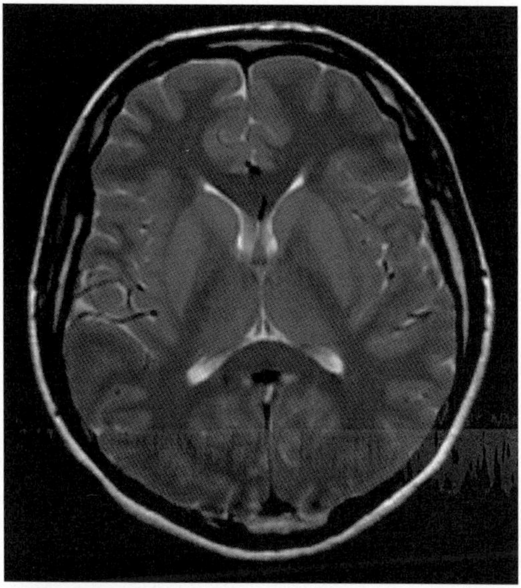

Figure 3.16 A sample PD weighted imaging of the brain.

(minimum time possible). When those conditions are met, the T1 component and T2 component of (3.5) will be very close to 1. Therefore, we will have a MR signal only proportional to the water concentration of proton density as shown in (3.5). This is what we call a PD weighted imaging or PD contrast imaging.

In a PD weighted imaging, the MR signal intensity for fat, WM, GM, and CSF ranges from lower to higher as shown in the sample PD weighted imaging in Fig. 3.16.

$$\text{MR signal} \propto \text{PD}. \tag{3.5}$$

T1, T2 and PD Weighted Imaging Parameter Guide

In this chapter, we discussed the T1, T2, and PD weighted imaging basis, mechanisms, and their relevance to clinical scanning. Especially for the new MR readers, we summarized user-defined imaging parameter's range and relative signal intentisities for reader's convenience in Table 3.1.

T1 and T2 Relaxation Values of the Tissues at Different Magnetic Field Strength

In this chapter, we talked a lot about the intrinsic tissue parameters, namely T1, T2, and PD properties. However, we also need to know those tissue parameters to be able to better appreciate the MR tissue signal differences. Among these parameters, T2* relaxation time is the one most sensitive external magnetic field. As a general guidance, Table 3.2 summarizes the main tissues and select pathologies with T1 and T2 relaxation time measurements in 0.2 and 1.5 T systems. Please note that the reported relaxation time measurements in literature can vary in a larger range and Table 3.2 is intended to provide a general guidance for the reader's own information.

Chapter 4

MRI Pulse Sequences

The Heart of MRI: Pulse Sequences

Arguably, one of the most important advantages of MRI is its ability to create multiple imaging contrasts such as T1, T2, and proton density. However, to understand what different type of MRI contrast means and how they are created, we will take a trip to the heart of MRI as called MR pulse sequences.

In general terms, MR pulse sequences are the computer software executing a series of commands to apply an rf pulse, gradients, data sampling windows, etc in a predefined timing window. Hence, there are quite a number of different pulse sequences that exist today, which are designed to acquire MR images. When we look closely to their origin, however, we can describe them as spin echo (SE) based and gradient echo based depending on the type of echo created. In addition, we can call them routine, fast, or ultrafast sequences. The naming or classification depends on the required time to run them and their spatial encoding design as either two dimensional (2D) or three dimensional (3D).

In this chapter, we will take a closer look at the most important pulse sequences in clinical use today to understand, what they are, why they are used, and how effective they are. Now, get ready to your voyage to the heart of MRI.

Spin Echo (SE) Pulse Sequences

A typical SE pulse sequence applies a number of rf pulses and gradients in a certain order as shown in Fig. 4.1. As shown in this diagram, we have a 90° and 180° rf pulses (typical of SE) required to create an SE. To excite and receive a signal from a region of interest, we apply a 90° rf pulse along with a slice selective gradient, $G_{\text{Slice Select}}$ (Gz). As the name hints, Gz is a gradient applied

M. Elmaoğlu and A. Çelik, *MRI Handbook: MR Physics, Patient Positioning, and Protocols*, DOI 10.1007/978-1-4614-1096-6_4,

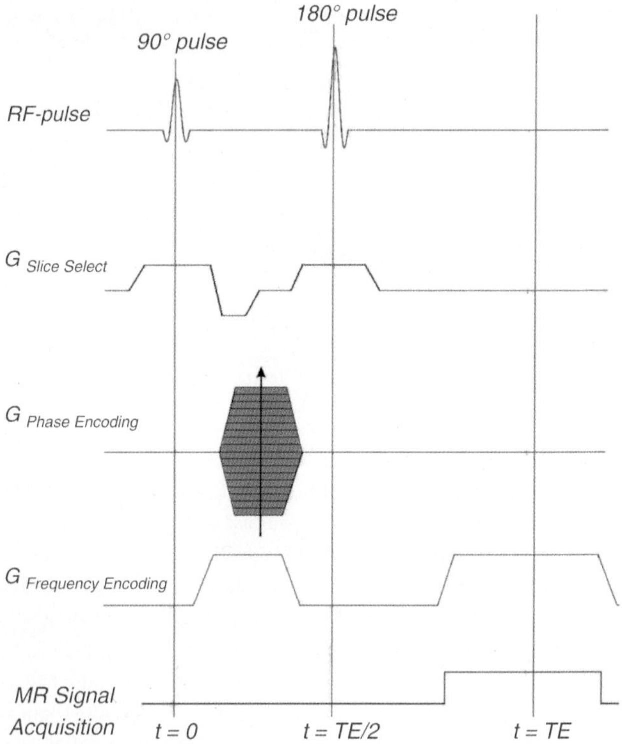

Figure 4.1 A typical spin echo pulse diagram.

with a certain amplitude to excite a slice with a defined thickness and its duration directly depends on the duration of rf pulse as well. Luckily, as a user, we do not have to interfere with amplitude and timings of these sequences directly. Today's MR scanners are smart enough to calculate them for you *when you enter your scan parameters* and *you will be notified politely if you try something out of range.* Other two gradients, as we call, frequency encoding (Gx) and phase encoding (Gy), are executed again in specific order to create an echo and acquire a line in raw data space (k-space). To collect the whole data, we need to repeat the phase encoding gradients (Gy) as many times as phase encoding matrix, so that we can acquire the signal for the whole raw data page. A small box at the bottom of this diagram indicates that we do record the MR signal at a certain time and for certain duration as called sampling time (Ts). The famous echo is formed during the sampling window at the echo time (TE), usually right at the center, and recorded to form an MR image later on. It may not be very clear from the diagram but the second 180° rf pulse is vital to the SE formation and one of the most important signatures of broader SE-based MR pulse sequences family. We can summarize the advantages and disadvantages of SE sequence as follows:

Advantages:

- Provides overall good-quality image.
- Provides optimal signal to noise ratio (SNR) and contrast to noise ratio (CNR).
- It is possible to obtain T1, T2, and PD contrast.
- It is one of the oldest sequences, and a broad range of literature is available for its clinical value.
- It is not very sensitive to susceptibility artefacts.

Disadvantages:

- MR acquisition time is quite long (12–20 min for T2 and PD, 4–7 min for T1 contrast).
- It deposits higher rf power compared to gradient echo sequences.

Fast Spin Echo (FSE) Sequences

Today, fast spin echo (FSE) and turbo spin echo (TSE) sequences are the most commonly used family of sequences. As the name indicates, they came from SE sequence base and their pulse diagram is somewhat similar to what we have shown in Fig. 4.1. However, to make them *much faster*, they do have a number of additional 180° rf pulses. Even though those rf pulses can be used to create separate images with different TE times (such as PD and T2) in one excitation as in the case for dual echo sequences, their sole use in FSE are to cover k-space with multiple phase encoding lines in a single excitation.

The number of 180° rf pulses in this case does have of significant value for image contrast and it is called as echo train length (ETL) or turbo factor. The most important advantage of this sequence type is that they enable us to acquire T1, PD, and T2 weighted images much faster than conventional SE sequence. As we mentioned above, this is achieved via filling up k-space by a factor proportional to the chosen ETL number. Ideally, the reader may think that the higher the ETL, the faster the MR acquisition. Even though this simple math logic is true, the chosen ETL has significant implication on the image contrast and image quality. As a general guideline, you can find the recommended range of key parameters in FSE (TSE) sequence family including TR, TE, and ETL for an optimal image contrast in Table 4.1 below. Please remember that these values are given based on 1.5 T MR systems, and they will differ somewhat in 0.2–3.0 T MR scanners available as today's clinical scanners.

To have a better idea of how fast are those FSE sequences, let's think about an FSE sequence with an ETL of 16. When we compare this sequence to an SE sequence for the same resolution and TR value, we can say that ETL of 16 speeds up MR acquisition by a factor of 16. Unfortunately, this is not the case in routine scanning due to additional factors such as number of slices to be covered within the same TR value. When we use FSE with a higher ETL factor, we also increase the scan time to collect 16 phase encoding lines for one single slice. Therefore, the number of slices we can acquire in a given TR value will also be reduced in FSE sequences. To compensate for the reduced number of slice acquisition in a given TR, we usually increase TR or acquire slices in *multiple groups or acquisitions*. As a result, we usually reduce the total scan time by a factor less than 16 in practical scanning. Nevertheless, we still achieve a very significant reduction in total scan time.

As shown in Table 4.1, the ETL factor for T1 weighted imaging is quite low (around 2–3) compared to PD and T2. Since the scan time reduction in T1 imaging is usually quite modest, we still use SE T1 imaging frequently in clinical scanning (typically for brain and musculoskeletal imaging) unlike T2 or PD weighted SE imaging. As a take-home message, we can summarize the advantages and disadvantages of FSE sequence as follows:

Table 4.1 Recommended range of parameters for FSE sequence is given for 1.5 T systems.

Contrast	TR (ms)	TE (ms)	ETL
T1	400–800	Minimum	2–3
T2	2,000 or higher	85 or higher	12 or higher
PD	2,000	20–25	6–8
PD–T2	2,000	40	6–9

Advantages:

- Provides overall good-quality image.
- Provides optimal SNR and CNR.
- It is possible to obtain T1, T2, and PD contrast much faster than conventional SE sequences.
- It is one of the oldest sequences and a broad range of literature is available for its clinical value.
- It is even less sensitive to susceptibility artefacts than SE sequences. The susceptibility artifacts are reduced with higher ETL factor.
- Reduction in scan time makes it more practical to acquire high resolution images.

Disadvantages:

- Images look more blurry than SE images.
- It deposits higher rf power compared to gradient echo sequences.
- T2 weighted FSE images show bright fat signal rather than darker fat signal due to J-coupling effect.

IR and STIR Sequences

Inversion recovery (IR) sequences are the broad range of sequences, which are used to suppress signal for a specific tissue or to enhance the contrast in certain applications. IR term is more general and can refer to any SE or gradient echo sequence with an additional inversion rf pulse as the first rf pulse of the sequence. STIR sequence is one of the best-known SE or FSE-based IR sequences.

STIR stands for Short Tau Inversion Recovery and one of the widely used IR sequences. The sequence design is almost identical to an SE or FSE sequence. However, before the 90° excitation rf pulse, we apply an 180° *inversion* pulse to *invert* the MR signal. The initial 180° *inversion* pulse places all the spins in the excited region of interest to – Z-axis and those spins slowly recover back to their original signal pointing to + Z-axis. From the user interface, when we choose a TI time (inversion time), which is equal to the 69% of the T1 value of a specific tissue, we can practically null or eliminate the signal from this specific tissue. In other words, we can make the signal from a specific tissue very dark. For example, if we want to eliminate fat signal, which has a T1 value around 230 ms, we need to choose a TI time around 160 ms (equal to 69% of 230 ms) to null or suppress the fat signal from resulting image. This sounds very easy and practical, right? Because of its simple design and efficient fat suppression, STIR sequence has been used since the beginning of modern clinical magnetic resonance imaging in almost all magnetic field strengths due to its inherent advantages. What if we choose a different TI value, let's say around 70 or 220 ms? In this case, we will get a different overall image and results can be quite interesting, as we will see later in the next chapter.

As the take-home message, we can summarize the advantages and disadvantages of STIR sequence and IR sequences in general as follows:

Advantages:

- Due to inversion pulse, the image quality perception is worse than SE or FSE images.
- It is possible to obtain T1 or T2 contrast.
- Provides very uniform fat suppression even in large FOV.
- Can be used in a broad range of magnetic field strengths.
- Varying TI can give us a different contrast or variable fat suppression.

Disadvantages:

- It usually takes longer to acquire.
- Due to longer scan time, the practical image resolution is lower than other sequences.
- Due to the inversion pulse, it is not recommended to be used in postcontrast acquisitions.

FLAIR (Fluid Attenuated Inversion Recovery) Sequences

Fluid attenuated inversion recovery (FLAIR) sequences are also part of IR sequence family. However, due to their widespread use, we discuss them in a separate section. The very well-known T2 FLAIR and less known T1 FLAIR sequences are the two main FLAIR sequences.

The main purpose of T2 FLAIR sequences is to null or suppress the cerebro spinal fluid (CSF) by choosing a right TI range (from 2,100 to 2,300 ms in 1.5 T) and a TR (from 8,400 to 9,200 ms). Please note that with the introduction of new 3D FLAIR sequences such as SPACE and CUBE from different manufacturers, the TI time and TR time can be lower due to the innovative approaches of 3D FLAIR imaging sequence. Suppressing CSF enables us a much better visualization of adjacent white matter (WM) tissues with possible lesions. Therefore, it is one of very essential sequences of any routine brain imaging.

The main purposes of T1 FLAIR sequences are to increase the T1 contrast and further reduce the CSF signal, which is already hypointense in T1 weighted imaging. Therefore, it is used in the brain to further improve the GM and WM contrast (especially in 3.0 T). It is also used in spine imaging, to improve the CSF and spinal cord contrast. For a good T1 FLAIR imaging, we recommend a TI time from 500 to 900 ms and a short TE time in the order of 20–30 ms.

Let's take a quick look at the main advantages and disadvantages of FLAIR sequences:

Advantages:

- Suppressing very bright CSF signal in T2 weighted images enables us much better contrast for WM lesions.
- It can improve the overall CNR in the brain and spinal cord.

Disadvantages:

- It usually takes longer to acquire.
- Due to longer scan time, the practical image resolution is lower than other sequences.
- Due to the inversion pulse, it is not recommended to be used in postcontrast acquisitions.

SSFSE (Single Shot Fast Spin Echo) or HASTE Sequence

SSFSE or HASTE sequence is one of the ultrafast sequences and it enables us to acquire whole MR data (k-space) in a single rf excitation or single shot. Here, the term *single shot* means a series of 180° rf pulses are applied following the initial 90° pulse and we do not repeat the 90° pulse excitation pulse again. This is simply due to the fact that we acquire the whole k-space needed to form an MR image in a long ETL in a very fast way. The number of 180° refocusing rf pulses is usually equal to the phase encoding matrix, and total scan time to form a single slice is on order of subseconds.

SSFSE sequences can have only T2 weighting due to its single shot design. If we divide this large number of ETL to smaller shots, we can produce a form of T1 weighted image, but this sequence cannot be called single shot anymore. Therefore, we should consider SSFSE or HASTE sequences as T2 weighted unless otherwise stated.

Let's take a quick glance of main advantages and disadvantages of SSFSE sequences:

Advantages:

- Their MR acquisition times are very fast.
- They can be used successfully for application requiring longer TE times such as MRCP, urography, myelograpy, etc.

- They are very efficient for fast MR imaging and breath hold localizer scans.
- Their sensitivity to susceptibility artefacts are very low due to very long ETL.

Disadvantages:

- Their overall image quality perception is usually quite low (they look blurry).
- They apply a significant amount of rf power and specific absorption rate (SAR) to body due to large number of repeated rf pulses.
- The resulting image looks quite blurry as a result of T2 filtering effect of large number of rf pulses.

Gradient Echo (GRE) Pulse Sequences

After SE family, the most commonly used sequences do belong to gradient echo (GRE) family. Even though the GRE and SE sequence diagrams are similar in terms of sequence structure, lack of the refocusing 180° rf pulse is the most striking difference between GRE and SE. In GRE sequences, there is also an initial excitation rf pulse with a flip angle that is equal to or smaller than 90° and we can call it theta (θ) in this book. As shown in Fig. 4.2, the pulse sequence diagram of a simple GRE sequence is almost identical to SE sequence with small differences on Gx gradient and missing 180° rf pulse. In fact, these seemingly *small differences* produce a so-called *gradient echo*. Hence, this sequence is called gradient echo sequence. As we may recall, the combination of *two rf pulses along with the gradients* creates SE.

In GRE sequence, the first negative Gx gradient dephases the MR magnetization vector in transverse plane and is called *dephasing gradient*. Right after the dephasing gradient, we apply the positive gradients to refocus (rephase) MR spins to create a perfectly centered gradient echo at TE time. The role of phase encoding (Gy) gradient is almost identical to SE, and it is executed to create an echo line in raw data space (k-space). Similarly, slice select gradient $G_{\text{Slice Select}}$ (Gz) is designed to excite a single slice of interest during the initial rf pulse. A small box at the bottom of this diagram indicates that we do record the MR signal at a certain time (around echo time) and for certain duration called as sampling time (Ts). The famous gradient echo is formed during the sampling window, usually right at the center, and recorded to form an MR image later on. In GRE sequences, we usually apply something called *rewinder* gradients at the end of each TR cycle (not shown in Fig. 4.2). The rewinder gradients serve the

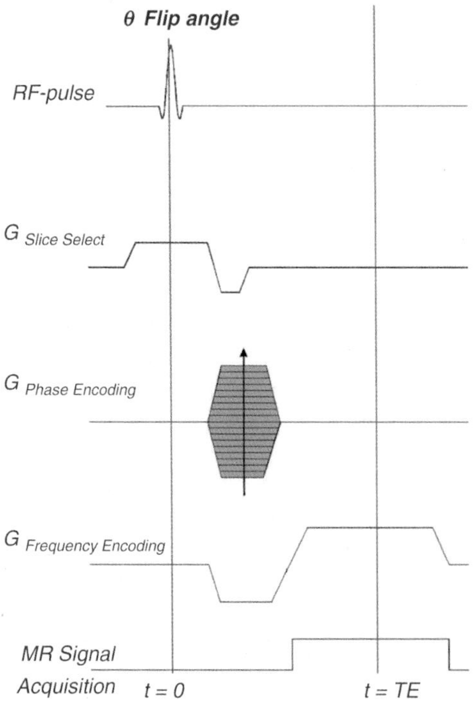

Figure 4.2 A typical gradient echo pulse diagram.

purpose of rewinding the MR magnetization, which is affected by the multiple gradients in three planes. The rewinding process can be achieved by applying overall symmetric gradient waveforms in a complete TR cycle and bringing the magnetization to the original state.

In general, a flip angle (θ), smaller than 90°, is applied in GRE sequences and usually shorter TRs are used as well. Smaller θ flip angle means that we end up with less signal in the transverse plane (a bad thing), but at the same time, the MR magnetization or signal can recover much faster (a good thing) since it is not fully tilted to transverse plane. Therefore, we can go or drive much faster with GRE sequences compared to SE sequences. If we make the θ very low and also choose a very short TR, MR magnetization reaches some form of steady-state (equilibrium) after a certain number of rf excitations and we can even create faster GRE sequence called as fast and ultrafast GRE sequences. These types of fast GRE sequences are used very frequently where we need the speed such as abdomen, musculoskeletal, and MR angiography applications.

GRE sequences can be divided into four main subgroups:

- T1 weighted spoiled gradient echo (SPGR) sequences
- T2* weighted refocused gradient echo pulses
- Ultrafast gradient echo sequences
- Balanced gradient echo sequences (SSFP)

Let's take a quick glance of main advantages and disadvantages of GRE sequences:

Advantages:

- It is possible to acquire T1, T2*, and PD weighted MR images very fast.
- They have greater sensitivity to blood flow and can be used for MR angiography.
- Due to low flip angle (smaller rf pulse), their SAR exposure is much less than SE family.
- Can be used for breath hold and dynamic acquisitions.

Disadvantages:

- Their SNR is usually lower than SE images.
- They can only produce T2* contrast but not T2 contrast as in SE.
- They are very sensitive to field homogeneity and susceptibility effects.
- They are noisier than SE sequences.

Fast Gradient Echo (Fast GRE) sequences

Fast GRE and GRE sequences are pretty similar sequences and mainly used for T2* weighted imaging. However, fast GRE sequences employ shorter duration rf pulses, partial echo (fractional echo), and higher receiver bandwidth to make them *fast*. Please note that receiver bandwidth (RBW) is one of the parameters we will be covering in the next chapter in more detail. In fast GRE sequences, the chosen TR value and flip angle are considerably smaller than the GRE sequences, and this reduction on TR gives us considerably shorter acquisition times. A fractional echo is a specific term used to indicate that we sample the echo during a smaller sampling window (Ts). Therefore, fractional echo can be used in fast gradient echo sequences to go faster instead of full echo.

Let's take a quick glance of main advantages and disadvantages of fast GRE sequences:

Advantages:

- Very short TR, partial signal averaging (NEX or NSA), and partial echo utilization make them very fast.
- Due to low flip angle (smaller rf pulse), their SAR exposure is much less than SE family.
- Due to shorter scan times, higher resolution can be reached.
- With the appropriate choice of TE, in-phase and out-of-phase images can be acquired easily.

Disadvantages:

- Due to short TR and low flip angle resulting in tissue signal saturation, SNR is usually lower.
- Partial NEX and fractional echo do further reduce the SNR.
- They are very sensitive to field homogeneity and susceptibility effects.
- They are noisier than SE sequences.

Spoiled Gradient Echo (SPGR) Sequences

SPGR sequences are the groups of sequences used to create mainly T1 weighted imaging. Here the word *spoil* refers to the sequence design feature used to *crush* or *spoil* any remaining magnetization at the end of each TR cycle. This can be achieved by applying the excitation rf pulse with a different phase in each TR cycle and/or applying quite strong crusher or spoiler gradients at the end of each TR cycle. These two methods can be used independently or together to spoil any remaining magnetization after data sampling in each TR. *This can be thought of erasing the blackboard (or whiteboard) in the classroom after each class, so that the new class can start their lecture with a new and clean board.* Similar to this analogy, spoiler creates a clean and erased blackboard for the new TR cycle. Why does that matter to us? Well, spoiling the magnetization at the end of TR cycle means that the previous history of applied gradients does not affect us (theoretically) and we can get a clean T1 weighting. Different manufacturers can call this sequence as SPGR, FLASH, SHORT, and T1-FFE.

Fast Spoiled Gradient Echo (Fast SPGR) Sequences

Fast SPGR and SPGR sequences are pretty similar sequences and mainly used for T1 weighted imaging. However, fast SPGR sequences may employ shorter duration rf pulses, partial echo (fractional echo), and higher receiver bandwidth to make them *fast*. Please note that RBW is one of the parameters we will be covering in the next chapter in more detail. In fast SPGR sequences, the chosen TR value and flip angle are considerably less than the SPGR sequences and this reduction on TR gives us considerably shorter acquisition times. We also can reach shorter TE times in fast SPGR. Shorter TEs can reduce susceptibility artefacts and increase the SNR.

Echo Planar Imaging (EPI) Sequences

Echo planar imaging (EPI) sequences, like SSFSE sequences, can be considered as one of the ultrafast sequences as well. This sequence has been designed in early 1990s with the development of more powerful MR hardware and utilizes very fast switching of gradients. After the initial rf excitation pulse, the gradients, especially in the frequency encoding direction, run almost nonstop until the whole k-space is covered, as shown in Fig. 4.3. Driving or running gradients almost nonstop with a very fast switching as shown in Fig. 4.3 is

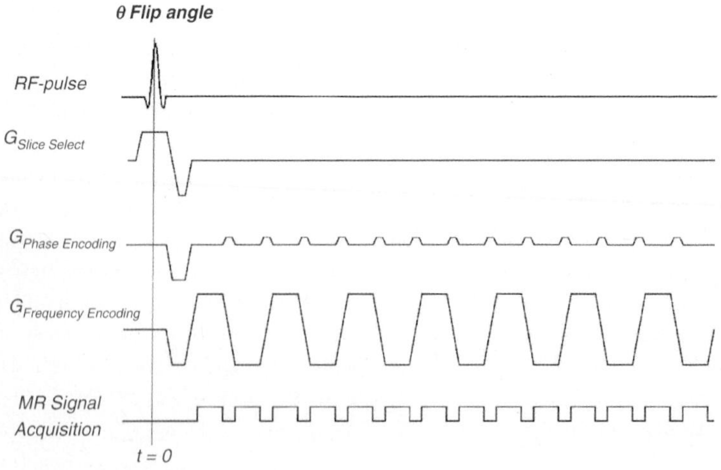

Figure 4.3 A typical gradient echo EPI pulse diagram.

very demanding on the MR hardware as you can imagine. However, new MR hardware and software are designed to enable this demand with state-of-art design and in some cases such as functional MRI (fMRI), EPI sequence can run quite a long time.

While the *trapezoidal* gradients in frequency encoding direction are applied to acquire one line of k-space, the small trapezoidal gradients (blips) in phase encoding direction take us to the next line of k-space with small increment, so that we can acquire the whole k-space line by line within a single cycle (single shot). Here the total number of positive and negative trapezoidal gradients on frequency encoding direction would be equal to phase encoding matrix. Similarly, total number of blips in phase encoding direction would also be equal to the defined phase encoding matrix. As a result of this powerful sequence, we can acquire a single slice in the order of 200 ms or more depending on the chosen matrix. As we can recall from SSFSE, EPI sequence is also a single shot sequence. Therefore, we can only produce a T2* weighted MR contrast from *gradient echo EPI* sequences. With an additional 180° rf pulse, we can produce a T2 weighted *SE EPI* sequence. We can also use multishot EPI sequences, which can enable us to create a form of T1 contrast with a significantly longer acquisition times. However, in this case, the resulting sequence will be more of a multi-echo gradient echo sequence rather than an EPI sequence. Therefore, I recommend that the reader assume that EPI sequences are either T2 or T2* weighted unless otherwise stated.

Let's take a quick glance of main advantages and disadvantages of EPI sequences:

Advantages:

- It is one of the fastest sequence in MR imaging.
- It is the base sequence for, very well-known diffusion weighted imaging (DWI) sequence.
- It is also the base sequence for diffusion tensor imaging (DTI), perfusion weighted imaging (PWI), and fMRI.
- It can provide the one of fastest T2* contrast imaging.

Disadvantages:

- Fast switching gradients require relatively new MR hardware. Therefore, it cannot be used efficiently at older MR scanners and some open MR scanners.

- Specific EPI artefacts and susceptibility artefacts may significantly degrade the image quality.
- Due to relatively low SNR, EPI imaging is performed at lower resolutions.
- It is not suitable for efficient T1 and PD contrast.
- Due to T2 filtering effect, resulting images are more blurry than conventional sequences.

Balanced Steady-State Free Precession (SSFP) Sequences

SSFP sequences were developed and introduced to clinical MRI during late 1990s and adapted quickly into routine imaging. SSFP sequences are based on the steady state magnetization principle. The term *balanced* is used mainly to indicate that the sequence design for this type of sequence requires that all gradients be applied in a way to rewind (or return back) them, so that we reach a zero phase after each excitation. SSFP sequence does have inherently very high SNR and is used with relatively low flip angle and very short TE and TR times. SSFP sequences can be called GRE, SPGR, Turbo FLASH, and FFE. On the other hand, different manufacturers can name the fully balanced SSFP sequences, which are the main interest here, as FIESTA, True FISP, or b-FFE.

Balanced SSFP sequences attract a great deal of attention because of two very important features: inherently high SNR and very short acquisition times. However, their contrast weighting is proportional to T2/T1 ratio rather than T1 or T2 itself. This somewhat unusual contrast weighting can be a great bonus especially when we want to see a high contrast between fluids and surrounding tissue. For example, balanced SSFP is used very commonly for cardiac applications where we like to have a good contrast between blood and myocardium. It can also be used for myelography, internal acoustic canal (IAC), coronary artery imaging, and certain noncontrast MR angiography. Nevertheless, T2/T1 ratio contrast can be a problem when we want to visualize various lesions with this type sequence. Why is it so? The main reason we can see lesions in MRI is that their T2, T1, or PD can be altered in disease states. Therefore, in a T2 and T1 weighted imaging can show a great difference between the lesion and normal tissue. However, T2 and T1 values of tissue cannot be altered independently even in disease state. So, the difference of normal tissue T2/T1 ratio and lesion T2/T1 ratio can be very small. Due to this small difference, we may not visualize the lesion well in balanced sequences even though it might be easily visible on a T2 weighted image.

Let's take a quick glance of main advantages and disadvantages of balanced SSFP sequences:

Advantages:

- One of the fastest sequences in MRI.
- They can be used very successfully for noncontrast MRA, cardiac MR, MRCP, myelography, and IAC applications.
- They do have inherently high SNR and short acquisition times.
- T2/T1 ratio contrast makes it possible to visualize vascular structure body fluids with great CNR.
- They can be designed and used for high resolution 2D or 3D MR imaging.

Disadvantages:

- Field in homogeneity can adversely affect the balanced state and create adverse artefacts.
- T2/T1 ratio contrast makes it difficult to visualize lesion with this sequence.
- They usually are noisier than most other sequences.

MR Spectroscopy Pulse Sequences

MR spectroscopy has been used extensively in chemistry for a long time and then introduced to clinical application to obtain cranial spectrum. Essentially, MR spectroscopy, also known as nuclear magnetic resonance (NMR) spectroscopy, is a noninvasive technique, which has been used to study metabolic changes in brain tumors, multiple sclerosis, Alzheimer, stroke, and other diseases affecting the brain. In the past, MR spectroscopy application was very time consuming since the user was supposed to do some manual steps to ensure a good spectrum. However, today, MR spectroscopy became much more easier to apply in clinical setting, thanks to advancement of MR hardware and software. Therefore, cranial MR spectroscopy applications are extended to body MR applications, including, but not limited to, breast, liver, prostate, and muscles.

MR spectroscopy technique is significantly different than MR imaging, and it will be great to look at those differences step by step:

- MR imaging provides spatial maps of water distribution in various tissues; MR spectroscopy provides spectral distribution of tissue metabolites as shown in Fig. 4.4.

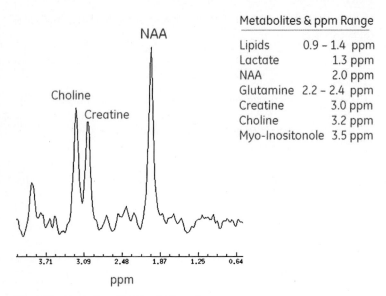

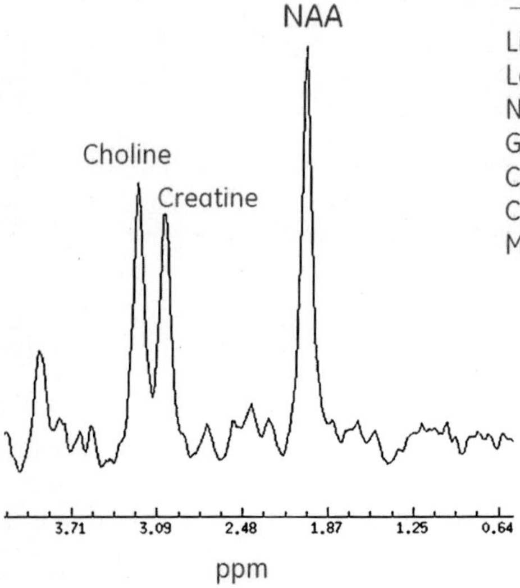

Metabolites & ppm Range	
Lipids	0.9 – 1.4 ppm
Lactate	1.3 ppm
NAA	2.0 ppm
Glutamine	2.2 – 2.4 ppm
Creatine	3.0 ppm
Choline	3.2 ppm
Myo-Inositonole	3.5 ppm

Figure 4.4 A typical long TE (144 ms) MR spectrum.

- The main purpose of proton MR spectroscopy is to obtain the concentration of major metabolites in the body while MR imaging is used to obtain morphological and functional information in the body.
- MR spectroscopy shows a spectrum graph, which is proportional to the concentration of metabolites, while MR images show a signal proportional to water content and relaxation properties of the tissues and lesions in the brain.
- MRS can be used to visualize *N*-acetyl aspartate, *NAA* (neuron activity marker), choline (cell membrane marker), creatine (energy metabolism), lipids (product of brain destruction), lactate (product of anaerobic glycolysis), myoinositol (glial cell marker, osmolyte hormone receptor), glutamine, and GABA (neurotransmitters). Alanine and few other metabolites can be visualized in different disease states as well.
- MRS graphs show the metabolite's spectral location in ppm (parts per million). This is essentially an indication of how far apart they are from the resonance frequency (chemical shift).

- The ppm location of metabolites visualized in MRS can be summarized below:
  - Lactate at *0.9–1.4 ppm*
  - Lipids at *1.3 ppm*
  - NAA at *2.0 ppm*
  - GABA at *2.2–2.4 ppm*
  - Creatine at *3.0 ppm*
  - Choline at *3.2 ppm*
  - Myoinositol *3.5 ppm*
  - Alanine at *1.48 ppm*

Single Voxel Spectroscopy (*SVS*): SVS is used to excite and receive spectrum signal from a small volume (typically 8 cm^3). For SVS data acquisition, either STEAM (stimulated echo acquisition mode) or PRESS (point resolved spectroscopy) technique can be used. PRESS sequence can provide higher SNR compared to STEAM sequence while STEAM sequence can show more metabolites. However, PRESS sequence is used more commonly in clinical practice, due to higher SNR, better stability, and lesser sensitivity to various artefacts.

Multivoxel Spectroscopy (*MVS*): MVS can be called as chemical shift imaging (CSI) as well to indicate that metabolites in the brain have a different chemical shift or resonance frequency with respect to each other. With MVS technique, larger region of interest can be covered. This large region of interest is divided into smaller voxels with an individual spectrum in them. The voxel size in MVS will be directly proportional to the matrix size used and will be much smaller than a typical SVS. In addition, MVS gives us opportunity to see spectrum from normal appearing tissue and lesion and makes it possible to do a quick comparison. Therefore, it is used quite commonly in clinical MRS practice.

Phase Contrast (PC) sequences

As we mentioned earlier, the MR signal we measure is a "complex signal" as it is called in engineering terms. The complex signal has two major components: magnitude and phase. Almost always, the magnitude of this complex signal is used to create an MR image. On the other hand, the phase component of this signal is simply ignored, because it does not give much information on morphology or the function of the tissues with few exceptions. Main applications we use in the phase information are 2D or 3D PC MRA, flow measurements, and recently developed susceptibility weighted imaging (SWI) applications.

PC MRA and flow measurements have been known and are used since the early days of MRI. PC techniques are based on the principle that *flowing blood or CSF in the body produces a different phase than stationary tissue and this phase is proportional to the direction and velocity of the flow*. Therefore, PC imaging is used to measure the blood flow and velocity even in very slow flow of CSF in the brain as well as major vessels of the body. In addition, PC angiography can be used to visualize arteries and veins of the brain by eliminating signal from stationary tissues in the background. However, in PC techniques, the user should check the literature and have an estimate of velocity of the vessels of interest for best image quality. This value, called as velocity encoding (venc), is required to optimize the dynamic range of phase information we will get with PC techniques. Due to more extensive flow measurements and renewed interest in noncontrast MR angiography applications, PC techniques have been used more commonly in clinical practice now.

Time-of-Flight (TOF) Sequences

Time-of-flight sequences are one of the most commonly used sequences among the noncontrast MRA sequences. 2D and 3D TOF technique is used to differentiate the stationary tissue and moving protons inside the blood vessels. This can be accomplished saturating the background signal in the slice that is to be imaged with rapid RF pulses. Since the fresh incoming blood supplies a significant amount of spins, which has not *seen* any of the rapid rf pulses, the blood vessels would have a quite bright signal while the stationary tissue signal is almost completely suppressed. TOF sequences use gradient echo pulse sequence family with relatively small flip angle to be able to create a series of *rapid rf pulses*. As it can be obvious to some of the readers, we can maximize the signal from blood if we choose the slice orientation perpendicular to the blood vessels. In this case, the time of travel (or time of flight) of protons in blood vessels will be the shortest and they will see only very few rf pulses during their travel within the slice. If we choose a slice orientation parallel to the blood vessel, the *time of flight* of blood spins will be the longest and they too will be saturated by the rapid rf pulses. By now, I am assuming that all the readers had understood where the seemingly unrelated name *Time of Flight* came from.

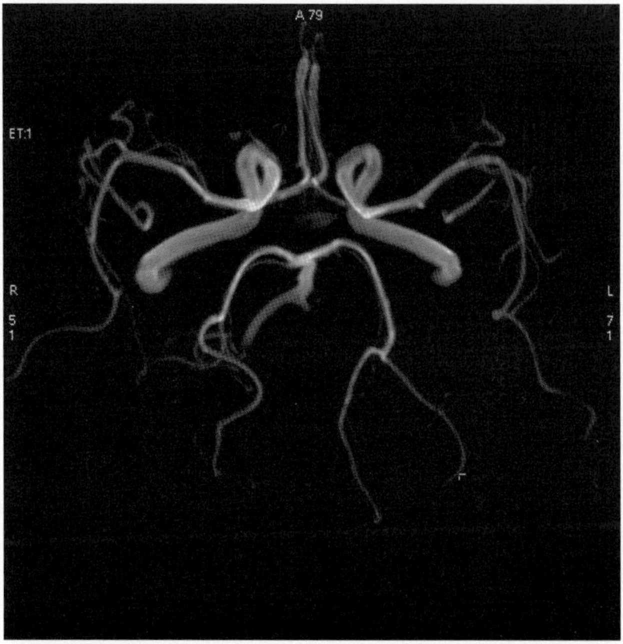

Figure 4.5 Circle of Willis MRA is a typical example of noncontrast 3D TOF.

One of the biggest advantages of TOF technique is that it can be used to visualize veins, arteries, or both. To selectively visualize arteries or veins, the user is requested to place a saturation band. For example, if you want to visualize Circle of Willis (COW) polygon as shown in Fig. 4.5, you need to put a saturation band superior to the 3D slab of interest.

Even though TOF technique has been used for quite a while now, it also suffers from some major drawbacks. TOF sequences usually require longer acquisition time and are sensitive to blood vessel orientation, susceptibility, and flow turbulences in stenosis or bifurcations. If the blood vessels are not exactly perpendicular to the slice, the stenosis can be overestimated easily. The readers should be aware of the potential pitfalls of TOF technique and interpret the results accordingly.

To optimize the MRA with TOF sequence, the user may be able to adjust some of the parameters. The main affect of the commonly used parameters can be summarized as follows:

- *Short TR*: The shorter TR results in further reduction of the background tissue signal while it also results in less SNR. This result should be intuitive: shorter TR means more rf pulses in a given imaging time, which in turn further saturates the stationary tissue.
- *Shorter TE*: Shorter TE reduces susceptibility and flow artefacts.
- *Flow Compensation*: Reduces blood flow–related ghosting artefacts.
- *Thin slices*: Thinner slices result in brighter blood signal but also reduce SNR.
- *Higher flip angle*: Further suppresses the stationary tissue signal.

Recent Sequences

The sequences mentioned above are the most commonly used sequences available almost on all the MR scanners. However, there are several new sequences, which came into the world of MRI within the last few years, and it is important to mention them here as well:

PROPELLER/BLADE/MULTIVANE: These sequences are available now by almost all major MR vendors and became available on most of new MR scanners. These types of sequences are developed to reduce the gross patient motion artefacts by acquiring the raw data in a rotating blade pattern (as the name indicates). In each rotation, a thick blade of k-space will be acquired to create a low-resolution image. At the end, the rotated k-space blades are combined with additional motion correction algorithms to create an almost motion-free high-resolution image. PROPELLER or BLADE image contrast can be T2, T2 FLAIR, T1 FLAIR, or T1 and mainly based on FSE sequence.

LAVA/VIBE/THRIVE: These 3D T1 gradient echo sequences are created by optimizing the k-space acquisition order and using parallel imaging techniques to accelerate the acquisition. They are mainly used for breath hold abdominal imaging applications (such as liver, pancreas, thoracs, and pelvis) and can be used to visualize the blood vessels and soft tissue at the same time.

VIBRANT/VIEWS/BLISS: These 3D T1 gradient echo sequences are created by optimizing the k-space acquisition order and using parallel imaging techniques to accelerate the acquisition. They are mainly used for breast imaging applications and can visualize both blood vessels and breast tissue at the same time. They are designed to utilize a number of efficient fat saturation techniques and regional focused shimming algorithms.

TRICKS/CENTRA/TWIST: The new sequences called as TRICKS, TWIST, or CENTRA are the 3D T1 weighted sequences designed to acquire MR angiographies very fast. By manipulating and dividing the k-space to a number of centric views and sharing the data from the views in consecutive acquisitions, they can collect a 3D MRA series on the order of 0.5 s while a conventional angiosequence takes about 15–20 s for a similar resolution. Therefore, they are rightly called as 4D MRA in some cases. In this type of sequences, the k-space can be divided into 2, 3, or 4 centric pieces as per design of the sequence. The user can choose as many repetitions (phases) as appropriate for their applications and run the sequence to create dynamic MRA (4D) series.

These sequences greatly reduce the need for timing of vessel filling and also provide dynamic enhancement of vessels with contrast injection applications.

Naming Conventions of MR Sequences by the Vendors

The fast pace of MR sequence development creates quite a bit of confusion on MR sequence naming. This is simply because that each developer or vendor comes up with a catchy and differentiating name for their new sequences. In the old good days, it was very easy to know and memorize few sequence names in each vendor. However, today, there are practically hundreds of sequences with a different name even though they might be somewhat similar to each other in their design. To ease the pain of multivendor users and to create a better communication among MR users, we prepared the cross naming convention table below. Simply because of the space limitation, we apologize not being able to include here more sequences and more vendors. With the recent increase of MR manufacturers, especially from Asia, we expect this list to grow soon and strongly recommend our users to update the list from various sources available on the Internet.

We would also like to remind you that each vendor designs their sequences with slightly different flavor. Therefore, the same sequence on a different MR manufacturer can give you quite a different image contrast and image quality. This list is intended for providing a general information on naming convention of similarly designed sequences for users and hoping that will fill a gap in clinical scanning. However, it does not indicate or imply that those sequences are identical to each other (Table 4.2).

Table 4.2 Naming convention for main MR pulse sequences for different vendors.

	GE	SIEMENS	PHILIPS	TOSHIBA
SPIN ECHO	SE, MEMP	SE	SE	SE
TURBO SPIN ECHO	FSE	TSE	TSE	FSE
SINGLE SHOT FSE	SSFSE	HASTE	Single shot TSE	FASE
FSE with FAST RECOVERY	FRFSE	RESTORE	DRIVE	FSE T2 pulse
GRADIENT ECHO	GRE	GRE	FFE	FIELD ECHO
INCOHERENT RF-SPOILED GRE	SPGR, FSPGR		T1 FFSE	FIELD ECHO
INCOHERENT GRAD-SPOILED GRE	MPGR	FLASH		FIELD ECHO
COHERENT GRE	GRASS	FISP	FFE	FIELD ECHO
BALANCED SSFP	FIESTA	True FISP	Balanced SSFP	True SSFP
DUAL EXCITATION BALANCED SSFP	FIESTA-C	CISS		
DOUBLE ECHO STEADY STATE		DESS		
MULTIECHO GRE	MERGE	MEDIC		
ULTRAFAST GRE	Fast GRE, fast SPGR	Turbo FLASH	TFE	Fast FE
VOLUME INTERPOLATED GRE	FAME, LAVA	VIBE	THRIVE	
T2 FLAIR	FLAIR	TURBO DARK FLUID	FLAIR	FLAIR
PARALLEL IMAGING	ASSET	iPAT	SENSE	RAPID
PROPELLER	PROPELLER	BLADE	MULTIVANE	
4D TIME RESOLVED MRA	TRICKS	TREAT, TWIST	CENTRA	
WATER and FAT SEPERATION	IDEAL, 3D-FLEX	VIBE-DIXON	mDIXON	

Chapter 5

MR Imaging Parameters and Options

MR Parameters

In MR imaging, there are somewhat a large number of parameters or factors affecting total exam time, signal to noise ratio (SNR), and contrast to noise ratio (CNR). Selection of right MR imaging parameters almost always results in better image quality and prevents the typical imaging artefacts seen on daily scanning. Therefore, it is very important to understand the working mechanism of those parameters for the best decision making.

In general, we can divide MR parameters into three main groups:

- MR imaging parameters
- MR pulse sequence parameters
- MR imaging options

In this chapter, we will take a detailed look on all the key parameters and will learn what they mean in everyday imaging, so that the reader can make educated decision on their optimization.

MR Imaging Parameters

This is the section where we will be defining the parameters we will be adjusting everyday such as field of view (FOV), imaging matrix, etc. The good news is that we will explain them with the real MR images, so that you can get a much better feeling on what they do. Let's start with FOV:

FOV (*Field of View*): FOV is given in cm or mm depending on the vendor and defines the length of MR image coverage in each plane. The FOV can be given as a single number such as 24 cm for square FOV or as 24 × 20 cm for

M. Elmaoğlu and A. Çelik, *MRI Handbook: MR Physics, Patient Positioning, and Protocols*, DOI 10.1007/978-1-4614-1096-6_5,

rectangular FOV. For 3D imaging, slab coverage in slice encoding direction can be given as well in addition to in-plane FOV. The rectangular FOV is chosen mainly to reduce the scan time and the smaller FOV almost always refers to the FOV in phase encoding direction. The effect of FOV on the resulting image is quite straightforward. The FOV is directly proportional to the SNR of the resulting image. If you double the FOV in frequency direction, then your image SNR will be 2 times better (doubled) as well. As shown in the figure below, if you halve FOV in both frequency and phase direction from 30 to 15 cm, then your SNR will be 4 times less. This remarkable reduction in SNR can also be confirmed visually with the more grainy or noisy image with smaller FOV. However, *this does not mean that small FOV is bad*. As an MR user, you need to choose the best FOV to fit into the region of interest and consult with the site radiologist for their preference, because smaller FOV can give you more detail by means of increased resolution as we will see in this section as well (Fig. 5.1).

Imaging Matrix: MR imaging matrix do not have any measurement units but it merely shows the number of how many sample points or measurements we are making during the acquisition. In the past, we had analog cameras to take pictures and now have digital cameras with a certain number of mega pixels. We can store those digital pictures on computer media. Now we are living in almost entirely digital world and we *sample* or measure everything by

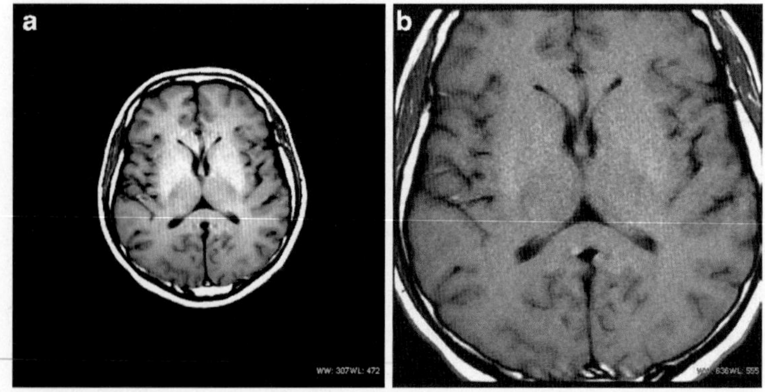

Figure 5.1 Sample images acquired with 30 cm (a) and 15 cm (b) FOV are shown on the same volunteer.

a finite (limited) number of points, so that we can store them in computers for a long time. If you see 512 × 512 imaging matrix, you can tell that this image was acquired with 512 points in frequency and phase direction. You can also commonly see rectangular imaging matrix such as 512 × 384. In this case, usually the lower imaging matrix will be applied in phase direction to reduce the total scan time. However, in some cases such as diffusion weighted imaging and balanced SSFP imaging, the frequency matrix can be lower than phase matrix to reduce the minimum echo time (TE), to increase SNR and to reduce geometric distortion and/or susceptibility artefacts.

The effect of imaging matrix on resulting image is inversely proportional to square root of the matrix factor. What does that mean? It simply means that if we double the matrix in one direction, SNR of the acquired image will decrease by the square root of 2, resulting in a 41% reduction in SNR. If we change our image matrix from 256 × 256 to 512 × 512, our SNR will be halved (square root of 4) since we double our matrix in two directions. Figure 5.2 shows the visual effect of image matrix change from 128 × 128 to 320 × 320. Please notice that while the higher imaging matrix results in noisier image, it has better resolution.

Let's now look at the resolution in more detail since it is directly connected to our discussion here.

Resolution: As we mentioned above, FOV and matrix selection are a natural part of resolution. However, due to its importance in MRI, it is very

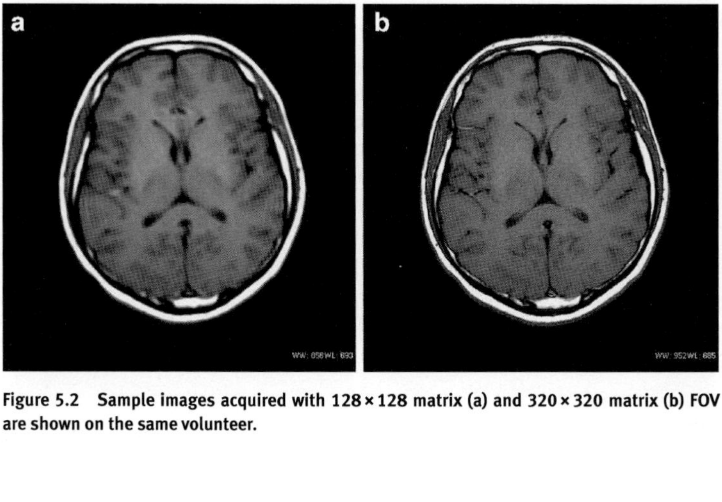

Figure 5.2 Sample images acquired with 128 × 128 matrix (a) and 320 × 320 matrix (b) FOV are shown on the same volunteer.

much needed to discuss resolution as a separate topic. Resolution in MRI can be defined as the ratio of FOV to matrix. If we assume a square matrix for a given FOV, then the image resolution will be in mm as shown below:

$$\text{Resolution} = \text{FOV} / \text{matrix in mm.}$$

If you have a rectangular matrix, then resolution can be stated as resolution in frequency and resolution in phase direction using the same exact formula as above. High resolution can be achieved either by reducing FOV or increasing by the matrix. Intuitively, lower resolution can be achieved by increasing the FOV and/or reducing the matrix. The resolution on slice direction can be defined directly by the slice thickness (TH). Resolution is directly related to SNR and one of the key but somewhat invisible parameters of MR imaging and a low resolution image almost always looks like a better image due to higher SNR.

Slice Thickness (*TH*): TH is defined in mm and determines the depth of your voxel on slice encoding direction. In simple words, it is the thickness of the slice you are imaging. The user-defined parameters in FOV, matrix, and TH are used by the MR scanner to calculate the exact rf gradient magnitude to be able to create a slice with the given thickness. In 2D imaging, the TH can be on the order of 4–8 mm for routine applications. For 3D imaging, the TH is usually much thinner and can vary from 0.5 to 5 mm depending on the application and coverage of anatomy. As shown below, the thicker the slice is, the higher the SNR becomes. However, the thicker the slice, the lower the resolution becomes. Therefore, TH selection also requires an educated decision by the user (Fig. 5.3).

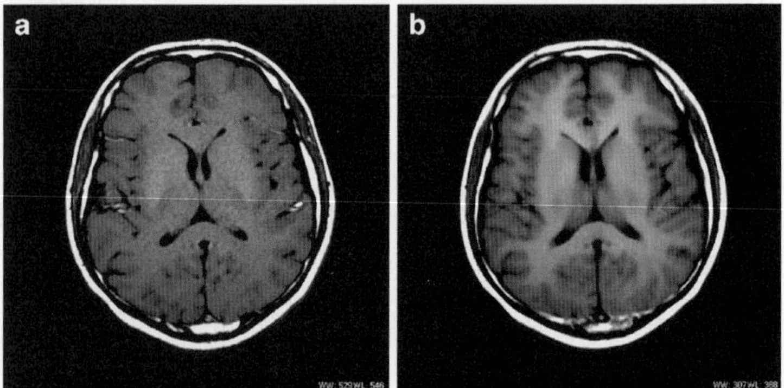

Figure 5.3 Sample images acquired with slice thickness of 3 mm (a) and 15 mm (b) are shown on the same volunteer.

Slice Spacing or Gap: Slice spacing or gap can be defined in mm or in percentage of the TH depending on MR manufacturers. Either in mm or in percentage, more than 25% slice spacing is recommend for routine 2D imaging. This spacing is needed to reduce the crosstalk artefacts caused by the excitation of neighboring slices with the application of imperfect slice selective rf pulse. However, with the advancement of MR technology and more frequent use of interleaved acquisition in routine imaging, you may be able to reduce slice spacing and even choose no spacing. Interleaved slice acquisition is a practical way of acquiring slices in a different acquisition order than sequential to minimize crosstalk issues. Please note that the crosstalk artefacts are not easily seen in most cases. Therefore, it is always better to check with your MR user guide or MR manufacturer for the recommended slice spacing for different protocols.

Number of Averages (*NSA, number of excitation* [*NEX*]): NSA is an indication of how many signal averages taken during an MR acquisition. This is usually achieved by repeating the acquisition in frequency direction and taking an average of the sampled signal. NSA is also called NEX or number of excitations. NEX or NSA is mainly used to increase SNR at the expense of increased acquisition time. SNR increase is directly proportional to the square root of NEX increase factor. For example, if we acquire an MR image with 2 NEX and 4 NEX rather than 1 NEX, we expect to see an SNR increase of 41 and 100%, respectively. In addition to the increased SNR, higher NEX would also give us smoother images by simply averaging the flow artefacts or typical ghosting artefacts coming from gross organ motion or breathing. A typical SNR increase is shown in the figure below. As we expect from the above discussion, SNR is doubled by simply increasing the NEX fourfold. Even though the resulting image looks much more pleasing to the eye, you have to remember that fourfold increase in NEX also means a fourfold increase in total scan time (Fig. 5.4).

Receiver Bandwidth (*RBW*): We would assume that RBW is one of the least known parameters of MR imaging and rarely used by the MR radiographers. We hope to shed some more light onto it, so that you can get a better feeling on what you are dealing with.

RBW is expressed in either hertz or kilohertz in MRI. Hertz is an engineering unit and can also be defined as 1/s. In MRI, if we choose a RBW of 32.5 kHz, it means that our sequence would acquire data up to this maximum RBW. Again here, we need to remember that we live in a digital world and can acquire signal in a relatively small number of point. For example, we can have only 256 sample points if we choose a frequency matrix of 256. The time duration between each sample points can be on the order of microseconds and

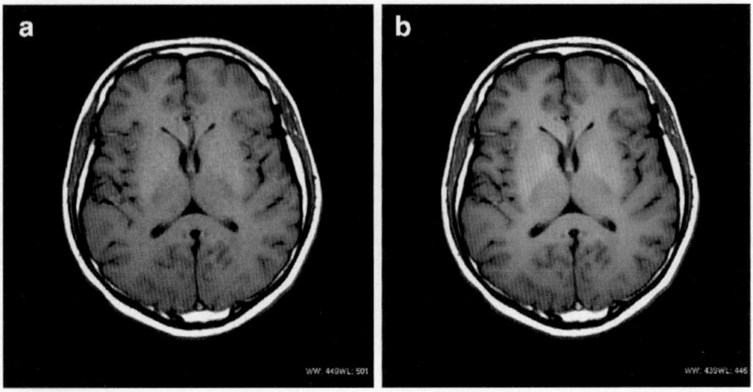

Figure 5.4 Sample images acquired with a NEX of 1 (a) and NEX of 4 (b) are shown on the same volunteer.

is defined as sampling time per pixel. From this sampling time and selected frequency matrix, you can calculate total RBW as follows:

$$\text{Total RBW} = \text{Frequency matrix} / \text{Ts (in seconds)}.$$

Of course as a user, you do not know what Ts in each case. However, if you choose a frequency matrix of 125 and RBW of 6.25 or 62.5 kHz, you can calculate your Ts as 20 or 2 ms, respectively. In some vendors, RBW can be expressed in Hertz per pixel. In this case, if you choose a RBW of 100 Hz and frequency matrix of 100, then your sampling time would be 10 ms. If you are wondering why we went into a confusing discussion on Ts, you are not alone but we will see why it is important and bear with me.

Very similar to NEX, SNR is also directly proportional to the square root of RBW change factor. As we have shown in the figure below, if we increase RBW tenfold from 6.25 to 62.5 kHz, we reduce SNR by square root of 10 (3.16). Even though this is a quite significant reduction in SNR, we also should know that higher bandwidth gives a much sharper image, reduces ringing artefacts (also called Gibbs ringing or truncation artefacts), and may also reduce the total scan time by means of faster data sampling. The increase of RBW has also one more benefit of reducing the typical chemical shift artefacts or fat displacement artefact. We can consider this as an added bonus for higher RBW. *However, we also have to remember that all these benefits come at the expense of reduced SNR* (Fig. 5.5).

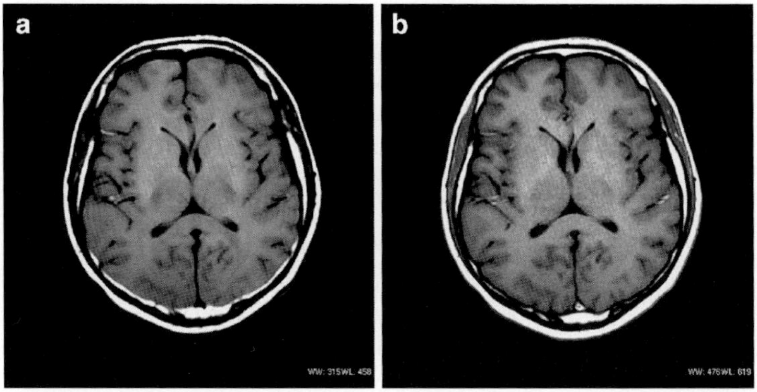

Figure 5.5 Sample images acquired with a receiver bandwidth of 6.92 kHz (a) and 62.5 kHz (b) are shown on the same volunteer.

Table 5.1 Effects of key parameters on SNR, resolution, and scan time.

Parameter	Direction of change	Resolution	SNR	Scan time
Slice thickness	If we decrease	Increases	Decreases	No change
FOV (frequency)	If we decrease	Increases	Decreases	No change
FOV (phase)	If we decrease	Increases	Decreases	Decreases
Matrix (frequency)	If we increase	Increases	Decreases	No change
Matrix (phase)	If we increase	Increases	Decreases	Increases
NEX (NSA)	If we increase	No change	Increases	Increases
RBW (bandwidth)	If we decrease	No change	Increases	No change

Summary of Key Parameter effects and tradeoff: Up to now in this chapter, we had touched some key parameters in MRI and discussed their effect on image quality. I feel that a simple tabular summary is going to make our understanding much more stronger. Hence, in the table below, we will show a quick summary of what would happen to SNR, resolution, and scan time if we *increase* or *decrease* a certain parameter (Table 5.1).

Frequency or Phase Direction Choice: For MR protocol optimization, artefact reduction, and scan time reduction, we sometimes have to decide on the frequency and phase encoding direction with respect to the anatomy of interest. For routine imaging, frequency direction should be chosen as the longer anatomical direction to eliminate folding or wrapping artefacts. For example, if you scan hips in axial plane, you should choose Right to Left (RL) as your frequency direction, so that you do not get wrapping in RL even if you choose a smaller FOV imaging. This decision is based on the fact that we almost never get a wrapping in frequency direction because of our very high sampling rate. So if we want to do let's say spine imaging in sagittal plane, we should choose head to foot (HF) or superior inferior (SI) as our frequency direction, right? Yes, this is right; however there is a catch here. If we choose SI as our frequency direction in sagittal spine imaging, we will be seeing significantly increased CSF flow and patient breathing artefacts in phase direction, which is anterior posterior (AP) in this case. Therefore, it will be wiser to optimize our protocol by choosing AP as our frequency direction, so that all these artefacts can be reduced very significantly. For brain imaging, we almost always choose RL for frequency direction in diffusion weighted imaging to reduce a different type of artefacts called susceptibility artefacts. For routine body imaging in axial plane, we choose RL as our frequency direction, so that we can reduce scan time by reducing the FOV in phase direction (phase FOV). If you understand the main logic of frequency and phase imaging direction selection, you can confidently apply it to more complicated and broader cases of oblique plane cardiac imaging, breast imaging, etc.

MR Pulse Sequence Parameters

Up to now we have discussed some key MR imaging parameters, which can be controlled by the user directly or indirectly. In this section, we will be looking at some additional MR pulse sequence parameters vital to SNR and CNR. As you can remember from Chap. 3, we already had a good exposure to some of those key parameters, and in this section, we will be reviewing them with more references to MR pulse sequences.

TR (*Repetition Time*): TR is given in milliseconds and defines the time interval between two consecutive 90° (or less) rf excitation pulses. However, for single shot spin echo (SSFSE, HASTE) or gradient echo (EPI) sequences, we apply a single rf excitation pulse, which can be 90° or less and TR definition becomes somewhat invalid. In this case, TR can be considered as very long and we can only get a T2/T2* contrast due to the long TR selection and single shot excitation. In spin echo–based sequences, TR and TE selection defines the image contrast weighting whether it is T1, T2, or PD. In gradient echo–based sequences, especially fast and ultrafast gradient echo techniques, TR, TE, and flip angle (FA) define the image contrast whether it is T1, T2*, or PD.

TE (*Echo Time*): TE is measured on milliseconds and defined as the time from the center of the initial excitation rf pulse (typically 90°) to the time where the signal (echo) reaches maximum. For a spin echo pulse sequence, the time can be defined as twice the time between 90° and 180° rf pulses. So how can we know all those timings? We do not have to. All the new MR systems are smart enough to adjust your gradients to create an echo at the time you entered manually on the user interface of the scanner and this makes things much easier for all of us. For FSE (or TSE), SSFSE, and EPI type multiecho sequences, there are some special cases due to the fact that we apply multiple refocusing 180° rf pulses (for spin echo–based sequences) or multiple rephasing gradients and can have an effective TE. We will discuss effective TE below for detailed information.

We can choose a higher TE value to create a T2 weighting. As we have shown in Fig. 5.6 below, we can have a T2 weighting by choosing either a TE of 80 or 175 ms. Like many other things in MRI, each choice will give us a different tradeoff. While the lower TE of 80 ms gives us relatively lower T2 weighting, it gives us remarkably higher SNR and a somewhat sharper image. On the other hand, higher TE value of 175 ms gives us more T2 weighting at the expense of significantly less SNR and blurrier image. If you can recall, in Chap. 3, we discussed the T2 decay of different tissue types and said that you can choose a TE time to optimize the image contrast (CNR) between different tissues. In the brain, GM and WM are the two main tissue types we are interested. If you use the formulas given in Chap. 3 using the real T1 and T2 values of WM and GM,

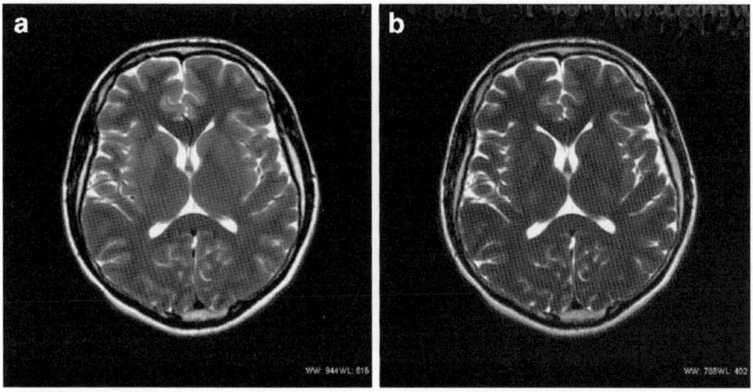

Figure 5.6 Sample images acquired with a TE time of 80 ms (a) and 175 ms (b) are shown on the same volunteer.

you can see that a TE time around 100 ms would give us the best CNR for a T2 imaging in SE or FSE sequence family for a long TR acquisition.

Effective Echo Time (*Eff TE*): For multiple echo images, the TE time can be selected by the user as well. However, specifically in FSE or HASTE type sequences, the TE time can be a multiplication of the time between two consecutive refocusing 180° rf pulses. This time is called as *Echo Spacing* and one of the invisible parameters created by the system. For example, if you enter a TE time of 100 ms for your T2 weighted FSE or TSE acquisition, you may end up getting an image with an effective TE time of 97.6 or 102 ms. The effective TE is usually annotated by the vendors just to state that it was the TE time, which can be achieved by the system. Echo spacing will depend on the system's gradient strength and slew rate. With the new systems and depending on the imaging parameters, it can be on the order of single digit milliseconds. As you can guess, the difference between the real and effective TE time is quite miniscule and may have no significant difference on the image quality.

Inversion Time, TI: Inversion time is also measured in milliseconds and defined as the time interval between the inversion 180° pulse and echo formation time.

TI time is used in some of older but essential pulse sequences including but not limited to STIR, T2 FLAIR, T1 FLAIR, the latest STIR DWI (DWIBS), and general FSE-IR or Gradient Echo-IR (GRE-IR) sequences. Depending on the application and pulse sequence, TI time can range from 50 ms to all the way up to 2,500 ms. For STIR or T2 FLAIR images, TI time is chosen to suppress fat and CSF signal, respectively. In T1 FLAIR and general GRE-IR sequences, it is used to enhance the T1 contrast of the resulting images. As we have seen in the previous chapter, TI time is chosen as the 69% of the T1 value of a specific tissue. Therefore, TI is chosen around 150 and 2,100 ms to suppress fat or CSF in the body, respectively. The sample STIR images below are acquired to give you a different perspective on what would happen if you experiment with different TI times. As you can see a short TI time of 70 ms gives an impressive image with almost no fat suppression while 145 ms TI time gives you a well-appreciated image with full fat suppression. The TI time of 270 ms reduced the signal from spinal vertebra, and fat signal comes back almost fully now. In certain cases like TI prepared body diffusion weighted imaging (STIR DWI), you can end up with a better image quality with a shorter TI time of 70–80 ms (Fig. 5.7).

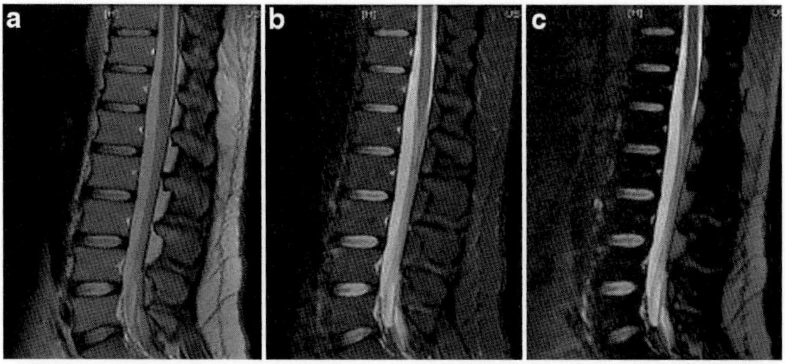

Figure 5.7 Sample images acquired with a TI time of 70 ms (a), 145 ms (b), and 270 ms (c) are shown on the same volunteer.

Echo Train Length (ETL) or Turbo Factor: ETL or turbo factor can be defined as the number of refocusing 180° rf pulses after the initial excitation rf pulse. FSE or TSE sequences with higher number of echoes are discovered after the initial spin echo pulses and reduced the MR image acquisition time significantly for T2 and PD weighted images. The higher ETL or turbo factor usually means a higher T2 weighting, shorter acquisition time, less number of slices, more motion artifact, and more blurry images. If that sounds like a typical tradeoff again, you are exactly right. In MR nothing comes for free.

Due to the greater advantages of FSE sequences, they are used very commonly in clinical scanning. ETL is usually chosen as 2–3 for a good T1 weighted image, 6–8 for a good PD weighted image, and 12–30 for a good T2 weighted image. It is important to know that modern MR scanners and additional pulse sequence design features reduced the adverse effects (blurring) of higher ETL and make them even more attractive. In the figure below, we have shown images acquired with an ETL of 8 and 24 while maintaining all other imaging parameters. When you carefully inspect those two images, you may get a slight impression that ETL of 24 gives a better T2 weighting for the same TE time and slightly more blurring. However, even for the trained eyes of our readers, it is very difficult to differentiate between these two sets of images. Therefore, you can choose an appropriate ETL as long as they are within the range given below to optimize your imaging protocol (Fig. 5.8).

Echo Spacing: As we mentioned in effective TE section, echo spacing is defined as the time between two consecutive refocusing 180° rf pulses. Echo

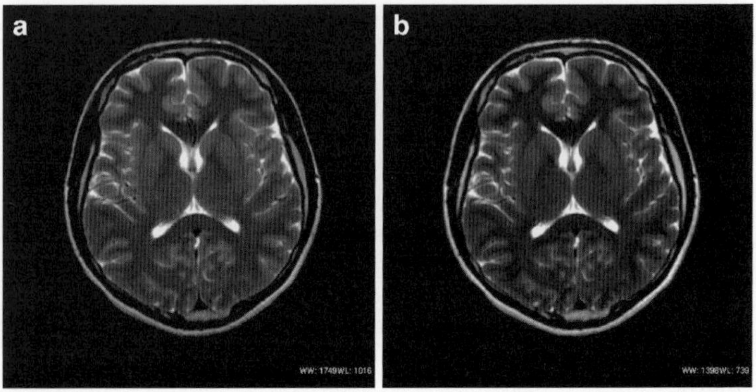

Figure 5.8 Sample images acquired with an ETL of 8 (a) and 24 (b) are shown on the same volunteer.

spacing is invisible to MR users. However, we can reduce echo spacing by reducing our resolution or increasing the RBW.

Flip Angle (*FA*): FA or tilting angle is defined by the initial rf excitation pulses and measured in degrees. It is an indication of how much of MR magnetization is pushed to the transverse (XY) plane. FA can be 90° for most of the spin echo–based sequences. It can vary from 5° to 90° for the broader gradient echo sequence family to create the desired image contrast and to accelerate the MR acquisition. It is one of the key parameters in gradient echo images affecting the resulting image contrast.

MR Imaging Options

In MR imaging, there are several imaging options used to enhance or alter the image contrast and to reduce the MR artefacts. The options such as fat saturation, cardiac gating, and flow compensation (FS) can be combined with certain pulse sequences depending on how they were designed and set up. Therefore, a good knowledge of those options, what they mean, and when they should be used is essential information for us. In this section, we will discuss a number of most important parameters and their use in MR imaging.

Fat Saturation (*FS*): Fat saturation option is one the most frequently used options in MR imaging. This option is also called chemical saturation due to its underlying principles. In the body, different metabolites can resonate at different frequencies. Water and fat resonate at around 220 Hz away from each other at 1.5 T and 440 Hz away at 3.0 T. Even though they resonate at different frequencies, we say that the frequency difference between fat and water is 3.5 ppm, independent of the field strength. The ppm can be calculated by dividing 220 Hz to 1.5 T resonance frequency (63.8 million) or 440 Hz to 3.0 T resonance frequency (127.6 million) and multiplying by million.

When we choose FS option, the scanner applies a narrow rf pulse just at the resonance frequency of the fat without affecting the water signal. In this case, we *excite* only the fat signal and produce a signal we do not want to use. By additional killer gradients, we practically kill (dephase) the fat signal. Afterward, we proceed with the routine pulse sequence to acquire the images without the fat signal. Therefore, we *saturate* the fat by means of a dedicated chemical saturation rf pulse. Fat saturation works pretty well in most cases. However, it may fail significantly in the following cases creating large field inhomogeneity:

- Large FOV scanning for whole body, abdomen, and pelvis exams
- Anatomically inhomogeneous structures such as neck and sinuses
- Around metallic implants

However, it also has the following advantages:

- Fat suppression technique can be applied with almost all the sequences
- Unlike STIR sequence, it does not alter the desired contrast mechanism of the pulse sequence

As an additional note, it is important to note that fat saturation pulses are designed only for fat excitation. However, due to the magnetization transfer (MT) effects resulting from an additional rf pulse applied off resonance, we will be losing some water signal as well and this decreases the overall signal.

Fat Suppression: Fat suppression technique is different than fat saturation by its inherent design and underlying principles. The fat suppression can be done with STIR imaging pulse sequences. Even though it is possible to create a somewhat T1 weighted and T2 weighted STIR image with an optimized TE choice, overall image contrast is altered by the initial inversion pulse here. Most of the radiographers and radiologists think that STIR images are noisy looking. However, the optimized protocol such as that given in this book improves the STIR image quality significantly when combined with the new state-of-art MR scanners and coils. Sample STIR images were shown in Fig. 5.7. The main advantage of STIR technique is its inherent insensitivity to magnetic field inhomogeneity. Therefore, it is used significantly in MSK imaging, whole body imaging, and neck imaging where inhomogeneity may become an issue.

Fat Separation: Fat separation is almost a new concept in routine imaging with the emergence of new pulse sequences separating water and fat. In late 1980s, three-point and two-point Dixon methods were used in research to separate water and fat using the inherent resonance difference of fat and water. As we can remember, fat and water have 3.5 ppm difference (fat has a lower resonance frequency). In three-point or two-point Dixon methods, the relevant numbers of slightly different TE times are applied to create a phase difference between fat and water. This means that we would have to repeat the same acquisition 2 or 3 times with the different TE times, so that we can measure the phase difference pixel by pixel and then make a separation between fat and water. This way we can get an efficient separation of water and fat image at the expense of 2 or 3 times longer acquisition time. These techniques have been used in low field routine clinical imaging for the last several years due to immense difficulties of getting a fat saturation. Recently, significantly improved and accelerated fat separation techniques have been developed (e.g., IDEAL, VIBE-Dixon, mDIXON, and LAVA-FLEX) for routine clinical imaging. They work as good as or better than STIR images and can enable us to create water (no fat), fat, in-phase, and out-of-phase images in a single acquisition.

Spectral inversion of lipids (*special*, *spir*, *spair*): Special or SPIR is a *special* technique combining fat suppression and fat saturation efficiently. In this case, a narrow rf inversion pulse applied only to invert the fat signal sparing the water signal. Then, routine scanning pulses were applied and signal is acquired at the TI time to eliminate fat signal more efficiently. Unlike STIR technique, SPECIAL fat sat technique does not alter the image contrast and is less susceptible to field inhomogeneties. Today, SPECIAL fat saturation is used mainly for gradient echo–based dynamic breast and liver imaging sequences and may be used more commonly in near future.

Flow Compensation (*FC*): MR imaging is a modality with many different types of image contrast and many different types of imaging artefacts. Blood flow– or general flow–related artefacts are one of the most common artefacts we may encounter in routine scanning. The flow artefacts result from the fact that the moving protons in the fluid will experience a different rf pulse due to a relatively longer TR time. Therefore, they will appear in a location different than their original location. FS option is designed to reduce the flow artefacts by means of application of additional gradients in the direction of FS.

The FC gradients can be first moment flow nulling (for a steady velocity) or second moment nulling (for acceleration). The second moment nulling techniques are very rare in routine imaging due to longer scan times required for those cases and almost always first moment nulling is used.

To give a better view of what FC is, we show a typical 3D T1 Gradient Echo pulse sequence in Fig. 5.9 with no FC. In Fig. 5.10, we show the same pulse diagram with FC. Additional FS gradients in frequency and slice encoding directions are encircled to show the main difference.

As shown in Fig. 5.10, FC requires additional gradient and increases the overall scan time. Therefore, we usually choose FC in one direction. As a general rule, FC is chosen in slice direction for axial plane imaging and is chosen

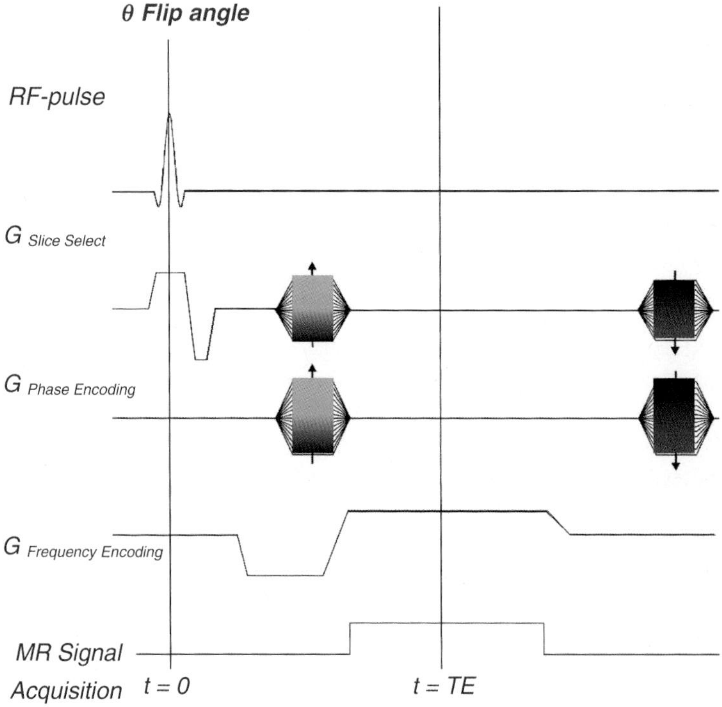

Figure 5.9 A typical 3D T1 fully rewinded gradient echo sequence with no flow compensation (FC).

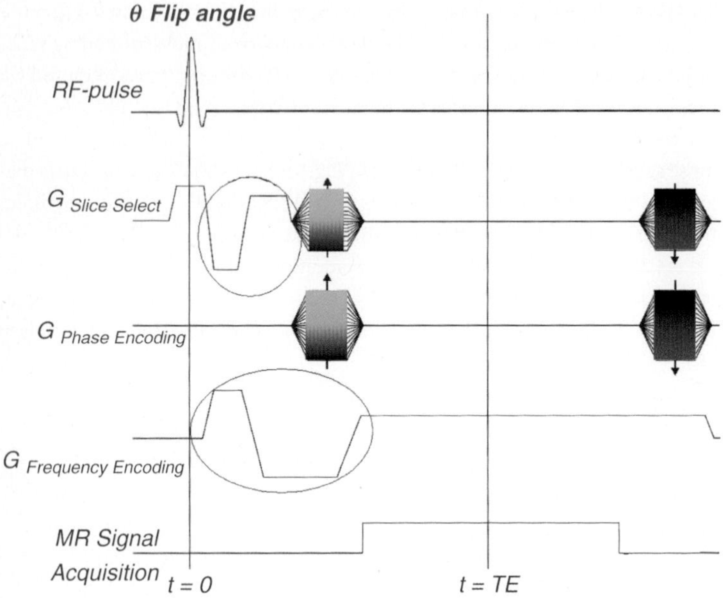

Figure 5.10 A typical 3D T1 fully rewinded gradient echo sequence with FC in frequency and slice direction.

in frequency direction in coronal or sagittal plane. Please note that the FC in phase direction is very rarely done because it requires a significant increase in scan time.

Saturation Bands (*SAT Bands*): SAT in MR are special rf pulses designed to be applied in any direction to significantly reduce the signal in region of application. We use them mainly to reduce the flow artefacts, gross patient motion artefacts (e.g., respiratory), cardiac motion artifacts, and involuntary body motion artefacts. In axial plane, superior or inferior SAT bands are applied to further reduce the fast flow artefacts of arteries. The so-called *concotenated SAT* bands can be linked with the axial slices to move in parallel to them, so that an efficient SAT can be maintained for the entire imaging region. In sagittal spine imaging, anterior or posterior rf pulses are applied to reduce cardiac, respiratory, and swallowing motion-related artefacts.

Respiratory Trigger (RTr): Respiratory triggering is an imaging option where we acquire data only in the expiration portion of breathing period. With this option, we image the body in a region with minimum respiratory motion. This option is usually compatible only with the long TR sequences such as T2 or PD imaging. In those cases, effective TR will depend on the patient breathing and number of respiratory intervals. Therefore, it cannot be used in combination with spin echo–based T1 or general gradient echo sequences. However, there are special sequences where we continuously scan with a fixed TR and also record respiratory waveform. Afterwards, we can sort the data to include data only from expiration period. Let's see a practical example of respiratory triggering:

Let's assume that our patient is breathing at a steady pace of 20 breaths per minute. In this case, our respiratory interval (RR interval) would be 3 s. Practically, about 30% of this RR interval, which is 900 ms, would be the time we can scan efficiently. As you can imagine, we can scan a limited number of slices within this time. If we want to acquire 30 slices and can do only 20 slices in 1 RR, then, we have to choose 2 RR to be able to cover all the slices we need. In this case, our effective TR will be 2 RR or 6 s. Respiratory trigger provides high SNR images and does not require patient to hold the breath.

Respiratory Compensation (RC): RC is one of the rarely used imaging options. In this case, the MR acquisition is performed without any trigger. Then the acquired data can be sorted retrospectively to reduce the breathing artefacts.

Navigator Triggering: Navigator triggering is quite similar to respiratory triggering option we explained above. With navigator technique, we do not use an external tool to view respiratory waveform. We simply apply a one dimensional navigator acquisition to monitor the diaphragm motion in real time. Based on the diaphragm motion, image is acquired in expiration. Navigator techniques may require longer acquisition times and more sensitive to patient motion during the acquisition. However, they work well with abdominal exams and also with cardiac exams, specifically for coronary imaging.

Cardiac Triggering/Gating: Cardiac gating option is very similar to respiratory triggering in its working base. With cardiac gating, the system detects the R peak and enables us to scan with a certain delay in time to significantly reduce the cardiac artefacts or make it possible to synchronize MR acquisition with cardiac waveform. Cardiac gating is a must for many of the cardiac imaging sequences such as fiesta, cardiac perfusion, viability, coronary imaging, black blood imaging, etc. However, we also use cardiac gating for blood flow, CSF flow, time-of-flight–based angiography techniques in the peripherovascular MR angiography applications.

Cardiac Compensation: Cardiac compensation option records cardiac waveform while acquiring the data continuously. Then the data are retrospectively sorted to minimize the cardiac motion. As we know, the diastolic phase of cardiac cycle is where the cardiac motion is minimum. With cardiac compensation option, phase encoding steps closer to the center of k-space is chosen from the diastolic cycle and edge of k-space is chosen from systolic cardiac cycle. Cardiac compensation works reasonably well but cannot be as good as cardiac triggering.

In-plane Matrix Interpolation (*ZIP* 512, *ZIP* 1024): These options are used to increase the *in-plane resolution* of the acquired image matrix through a mathematical interpolation. These options cannot change the initial resolution but can be effective showing more details with the somewhat artificial resolution increase. If you have acquired images up to 256 matrix size, you can choose ZIP 512 option to create images with interpolated 512 × 512 matrix. If you acquire images with a true resolution up to 512 in any plane, you can choose ZIP 1024 to create interpolated 10124 × 1024 image matrix. We do not recommend choosing ZIP 1024 for an image matrix up to 256 since you may start seeing visible artefact due to significant amount of interpolation. ZIP options increase the data space. However, they can be used in routine imaging to improve the overall image quality with no SNR or time penalty.

Slice Interpolation (*ZIP* 2, *ZIP* 4): A 3D MR acquisition considers the slice direction as a third encoding axis and it is commonly called *slice encoding*. The slice direction volume or slab is encoded to create a certain TH in each 3D slice. Similar to in-plane matrix interpolation, we can interpolate TH with the options of ZIP 2 or ZIP 4. Let's assume that we acquire a 3D brain T1 image with a TH of 2 mm and 40 slices. If we choose ZIP 2 option during the acquisition, we will end up having 80 slices with an interpolated 1-mm TH. If we choose ZIP 4 option during the acquisition, we will end up having 160 slices with an interpolated 0.5-mm TH. These options cannot change the original resolution but can be effective for showing more details in the multiplanar reformatted images and can give a higher resolution impression. Even though they increase the true number of slices by a factor of 2 or 4, they can be used in routine 3D imaging to improve the overall image quality with no SNR or time penalty.

Magnetization Transfer (MT): In MRI, we can define a resonance frequency of water protons by the Larmor equation as we have shown in Chap. 2. This resonance frequency may seem to be a single peak centered perfectly at this resonance frequency. However, in the tissue, we can have bounded and unbounded water protons. Bounded water protons usually have a large protein concentration and can have a larger frequency bandwidth. There is also a continuous water exchange between the bounded and unbounded water. MT option applies an off-center rf pulse away from the resonance frequency somewhere from 800 to 1,600 Hz. This off-center MT pulse saturates the bound water with significant amount of proteins. The saturation of bound water significantly increases the contrast between unbound water and tissues with bound water. MT option is used mainly for brain MRA to better delineate the blood vessels. Recently, it has been used for MS protocols as well and to create what is called a MT ratio in MS patients as well.

No Phase Wrap (NPW), Foldover Suppression: Phase wrap, aliasing, or fold over are the common names of folding artefacts seen in MRI in phase encoding direction. NPW, antialiasing, or fold over suppression are the options to eliminate this artefact. It is one of the most well-known options for MR users. Depending on the vendor, the fold over elimination design may differ. However, in general, NPW option doubles the FOV and matrix in phase direction while halving the NEX during the acquisition, so that the acquisition time remains the same. Then, only the original FOV is reconstructed and displayed in the final image.

Smartprep, Bolustrack: Contrast enhanced MR angiography has some specific user-friendly options to make it much easier to catch and scan the MR images on the right time. For this purpose, smartprep or bolustrack options can be used. With these options, the user chooses a larger vessel of interest and places a small *tracker* inside the vessel. During the actual acquisition, MR system starts measuring the signal from this area and start the MRA acquisition when it detects the contrast agent presence in the vessel by means of increased signal intensity. These options provide greater ease of use but may be prone to typical patient motion.

Fluora Trigger (FTr): Contrast enhanced MRA is done automatically by the scanner if you choose the smartprep option and the user has almost no control. Fluoratrigger or bolustrack MRA is designed to display a user selected slice location in almost real time, so that the user can see the contrast arrival and vessel filling on the screen. Then, he can start the MRA in the desired time point. This option gives the full decision power to the user with the real-time monitoring of the contrast arrival.

Parallel Imaging: With the advancement of MR imaging in multielements and multichannel systems, parallel imaging became a vital part of MR imaging. Parallel imaging enables the MR signal to be acquired by multiple coil elements by a user-defined acceleration factor, then the acquired image is processed to create an MR image. With parallel imaging, it is possible to reduce the MR acquisition time by a factor of 2, 3, 4, or even 10 depending on the coil design. However, the SNR is also reduced by a square root of parallel imaging factor. It is also difficult to combine parallel imaging with small FOV where the region of interest is larger than the FOV (pelvic imaging, etc.). There are several types of parallel imaging methods. Some of those may require a so-called calibration scan to create a sensitivity map of each coil elements. Others create a calibration map from the original data acquisition. In any case, parallel imaging can create their own artefacts and users should follow the guidelines given by their vendors for their imaging applications.

Naming Conventions of MR Parameters by the Vendors

MR imaging parameters can differ from vendors to vendors by design and naming convention can be also quite confusing. The naming convention table below is created to give a better understanding of those parameters for the users using MR scanners by different vendors (Table 5.2).

Table 5.2 Cross names of commonly used MR parameters.

	GE	SIEMENS	PHILIPS	TOSHIBA
PRESATURATION	Spatial SAT	Pre sat	REST	Pre sat
CHEMICAL FAT SAT	FAT SAT, SPECIAL	FAT SAT	SPIR, SPAIR	FAT SAT
MOVING SAT BANDS	CONCAT SAT	Travel SAT	Travel REST	Travel SAT
RAMPED RF PULSE	RAMP PULSE	TONE	TONE	TONE
SLICE SPACING	SPACING	Distance factor in percent	Slice gap	Slice gap
MAGNETIZATION TRANSFER	MTC	MTC/MTS	MTC	SORS-ST
FLOW COMPENSATION	FC	FC	FC	FC
RESPIRATORY TRIGGERING	RTr/RC	Resp gated	PEAR/Resp trigger	Resp gated
ECG GATING	Card. gated triggered	ECG triggered	ECG, VCG triggered	Card. gated
AUTOMATIC MR CONTRAST TRIGGERING	Smart Prep/fluora trigger	Care bolus	Bolustrack	Visual Pro
ECHO TRAIN NUMBER	ETL	Turbo factor	Turbo factor	ETL
TIME BETWEEN ECHOES	Echo spacing	Echo spacing	Echo spacing	Echo spacing
OVERSAMPLING in PHASE DIRECTION	No phase wrap (NPW)	Phase oversampling	Fold over suppression	Phase wrap suppression
RECEIVER BANDWIDTH	Receiver bandwidth (RBW) kHz	Bandwidth, Hz/pixel (hertz per pixel)	Water/fat shift (Hz)	Bandwidth

Part II

MR Safety, Patient Positioning, Protocol Design, Graphical Prescription and MR Applications for Anatomical Regions

Chapter 6

Introduction to Safe Clinical Scanning

MR Safety, Patient Positioning, and Protocol Setup Guidance

We sincerely want to congratulate all our readers, who succeeded reading the first 5 chapters to understand the theoretical basis of MR imaging. We can assure that the time you spent is well worthed and you will be able to understand the following chapters better.

In this and following chapters, we will focus on clinical MR applications, patient preparation, patient positioning, and graphical prescription. Additionally, we will provide some examples of optimized MR protocols. The graphical prescription guidance given in this book is based on our collective experience working with many different multinational radiologists, and it is fairly applicable to any vendor. We strongly encourage you to try the given graphical prescription guidance in order to obtain diagnosable images. The patient positioning and MR protocol samples may vary depending on the vendors, coil design, and type of pulse sequences. Therefore, you may have to do appropriate modifications to get the optimal image quality in your institute.

Please always remember that whatever you do, patient safety is the most important single topic you have to focus at all times. In the following section, we will focus MR safety for everyday scanning. However, we strongly suggest you to regularly follow MR safety updates on multiple sources.

MR Safety

Magnetic resonance imaging is one of the safest imaging techniques as of today, which is its great strength. However, non-MR personnel, patients, and legal

M. Elmaoğlu and A. Çelik, *MRI Handbook: MR Physics, Patient Positioning, and Protocols*, DOI 10.1007/978-1-4614-1096-6_6,

guardians should be aware of the strong magnetic field present at all times. This strong magnetic field can be dangerous at times if it is ignored.

As we mentioned above, MR safety is a broad and dynamic subject. There are textbooks and electronic sources devoted to MR safety. We suggest our readers to check specifically www.mrisafety.com web page and books on MRI safety for additional reading. It is also important to remember that MR safety facts can vary depending on the field strength. If you are scanning with both 1.5T and 3.0T systems, you should always remember that 1.5T and 3.0T safety standards are different for different type of patients with implants. Again, do not assume but always verify facts from up-to-date credible sources.

In this section, we will be discussing the fundamental components of MR safety in daily clinical practice. Let's look at the three main components of MR safety:

- MR Personnel Safety
- Patient and Non-MR Personnel Safety
- MR System Safety
- Other Considerations

MR Personnel Safety

MR safety training for MR personnel is usually provided or supported by employers. MR safety trainings should be prepared by legally authorized institutions. Also it should be done for all new members joining the team and should be repeated on regular basis. These trainings should include anyone who may be involved with MR scanner or room at certain points, including, but not limited to, janitors, firewardens, security guards, nurses, physicians, and hospital maintenance staff.

Additionally, MR radiographers should receive proper MR safety training (dedicated to their equipment) from the MR vendors during the MR application training and receive the additional information on the form of user manuals and safety manuals. MR safety information should be updated from audio, video, and web-based sources. Even though there are a number of web pages you can consult for MR safety information, we suggest you to check www.mrisafety.com and www.imrser.org web pages regularly for updated MR safety issues.

It is always the best practice to put reminder signs, posters, and pictures in a visible corner of the MR room. It is also important for the MR radiographers to sit in a place with direct view of the MR room entrance. As experienced MR experts, you are literally the gate keepers.

Patient and Non-MR Personnel Safety

Patient safety is our most important priority and it should be treated accordingly. For any MRI scan, both patient and legal guardian should fill out a so-called "patient consent form or informed consent" separately and state any surgical procedures, implants, relevant work, and health history. In some countries, this form might be a legal requirement to enter the scan room. However, patient and legal guardians should be informed that they have right to cancel MRI exam at any point of scanning.

The sample patient consent form can be obtained from multiple sources. However, the institute can do appropriate additions based on the demographics of the institute. After the form is filled out by the patient, MR staff should go over the responses to clarify any misunderstandings communicating directly with the patients and confirm the form prior to the exam. The MR scanning environment, approximate duration, and potential effects (peripheral nerve stimulation (PNS), noise exposure, etc.) should be explained.

Non-MR personnel are subject to exactly the same rules applied to patients. The basic rule is: Rather than MR personnel, No one is permitted to enter MRI scan room without being screened by MR personnel.

Things to Do Before the MRI Exam at the Waiting Room

- Take your time to talk to the patient to explain the form and how to fill it.
- Review the form with the patient and ask additional questions if they do have any stimulator (neuro, bone, etc.), aneurysm clips, cardiac valves, pacemakers, and any type of metallic implants such as cochlear (hearing aid) or ocular.
- If the patient is pregnant or suspecting pregnancy, consult with the radiologist before performing the MRI exam. The decision makers are patients or legal guardians, but the potential advantages and risks must be explained to patient or legal guardians prior to the exam by physicians or radiologists.
- If the patient has been or had been held a relevant job such as working in a metal factory, be extra cautious and question the patient regarding any work-related accidents.
- Ask patient to change clothes with MR gown and remove any metallic objects including jewelry, hair pins, watch, mobile devices, etc.
- Scan the patient with a metal detector one more time before taking them into the MR room to make sure that there are no loose metallic objects.

- Intensive care or emergency room (ER) patients should be transferred to an MR compatible stretcher or MR scanner table outside the MR room. The patient should be screened carefully to remove any metallic objects such as oxygen tubes and monitoring devices incompatible with MR.

Things to Do During the MRI Exam at the MR Scanner Room

When you finish screening the patient in the waiting room, please consult with your radiologist if there are any questions or worries. If the patient has a type of implant, do not take him/her to MR room until the implant's MR safety is confirmed. If it is safe to scan the patient, we can follow the steps given below.

- Lower the MR table and ask the patient to lie down.
- Place protective pads between the coil and anatomy of interest.
- Give and instruct the patient how to insert MR compatible spongy ear plugs to reduce the noise experienced by the patient. We recommend to give an additional head phone with a relaxing music for patient comfort.
- Ask the patient to close the eyes when laser lights are turned on to landmark the region.
- Place safety pads between the patient body and magnet bore in order to eliminate RF burning risk.
- When you place coil, straighten the cables to avoid any loop and avoid direct contact between the cable and bare skin.
- Give the patient the patient alarm bell and explain them that they should press whenever they feel like they need it (burning sensation, claustrophobia, pain, nausea, etc.). Test the buzzer with the patient prior to scanning to make sure that it is working well.
- To reduce the potential PNS in MRI, avoid any closed circuits or loops in patient body resulting from crossing the legs or holding hands above the head.

Things to Do to Ensure MR System Safety

Obviously, patient and MR personnel safety is our top priority for MR scanning. We would like to add up the following check points for MR system safety to this list, which is somewhat connected to general safety precautions:

- MR scanner room and the critical five Gauss lines should be clearly marked within the hospital with the easy to understand signs.

- MR scan room door and its floor should have large and very visible and catchy signs showing the strong magnetic field and warning against unauthorized access.
- MR radiographers should have a clear and unobstructed view of the MR room door at all times.
- Any related medical personnel, maintenance department, and security staff should be trained on the hazards of ever present magnetic field to ensure the safety.
- For superconducting magnets, MR quench button should be in an easily accessible location and direct MR staff should be trained on the presences and usage of this button.
- MR power cutoff button should be in an easily accessible location and direct MR staff should be trained on the presences and usage of this button.
- Certain key technical specs such as MR power supply quality, temperature, helium level, should be monitored periodically to ensure the system safety.
- Any device incompatible with MR should not be in the MR room. The obvious dangerous ferromagnetic equipment such as oxygen tubes and wheelchair should always be outside the MR room.

Some Important Considerations

MR safety is quite a dynamic topic and direct MR staff (radiographers, radiologists, and supervisors) should periodically follow the new developments in this field. Parallel to more extensive MRI applications in clinical practice, new implants become safer or even completely compatible with MR imaging. However, there is no room for guessing MR compatibility. We are directly responsible to document any type of implants and validate their safety before admitting the patient to MRI. In this section, we would like to touch base with several important points to remind you the contraindications of MRI:

- *Contraindicative Implants*: Electrically, mechanically, or magnetically activated implants such as cardiac pacemakers, nerve stimulators, cochlear implants, and metallic splinters in the eye. Even though some specialized MR centers scan the patients with cardiac pacemakers on rare occasions, you should treat cardiac pacemakers as an absolute contraindication for MRI. Similarly, cochlear implants may not be an absolute contraindication for MRI. However, there is a strong chance of interference and damage on the implant due to strong field. Higher field strengths pose more treat to patients with implants.

- *Relatively Contraindicative Implants*: A growing list of safer implants is in development for patients today. However, all implants, such as hemostatic body implants, insulin pumps, non-ferromagnetic metallic implants, type, and location, should be verified for safety before the MR examination. You should keep one of the latest editions of MR safety books to check the implants MRI compatibility. If the patient does not know the type of implant or not so sure, you need to check with the doctor operated to get the accurate information.
- *Pregnancy*: As of today, there are no strong results putting pregnancy as a contraindication for MRI. However, as a safety precaution, MR scanning is avoided within the first 3 months of pregnancy. Afterwards, MR scanning can be performed only if the clinical needs outweigh the potential risks of MR scanning. Same discussion above is also directly applicable to pregnant MR personnel. They should also avoid entering MR room and staying in MR room during actual scanning as much as possible. In case of scanning pregnant patients, the MR scan should be done as fast as possible to minimize the potential risks and contrast injection should be avoided. After all these information, we can provide following checklist for pregnant patients:
  - If there is a high risk of mother's life due to serious clinical condition
  - If other nonionizing forms of diagnostic imaging are inadequate
  - If the MR examination provides vital information for the patient and the fetus life that would otherwise require exposure to ionizing radiation
  - If the patient clinical symptoms look like brain and spine disease
  - In the case of dangerous diseases such as cancer
  - If termination of pregnancy is considered
  - MR contrast agents should not be used routinely in pregnant patients. Each case must be analyzed individually. The decision to administer MR contrast agent to pregnant patients should be accompanied by a well-documented and thoughtful risk-benefit analysis (ACR guidance, 2007)
- *Contrast Agents*: According to ACR guidance cleared in 2007, no patient is to be administered prescription MR contrast agents without orders from a duly licensed physician. Only qualified physicians and radiologist can decide for administration of legally approved MR contrast agents by commenting thoughtful risk-benefit ratio analysis. However, the potential risks and benefits must be explained to patient or legal guardian and informed consent must be taken prior to the injection.

- *Gadolinium-based Contrast Agents and Nephrogenic Systemic Fibrosis (NSF)*: It has been recently appeared that there might be serious effect of gadolinium-based contrast agents for development of NSF in patients with severe renal dysfunction. According to latest publications and announcements of international committees (such as ACR and IMRSER), prescreening of renal function assessment by glomerular filtration rate (GFR) test is essential for patient with any kidney-related disease or trauma (age > 60).

For more information, please refer to updated MR safety web pages such as:
www.mrisafety.com
www.acr.org
www.fda.gov/default.htm
www.imrser.org/Default.asp

Patient Positioning

Correct patient positioning is key to an accurate diagnosis for all imaging modalities. In computed tomography, we are practically limited to axial plane, and patient positioning becomes much easier. Especially in MRI, patient positioning has direct effect on image quality and appropriate diagnosis. However, there are various approaches for patient positioning in relation to anatomical reference and/or pathology. In this book, the later chapters explain correct patient positioning with detailed pictures. We strongly believe that there will be a significant improvement in your resulting image quality and you can eliminate the artifacts occuring due to inappropriate patient positioning if you strictly follow the patient positioning that we provide in following chapters.

In this section, we would like to emphasize some general rules to be remembered when positioning the patient in an MR scanner:

- The anatomy of interest should be placed at the center of the coil to optimize the MR signal.
- The anatomy of the interest should be centered at the magnet isocenter as much as possible.
- The anatomical position should be in the correct radiological reference position.
- If your magnet has multiple coils for the same anatomy, choose the best fitting coil for the patient's anatomical size.
- *Coil:* Additional accessories created for MRI in different sizes and properties to transmit and/or receive the signal from different anatomical structures.

Protocol Creation

An MRI protocol can be defined as the set of pulse sequences and parameters preferred by the radiologist based on his expert opinion. Therefore, the MR protocol creation and selection is the key to acquiring the complete information for an accurate diagnosis.

A typical protocol for each anatomy would have a number of pulse sequences in multiple orientations (e.g., axial, sagittal, and coronal). The exact type and number of sequences to be prescribed can vary significantly for each country and institution. It is also not unusual to have slightly different protocols within the same hospital for different radiologists for the same anatomy. This is simply due to the fact that there is "single correct protocol for a specific anatomy of interest." The protocol creation decision should be left to the radiologist and should not be changed by radiographers.

In this book, we will give sample protocols for the anatomy of interest and possible disease states. Those protocols are *sample protocols* based on our collective experience and direct communication with the radiologists' expectations in a relatively vast region of the world. In this book, we also made a great effort to provide you the exact pulse sequence imaging parameters and options. Even though these parameters can vary for different vendors, coils, and pulse sequences, it is important to have reference parameters we can relate to.

The readers of this book are welcome to test and use those protocols as they like. However, it is their responsibility to create the best protocols for their own education, training, and experience.

Graphical Prescription

MRI is known superior to other imaging modalities because of multiplanar capability. The graphical prescriptions in MRI are named as axial, coronal, and sagittal views with their oblique definitions. We assume that you are quite familiar with these terms. However, we will define them below for our readers who are new to MRI:

- *Axial plane* is also called transverse or horizontal plane. It is an imaginary plane dividing the body into superior and inferior slices as shown in Fig. 6.1. Axial plane is exactly perpendicular to sagittal and coronal planes.
- *Coronal plane* is also called frontal or vertical plane. It is an imaginary plane dividing the body into anterior (ventral) and posterior (dorsal) slices as shown in Fig. 6.2. Coronal plane is exactly perpendicular to axial and sagittal planes.

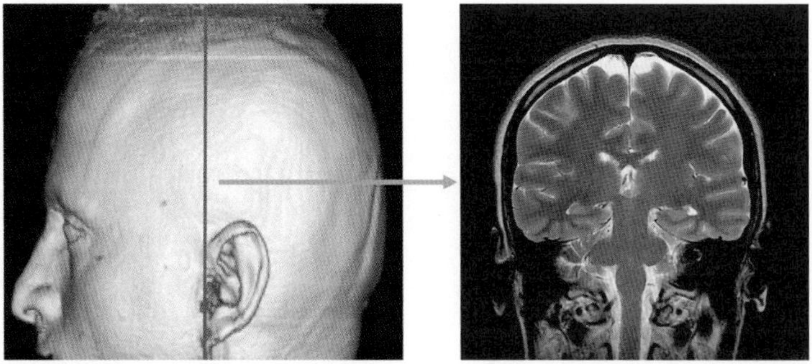

Figure 6.1 Axial plane is a *horizontal* imaginary plane (shown in *red*) dividing the cranium into superior and inferior slices.

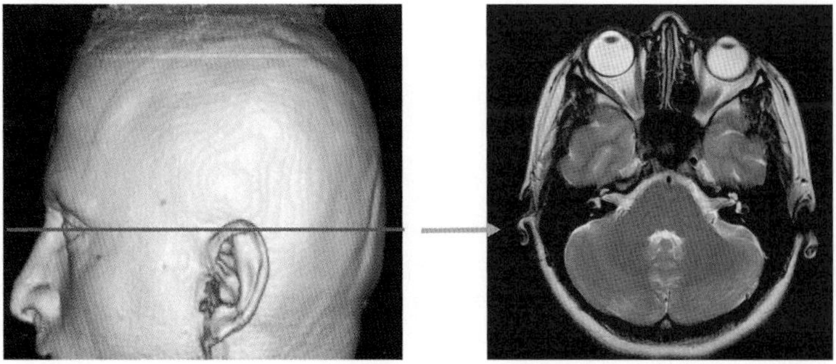

Figure 6.2 Coronal plane is a *vertical* imaginary plane (shown in *red*) dividing the cranium into anterior and posterior slices.

- *Sagittal plane* is an imaginary plane dividing the body into right and left slices as shown in Fig. 6.3. Sagittal plane is exactly perpendicular to axial and coronal planes.
- *Oblique plane* is a term used frequently in MRI to state that the acquisition plane has on obliquity and angulation with one of the orthogonal planes. Depending on the angle of the plane with each perpendicular planes, we can call it oblique-axial, oblique-coronal, or oblique-sagittal.

We will be using the "graphical prescription" term for slice positioning in these planes. The direction of slice positioning might be differing for each

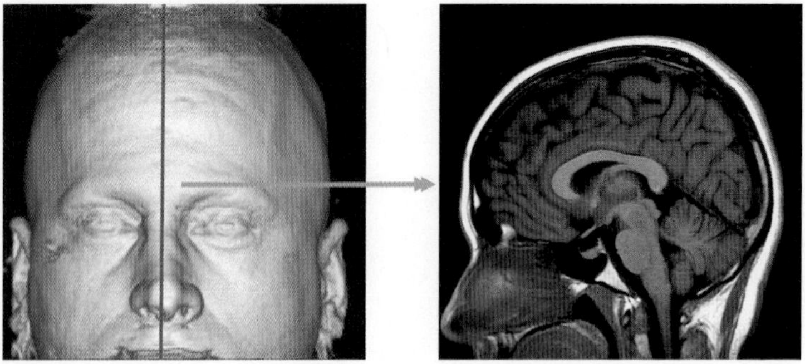

Figure 6.3 Sagittal plane is an imaginary plane (shown in *red*) dividing the cranium into left and right slices.

institute or clinics, but it is important to follow a standard slice prescription in order to get oriented with the MR images easily. Even though there is no universal slice acquisition order, in this book, we prescribe slices as shown below to be *consistent* throughout the book:

- *Axial slice* acquisition starts from superior to inferior (S–I) or head to feet (H–F)
- *Coronal slice* acquisition starts from anterior to posterior (A–P)
- *Sagittal slice* acquisition starts from right to left (R–L)

Graphical MR slice prescription for the anatomy of interest should be consistent between different patients and among different radiographers. For example, when prescribing axial, sagittal, or coronal brain slices, we identify specific landmarks and place our slices with respect to the landmarks (e.g., corpus callosum and mid-brain), so that we end up getting almost the same slice location for different patients. Since misaligned or incorrect slice prescription may lead to significant diagnostic problems, graphical prescription is one of the most important aspects of MR imaging. Due to greater importance of correct slice prescription, today, there are several automatic graphical slice prescriptions available for brain, spine, and knee imaging. In addition, automatic slice prescription software for more complex anatomies such as cardiac imaging is under development. All these automatic software are recently introduced to MR community to reduce slice prescription variations for regular patient follow-up and increase the slice prescription consistency. New 3D volume imaging acquisition sequences will reduce the need for the precise graphical prescription demand provided by the software. However, we recommend you to take advantage of the new technology coming into MR community.

MR Applications for Anatomical regions

We can divide human body into five major anatomical regions for MR imaging applications. These are *central nervous system imaging, musculoskeletal imaging, body imaging, cardiovascular imaging*, and *breast imaging*. In this book, the chapters are organized as per this division of anatomical regions. Each chapter contains subtitles called patient preparation, protocol samples, and graphical prescriptions, which are given for the region of interest and different diseases. For example, brain imaging chapter includes multiple section such as routine imaging, epilepsy, stroke, etc. to optimize the general scanning tips better for more specific cases. We feel that this is a more efficient and productive way of teaching and hope that you feel the same as well.

If you are ready, let's dive into the depths of MR clinical applications.

Chapter 7

Central Nervous System: MRI Protocols, Imaging Parameters, and Graphical Prescriptions

Central nervous system clinical applications are one of the most important and most common MRI imaging procedures as of today according to number of requests. Central nervous system can be divided to *head, neck* and *spine* applications. In this chapter, central nervous imaging applications will be covered in the same order for easier organization and follow up. For each section, we will discuss patient preparation, patient positioning, routine imaging protocols, additional imaging protocols for specific needs, graphical prescriptions and MR imaging protocol parameters.

Head Imaging

A step-by-step approach to head and brain MR imaging is given below:

Patient Preparation: The patient consent form should be given to the patient with a detailed explanation on the content. The form should be carefully read, all questions must be answered with clear answers such as "YES" or "NO," and additional clarifications should be written. It must be signed by the patient or legal guardians and confirmed by MR personnel. If there are any surgical implants, radiologist on duty has to make a decision based on implant type and MR compatibility. *If there is any suspicion or lack of information on the implant, do not take any risk with the patient safety and do not scan the patient.* If the form is complete with all the information, the patient should change to MR gown and remove any clothing with any metal. It is always a good practice to remove the

M. Elmaoğlu and A. Çelik, *MRI Handbook: MR Physics, Patient Positioning, and Protocols*, DOI 10.1007/978-1-4614-1096-6_7,

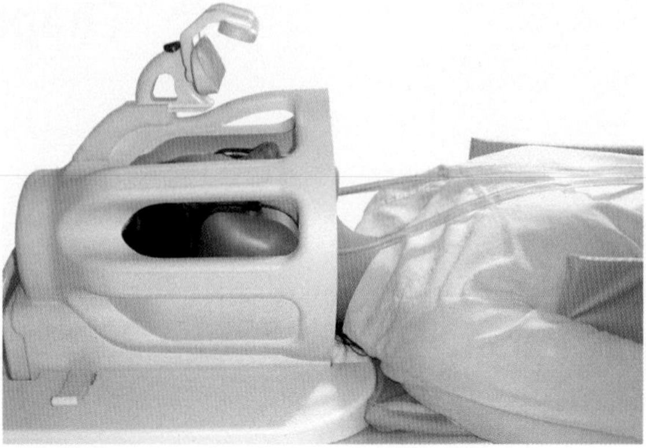

Figure 7.1 A sample patient positioning in an eight channel brain coil.

jewelry as well. As the last line of patient safety, it is also a good practice to scan patient with a handheld metal detector before taking the patient to MRI room.

Patient Positioning: Patient head should be centered at the brain coil, chin pointing upward as shown in the figure below. Patient should use earplugs for hearing protection with additional headsets and/or immobilization pads should be placed around the head to reduce the noise and gross patient motion. The head should also be fixed with additional straps for further patient motion reduction while keeping patient safety and comfort as a priority. We also recommend placing the leg support pads for patient comfort. Alarm bell should be given to patient and tested. After landmarking the center of the brain coil or just below the eyes using laser marker lights (while the eyes are closed) or touch sensors, you can send the patient in and start the exam (Fig. 7.1).

Let's take a look at the most frequently used protocols and graphical prescriptions:

Routine Brain

Sample Imaging Protocols

Routine brain imaging is used for the patients referred to MRI without any specific diagnosis and it can be applied for general nonspecific headache, check-up, or similar control purpose scanning (Table 7.1).

Tips and Tricks

- Sagittal T1 can be replaced by a sagittal T2 sequence that might be more informative for visualizing craniocervical lesions (e.g., MS plaques, Chiari

Table 7.1 Routine brain protocols and prescription planes.

Sequences	Comments	Slice order
Three plane localizer	Acquire 1–3 slices minimum in each plane	
Axial T2	Parallel to anterior and posterior tips of corpus callosum (CC)	S-I
Axial T1	Parallel to anterior and posterior tips of CC	S-I
Axial T2 flair	Parallel to anterior and posterior tips of CC	S-I
Sagittal T1	Parallel to midbrain line and orthogonal to axial and coronal slice prescription	R-L
Coronal T2	Choose the middle sagittal slice and prescribe slices parallel to brain stem	A-P
Postinjection	*If you decide to inject*	
Axial T1	Same as axial slice prescription as above	S-I
Coronal T1	Same as coronal slice prescription as above	A-P
Sagittal T1	Same as sagittal slice prescription as above	R-L

malformations). Recently, diffusion weighted imaging (DWI) has been added to routine brain imaging as well. It can also be routinely acquired for older patients.

- It is also important to remind that T1 flair as an alternative to T1 imaging can be used for routine brain imaging. T1 flair sequence provides better gray-white matter contrast and has shorter acquisition times due to higher echo train length. It also further suppresses the CSF resulting in better image quality. However, due to inversion pulse associated with the T1 flair sequence, there are considerable worries regarding postcontrast use of T1 flair sequence.

Sample Imaging Parameters

These imaging parameters are given to provide an optimum tradeoff between higher resolution and shorter scan time.

1.5 T Parameters (Table 7.2).
3.0 T Parameters (Table 7.3).

Graphical Prescription

Axial, sagittal, and coronal imaging protocols are given below. The slice coverage in each image is shown in white color and reference landmarks are shown in red for easy follow-up (Figs. 7.2–7.4).

Table 7.2 Routine imaging parameters for an eight channel brain coil.

	T2	T2 flair	T1	T2	T1 flair	T2	Diffusion
Plane	Axial	Axial	Axial	Coronal	Sagittal	Sagittal	Axial
Sequence type	FRFSE	FSE	SE	FRFSE	FSE	FRFSE	EPI
TE	85	150	14	85	MinFull	85	Min
TR	3,360	8,000	460	4,680	2,384	4,860	6,000
ETL	16	Auto		18	7	22	
BW	31.25	31.2	19.2	31.2	27.8	41.67	250
Slice thickness	5.5	5.5	5.5	5.5	5	4.0	5.5
Slice spacing	1.5	1.5	1.5	1.5	1.5	1.0	1.5
FOV	24	24	24	24	24	22	24
Matrix	416 × 416	352 × 224	320 × 224	416 × 384	320 × 224	352 × 352	128 × 128
NEX/NSA	2	2	2	1	2	2	2
Freq Direction	A-P	A-P	A-P	S-I	S-I	S-I	R-L
TI/b value		2,000			750		1,000

Table 7.3 Routine brain imaging parameters for an eight channel brain coil.

	T2	T2 flair	T1	T2	T1 flair	T1 flair	Diffusion
Planes	Axial	Axial	Axial	Coronal	Sagittal	Axial	Axial
Sequence type	FRFSE	FSE	SE	FRFSE	FSE-IR	FSE-IR	EPI
TE	85	125	MinFull	85	MinFull	Minfull	Min
TR	4,000	9,000	875	3,050	2,400	2,500	8,000
ETL	20	Auto		24	7	7	
BW	62.5	31.2	31.25	41.67	62.5	62.5	250
Slice thickness	5	5	5	5	5	5	5
Slice spacing	1.5	1.5	1.5	1	0.5	1.5	1.5
FOV	24	24	24	24	24	24	24
Matrix	512 × 512	352 × 224	384 × 224	416 × 416	384 × 256	480 × 288	192 × 192
NEX/NSA	1	1	1	1	1	1	1
Freq Direction	A-P	A-P	A-P	S-I	S-I	A-P	R-L
TI/b value		2,250			920	920	1,000

Stroke Protocol

Sample Imaging Protocols

Sample protocol for acute or chronic stroke patient is given below. For stroke patients, DWI sequence is one of the most important sequences. Therefore, DWI sequence is prescribed right after the localizer images before potential gross patient motion makes the MR imaging very difficult (Table 7.4).

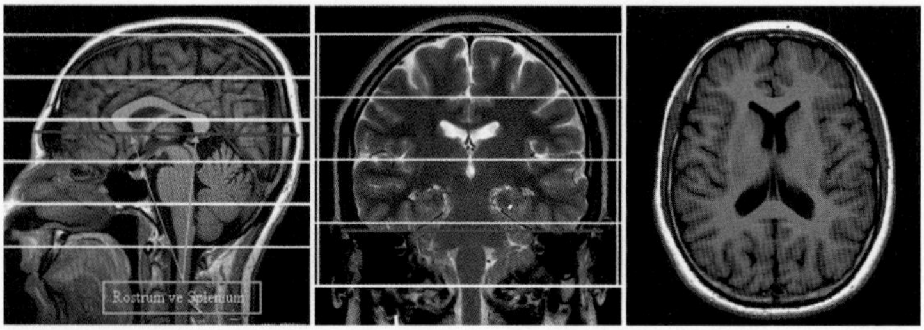

Figure 7.2 Axial brain planning from sagittal and coronal images.

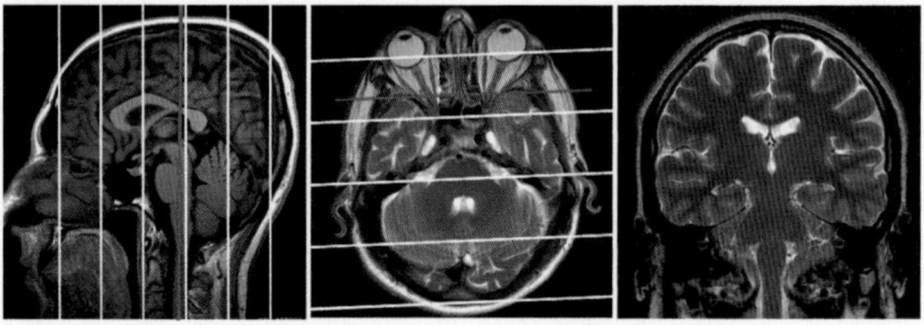

Figure 7.3 Coronal brain planning from sagittal and axial images.

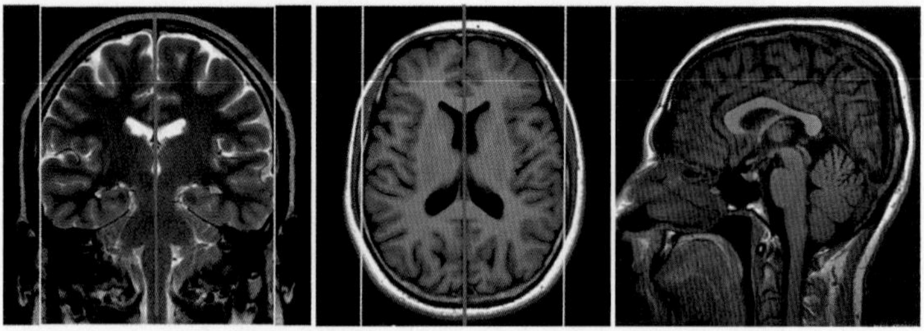

Figure 7.4 Sagittal planning from coronal and axial images.

Table 7.4 Brain stroke protocols and prescription planes.

Sequences	Comments	Slice order
Three plane localizer	Acquire 1–3 slices minimum in each plane	
Axial diffusion	Typically a *b* value of 1000 mm^2/sec is chosen for DWI	S-I
Axial T2	Parallel to anterior and posterior tips of CC	S-I
Axial T2 flair	Parallel to anterior and posterior tips of CC	S-I
Axial T2* GRE	Parallel to anterior and posterior tips of CC	S-I
Coronal T2	Choose the middle sagittal slice and prescribe slices parallel to brain stem	A-P
Sagittal T1 flair	Parallel to midbrain line and orthogonal to axial and coronal slice prescription	R-L
Axial 3D TOF	Prescribe for Circle of Willis and make it as short as possible	S-I
Postinjection	*If it is decided to inject*	
Perfusion EPI	EPI GRE T2* sequence prescribed to cover the whole brain with a 5–7 mm slice thickness and 1.5–2.0 s scan time per phase (total of 40 phases)	S-I
Axial T1	Same as axial slice prescription as above	S-I
Coronal T1	Same as coronal slice prescription as above	A-P
Sagittal T1	Same as sagittal slice prescription as above	R-L

Tips and Tricks

- GRE is T2* weighted sequence is very sensitive to local magnetic field inhomogeneities induced by iron in the blood and blood-breakdown products. Therefore, it is preferred in stroke cases for detecting acute or chronic hemorrhage. To take this advantage and further reduce the total scan time, coronal T2* can be prescribed instead of coronal T2.
- Parallel MR imaging is recommended at least for DWI imaging to reduce the susceptibility artifacts around posterior fossa. If it is available, non-EPI–based diffusion imaging techniques (e.g., PROPELLER DWI) can be used to further reduce the susceptibility artifacts as shown in Figs. 7.5 and 7.6.
- *Perfusion MRI*: Perfusion imaging can be performed either with gradient echo–based (GRE) EPI sequences or spin echo (SE)–based EPI sequences. Perfusion imaging, combined with DWI, is used to define ischemic core and ischemic penumbra. In addition, there is a large volume of research indicating that it can be used for tumor grading as well. From perfusion imaging, it is also possible to calculate hemodynamic maps such as cerebral blood volume (CBV), cerebral blood flow (CBF), mean transit time (MTT), and time to peak (TTP).

Sample Imaging Parameters for 1.5 T

See Table 7.5

Graphical Prescription

Axial, coronal, and sagittal planning is same as routine brain as you can expect. The slice coverage and orientation for the 3D TOF sequence is shown below.

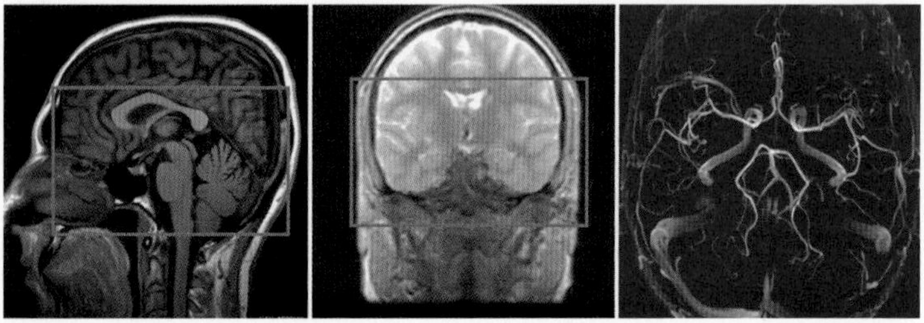

Figure 7.5 Axial 3D TOF MR angiography planning from sagittal and coronal images is shown.

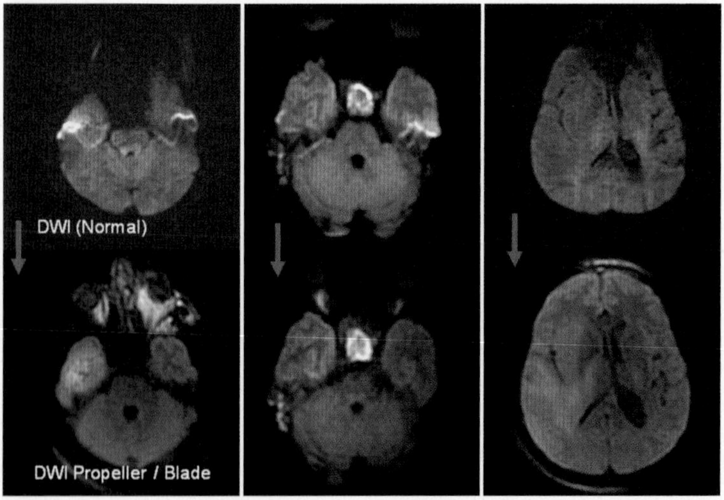

Figure 7.6 Comparison of EPI DWI and non-EPI DWI (PROPELLER DWI) images shows significant reduction in MR susceptibility artifacts.

Table 7.5 Brain stroke imaging parameters for an eight channel brain coil.

	Diffusion	Fast T2	T2 flair	T2*	T2	T1 flair	3D TOF	Perfusion
Planes	Axial	Axial	Axial	Coronal	Coronal	Sagittal	Axial	Axial
Sequence type	EPI	FRFSE	FSE	GRE	FRFSE	FSE	TofSPGR	EPI
TE	Min	85	150	25	85	MinFull	Min	40
TR	6,000	4,040	8,000	725	4,680	2,384	Min	1,500
ETL		27	Auto		18	7		
BW	250	62	31.2	10.0	31.2	27.8	20.0	Auto
Slice thickness	5.5	5.5	5.5	5.5	5.5	5	1.2	5.5
Slice spacing	1.5	1.5	1.5	1.5	1.5	1.5	−0.6	1.5
FOV	24	24	24	24	24	24	24	27
Matrix	128 × 128	352 × 352	352 × 224	288 × 224	416 × 384	320 × 224	352 × 224	128 × 128
NEX/NSA	2	1	1	1	1	2	1	1
Freq Direction	R-L	A-P	A-P	S-I	S-I	S-I	A-P	R-L
TI/b value/FA/Zip	$b = 1{,}000$		$b = 2{,}000$	FA: 25		TI: 750	Zip2	

Epilepsy

Epilepsy is a somewhat common neurological disorder characterized by sudden unprovoked seizures. Several disorders, such as trauma, cysts, tumors, arteriovenous malformations, which can cause epilepsy, can be visualized reliably with MR imaging. However, if there is no obvious disorder, MR imaging should be done in a specific way to better visualize the temporal love structures in oblique coronal view. In those cases, we recommend starting the MR imaging with sagittal plane rather than axial to save time and better plan the oblique coronal prescriptions. After the sagittal plane, routine axial plane images and high resolution oblique coronal images are prescribed.

Sample Imaging Protocols

See Table 7.6

Table 7.6 Sample sequences for brain epilepsy protocol.

Sequences	Comments	Slice order
Three plane localizer	Acquire 1–3 slices minimum in each plane	
Sagittal T1 flair	Parallel to midbrain line and orthogonal to axial and coronal slice prescription	R-L
Axial T2	Parallel to anterior and posterior tips of CC	S-I
Axial T2 flair	Parallel to anterior and posterior tips of CC	S-I
Axial T1 flair	Parallel to anterior and posterior tips of CC	S-I
Coronal T2 flair	Perpendicular to temporal lobes, specifically to hippocampus with a 3–4 mm slice thickness	A-P
Coronal T2-IR	Perpendicular to temporal lobes, specifically to hippocampus with a 3–4 mm slice thickness	A-P
Coronal T2	Perpendicular to temporal lobes, specifically to hippocampus with a 3–4 mm slice thickness	A-P
Coronal 3DT1-IR	Whole brain is scanned with the same coronal angle as above with 2–3 mm slice thickness	A-P
Postinjection	***No injection is needed if there is no lesion***	
Axial T1	Same as axial slice prescription as above	S-I
Coronal T1	Same as coronal slice prescription as above	A-P
Sagittal T1	Same as sagittal slice prescription as above	R-L

Sample Imaging Parameters for 1.5 T

The imaging parameters for the epilepsy protocol are shown below for a 1.5-T system. Please note that the protocols that are same as the routine brain imaging are not shown in Table 7.7.

Graphical Prescription

Axial and sagittal brain prescriptions are same as routine brain, and oblique coronal imaging prescription planes should be perpendicular to hippocampus as shown in Fig. 7.7.

Hemorrhage

Sample Imaging Protocols

It is important to complete the MRI scan for hemorrhage patients. Therefore, only the most critical sequences are prescribed in as short scan time as possible. If you plan to run MR angiography, please remember that hemorrhage looks hyperintense on time-of-flight (TOF) technique and it can be quite difficult to visualize vascular structure in hemorrhagic regions. Therefore, we recommend phase contrast (PC)–based MRA sequences with a proper velocity encoding (venc) in order to visualize the flowing protons only.

Sample protocols for hemorrhagic patients are shown in Table 7.8.

Sample Imaging Parameters for 1.5 T

See Table 7.9

Graphical Prescription

All the graphical prescriptions are same as routine brain imaging.

MS (Multiple Sclerosis) and Demyelination Diseases

Sample Imaging Protocols

Multiple sclerosis or the broader demyelinating diseases are the diseases of nervous system in which the myelin sheath around the neurons has been damaged. Unfortunately, the demyelinating diseases are on the rise globally and there is a strong chance that you will be scanning patients suffering from this type of disease using MR imaging. MRI examination on those patients usually includes contrast agent injection and postcontrast scanning in a later time (5–10 min after the injection). For MS patients, in addition to routine brain imaging, magnetization transfer (MT) pulse applied T1 sequence can

Table 7.7 Epilepsy protocol imaging parameters for an eight channel brain coil is shown.

	T2 flair	T2-IR	3DT1-IR	T2	T1 flair	T1 flair	Diffusion
Plane	Coronal	Coronal	Coronal	Coronal	Sagittal	Axial	Axial
Sequence type	FRFSE	FSE-IR	FSPGR	FRFSE	FSE	FSE	EPI
TE	150	35	MinFull	85	MinFull	Minfull	Min
TR	8,002	3,840	Min	4,680	2,384	2,366	6,000
ETL	Auto	8–12		18	7	7	
BW	31.2	41.67	15.63	31.2	27.8	27.8	250
Slice thickness	4	4	2	4	5	5.5	5.5
Slice spacing	0.5	0.5	−1	0.5	1.5	1.5	1.5
FOV	22	22	22	24	24	24	24
Matrix	288 × 224	352 × 320	288 × 288	416 × 320	320 × 224	320 × 224	128 × 128
NEX/NSA	2	2	1	4	2	2	2
Freq Direction	S-I	S-I	S-I	S-I	S-I	A-P	R-L
TI/b value/FA	TI: 2,000	TI: 120–200	TI: 400 FA: 12		TI: 750	TI: 750	$b=1{,}000$

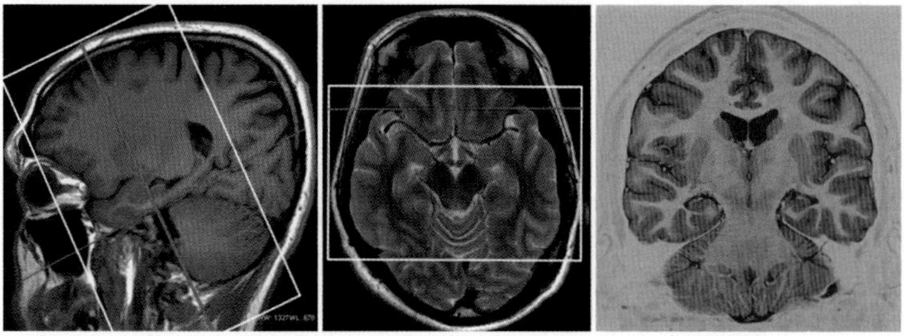

Figure 7.7 Oblique coronal imaging prescriptions for temporal lobe are shown.

Table 7.8 Sample protocol for hemorrhage patients.

Sequences	Comments	Slice order
Three plane localizer	Acquire 1–3 slices minimum in each plane	
Axial diffusion	Parallel to anterior and posterior tips of CC	S-I
Axial T2 fast	Parallel to anterior and posterior tips of CC	S-I
Axial T2 flair	Parallel to anterior and posterior tips of CC	S-I
Coronal T2*GRE	Choose the middle sagittal slice and prescribe slices parallel to brain stem	A-P
Sagittal T1 and PD	Parallel to midbrain line and orthogonal to axial and coronal slice prescription	R-L
Axial PCA	A proper venc selection is important for PC techniques	S-I

be added as well. MT pulse is a longer duration and off resonance (1,000–2,000 Hz away from resonant frequency) suppresses the proteins in the brain and delineates the MS plagues with a very good contrast. Since postcontrast scanning may lead to enhancement of different lesions, we recommend scanning MT T1 precontrast as well. It is also important to remember that MS and demyeliniating diseases are an active area of clinical research and you may add new sequences to your routine based on the slid information from recent literature.

The recommended protocols for MS and demyelinating diseases are given in sample protocol I and II, respectively.

Table 7.9 Hemorrhage protocol parameters for an eight channel brain coil are shown.

	Diffusion	Fast T2	T2 flair	T2*	PD	T1 flair	3D PC Art/Ven
Planes	Axial	Axial	Axial	Coronal	Sagittal	Sagittal	Axial
Sequence type	EPI	FRFSE	FSE	GRE	FSE	FSE	PC
TE	Min	85	150	25	MinFull	MinFull	Min
TR	6,000	4,040	8,000	725	1,500	2,384	20
ETL/VENC		27	Auto		5	7	10–60
BW	250	62	31.2	10	41	27.8	15.63
Slice thickness	5.5	5.5	5.5	5.5	5.5	5	3
Slice spacing	1.5	1.5	1.5	1.5	1.5	1.5	0
FOV	24	24	24	24	24	24	22
Matrix	128 × 128	352 × 352	352 × 224	288 × 224	416 × 384	320 × 224	256 × 192
NEX/NSA	2	1	1	1	1	2	1
Freq Direction	R-L	A-P	A-P	A-P	S-I	S-I	S-I
Gating/Venc							PG: 80/20
TI/b value/FA	1,000		2,000	25		750	FA: 20

Protocol I for MS patients
See Table 7.10

Protocol II for general demyelinating diseases
See Table 7.11

Table 7.10 A sample protocol for MS patients is given.

Sequences	Comments	Slice order
Three plane or scout	Acquire 1–3 slices minimum in each plane	
Axial T2	Parallel to anterior and posterior tips of CC	S-I
Axial T2 flair	Parallel to anterior and posterior tips of CC	S-I
Axial T1 flair	Parallel to anterior and posterior tips of CC	S-I
Axial T1 MT	Should be same as axial T2 prescription	S-I
Sagittal T2 flair	Parallel to midbrain line and orthogonal to axial and coronal slice prescription	R-L
Coronal T2	Choose the middle sagittal slice and prescribe slices parallel to brain stem	A-P
Postinjection	*If it is decided to inject, start scan 5 min after the injection*	
Axial T1 MT	Same as axial slice prescription as above	S-I
Coronal T1	Same as coronal slice prescription as above	A-P
Sagittal T1	Same as sagittal slice prescription as above	R-L

Table 7.11 Sample protocols MS and other demyelinating diseases.

Sequences	Comments	Slice order
Three plane or scout	Acquire 1–3 slices minimum in each plane	
Axial T2 flair	Parallel to anterior and posterior tips of CC	S-I
Axial T1 SE	Parallel to anterior and posterior tips of CC	S-I
Injection	*If it is decided to inject, scan at least two different planes*	
Sagittal T2	Parallel to midbrain line and orthogonal to axial and coronal slice prescription	R-L
Axial T2	Parallel to anterior and posterior tips of CC	S-I
Coronal T2	Choose the middle sagittal slice and prescribe slices parallel to brain stem	A-P
Coronal T1 SE	Same as coronal slice prescription as above	A-P
Axial T1 SE	Same as axial slice prescription as above	S-I

Tips and Tricks

- T2 flair: T2 FLAIR sequence is one of the most important sequences for MS patients. We recommend running T2 flair with interleaved acquisitions. This way, the slice crosstalk and CSF flow artifacts can be reduced further.
- 3D T2 Flair sequence may provide more details compare to 2D Flair sequence. Some of the recent studies showed that smaller WM lesions can be easily detected by using 3D T2 Flair with Fat Saturation.
- Injection time: In the second protocol, injection is done right after T1 weighted sequences to extend the time for postcontrast T1 sequences. However, the effect of contrast on sagittal and coronal T2 is negligible.

Sample Imaging Parameters for 1.5 T

See Table 7.12

Graphical Prescription

All the graphical prescriptions are same as routine brain imaging.

Trigeminal Neuralgia (TN)

Sample Imaging Protocols

The protocols for the patients referred to MRI for trigeminal neuralgia are almost similar to routine brain imaging. However, additional thin slice 2D T2 and T1 or 3D volume acquisitions should be added for trigeminal nerves. Even though most of the new MRI systems have quite impressive 3D balance GRE sequences, we recommend the imaging protocols with 3D sequences (Protocol I) and without 3D sequences (Protocol II) to cover all systems.

Protocol I using 3D Volume Imaging Sequences

See Table 7.13

Protocol II using only 2D Imaging Sequences

See Table 7.14

Sample Imaging Parameters for 1.5 T

See Table 7.15

Graphical Prescription

All the graphical prescriptions are same as routine brain imaging. Thin slice 2D and 3D sequences should be planned specifically for trigeminal nerves as shown in Figs. 7.8 and 7.9a.

Table 7.12 MS protocol imaging parameters for an eight channel brain coil is shown.

	T2	T2 flair	T2	T2 flair	T1 MT	T1	T2
Planes	Sagittal	Sagittal	Axial	Axial	Axial	Axial	Coronal
Sequence type	FRFSE	FSE	FRFSE	FSE	SE	SE	FRFSE
TE	85	150	85	150	MinFull	14	85
TR	6,040	8,000	4,680	8,800	500	460	4,680
ETL	22	Auto	23	Auto			18
BW	41	31.2	41.7	31.2	31	19.2	31.2
Slice thickness	4	4.0	5.5	5.5	5.5	5.5	5.5
Slice spacing	0.5	0.5	1.5	1.5	1.5	1.5	1.5
FOV	22	24	24	24	24	24	24
Matrix	352 × 352	352 × 224	416 × 416	352 × 224	320 × 224	320 × 224	416 × 384
NEX/NSA	2	1	2	2	2	2	1
Freq Direction	S-I	A-P	A-P	A-P	R-L	A-P	S-I
SAT band/zip							
TI/b value/FA		TI: 2,000		TI: 2,200	FA: 72		

Table 7.13 Sample TN protocols using 2D and 3D sequences.

Sequences	Comments	Slice order
Three plane localizer	Acquire 3–5 slices minimum in each plane	
Axial T2	Parallel to anterior and posterior tips of CC	S-I
Axial T2 flair	Parallel to anterior and posterior tips of CC	S-I
Axial 3D fiesta/CISS	Use 1–2 mm slice thickness and include posterior fossa	S-I
Axial 3D T1	Use 1–2 mm slice thickness and include posterior fossa	S-I
Sagittal T2	Parallel to midbrain line and orthogonal to axial and coronal slice prescription	R-L
Coronal 3D fiesta	Choose the middle sagittal slice and prescribe slices p arallel to brain stem	A-P
Postinjection	*If it is decided to inject!*	
Axial 3DT1	Same as axial 3D slice prescription as above 1–2 mm	S-I
Coronal T1	Same as coronal slice prescription as above	A-P

Table 7.14 Sample TN protocols using only 2D sequences.

Sequences	Comments	Slice order
Three plane localizer	Acquire 3–5 slices minimum in each plane	
Axial T2	Parallel to anterior and posterior tips of CC	S-I
Axial T2 flair	Parallel to anterior and posterior tips of CC	S-I
Axial T2 thin slice	Use 2–3 mm slice thickness and include posterior fossa	S-I
Axial T1 thin slice	Use 2–3 mm slice thickness and include posterior fossa	S-I
Sagittal T2	Parallel to midbrain line and orthogonal to axial and coronal slice prescription	R-L
Postinjection	*If it is decided to inject!*	
Axial T1 thin slice	Same as axial slice prescription as above	S-I
Coronal T1 thin slice	Same as coronal slice prescription as above	A-P

Brain Tumors (TM)

Sample Imaging Protocols

There are several types of brain tumors and MRI scanning should provide as much information as possible for the type and size of the tumor. Therefore, it is important to scan multiple planes to better visualize the tumor particularly postinjection of contrast agent. The protocols given below are used to provide as much detail as possible for the clinicians in relatively shorter scan time. Please note that we provided two different commonly used protocols for tumor

Table 7.15 Hemorrhage protocol imaging parameters for an eight channel brain coil is shown.

	T2	T2	T2 flair	3DT2	3DT1	T2	T1
Planes	Sagittal	Axial	Axial	Axial	Axial	Axial	Axial
Sequence type	FRFSE	FRFSE	FSE	Fiesta	FSPGR	FRFSE	FSE
TE	85	85	150	Min	MinFull	120	MinFull
TR	6,040	4,680	8,800	Auto	Auto	3,080	660
ETL	22	23	Auto			22	3
BW	41	41.7	31.2	83	15	31.2	31.2
Slice thickness	4	5.5	5.5	1.2	1.6	2.5	2.5
Slice spacing	0.5	1.5	1.5	−0.6	−0.8	0.5	0.5
FOV	22	24	24	22	18	18	18
Matrix	352 × 352	416 × 416	352 × 224	384 × 384	256 × 256	288 × 288	288 × 256
NEX/NSA	2	2	2	4	1	6	3
Freq Direction	S-I	A-P	A-P	A-P	A-P	A-P	A-P
SAT band/zip				Zip2	Zip2		
TI/b value/FA			2,200	FA65	Auto/15		

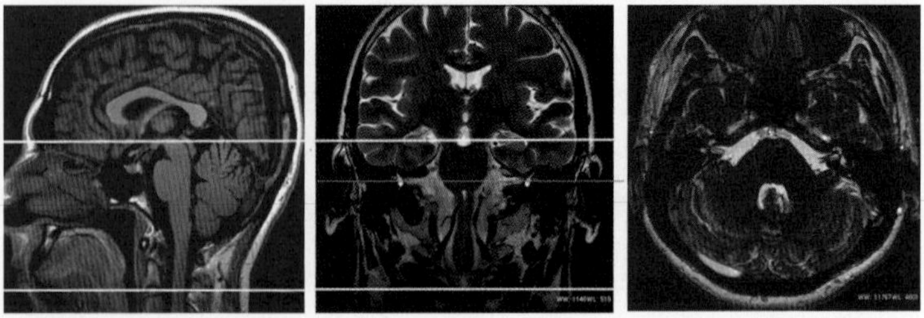

Figure 7.8 Thin slice axial prescription for trigeminal nerves is shown.

Table 7.16 A standard brain tumor protocol is given.

Sequences	Comments	Slice order
Three plane localizer	Acquire 1–3 slices minimum in each plane	
Axial T2	Parallel to anterior and posterior tips of CC	S-I
Axial T2 flair	Parallel to anterior and posterior tips of CC	S-I
Axial T1	Parallel to anterior and posterior tips of CC	S-I
Coronal T1	Choose the middle sagittal slice and prescribe slices parallel to brain stem	A-P
Post injection	***Scan at least in two planes post contrast***	
Axial T1	Same as axial slice prescription as above	S-I
Coronal T1	Same as coronal slice prescription as above	A-P
Sagittal T1	Parallel to midbrain line and orthogonal to axial and coronal slice prescription	R-L

patients. We also encourage our readers to explore the recently developed Fast Spin Echo 3D T2 and Fast Spoiled GRE T1 weighted protocols as alternative or additional information to 2D protocols in use today.

Protocol I
See Table 7.16

Protocol II
See Table 7.17

Sample Imaging Parameters for 1.5 T
See Table 7.18

Table 7.17 Imaging parameters for an eight channel brain coil is shown.

	T2	T2 flair	T1	T1	T1 flair	T2 flair	Diffusion
Plane	Axial	Axial	Axial	Coronal	Sagittal	Coronal	Axial
Sequence type	FRFSE	FSE	SE	SE	FSE	FSE	EPI
TE	85	150	MinFull	MinFull	MinFull	150	Min
TR	4,680	8,800	420	420	2,384	8,000	6,000
ETL	23	Auto			7	Auto	
BW	41.7	31.2	27	27	27.8	31.2	250
Slice thickness	5.5	5.5	5.5	5.5	5	5.5	5.5
Slice spacing	1.5	1.5	1.5	1.5	1.5	1.5	1.5
FOV	24	24	24	24	24	24	24
Matrix	416 × 416	352 × 224	384 × 224	320 × 224	320 × 224	352 × 224	128 × 128
NEX/NSA	2	2	3	2	2	2	2
Freq Direction	A-P	A-P	A-P	S-I	S-I	S-I	R-L
TI/b value/FA		2,200			750	2,000	1,000

Table 7.18 An additional brain tumor protocol is given.

Sequences	Comments	Slice order
Three plane localizer	Acquire 1–3 slices minimum in each plane	
Axial T2	Parallel to anterior and posterior tips of CC	S-I
Axial T1	Parallel to anterior and posterior tips of CC	S-I
Coronal T2 flair	Choose the middle sagittal slice and prescribe slices parallel to brain stem	A-P
Post injection	*Scan at least in 2 planes post contrast*	
Axial T1	Same as axial slice prescription as above	S-I
Coronal T1	Same as coronal slice prescription as above	A-P
Sagittal T1	Parallel to midbrain line and orthogonal to axial and coronal slice prescription	R-L

Tips and Tricks

- 3D T2 and T1 weighted isotropic sequences are valuable in brain TM imaging if they are available in your system.

Graphical Prescription

All the graphical prescriptions are same as routine brain imaging.

Orbits

Patient Preparation and Positioning

Patient Preparation: In addition to patient preparation for brain imaging, please make sure you remove any removable metallic dental implants, piercing and remove the makeup, especially eyeliner.

Patient Positioning: If you have only the brain coil, the patient positioning will be identical to routine brain imaging (see Fig. 7.1). However, if your site has loop coil with the setup attachment (also called as TMJ coil), you position the coil as close as possible to orbits and make sure that each loop is well centered as shown in the figure below. Please note that the loop coils usually have shorter signal penetration depth but remarkably higher SNR than a general brain coil (Figs. 7.9b,c).

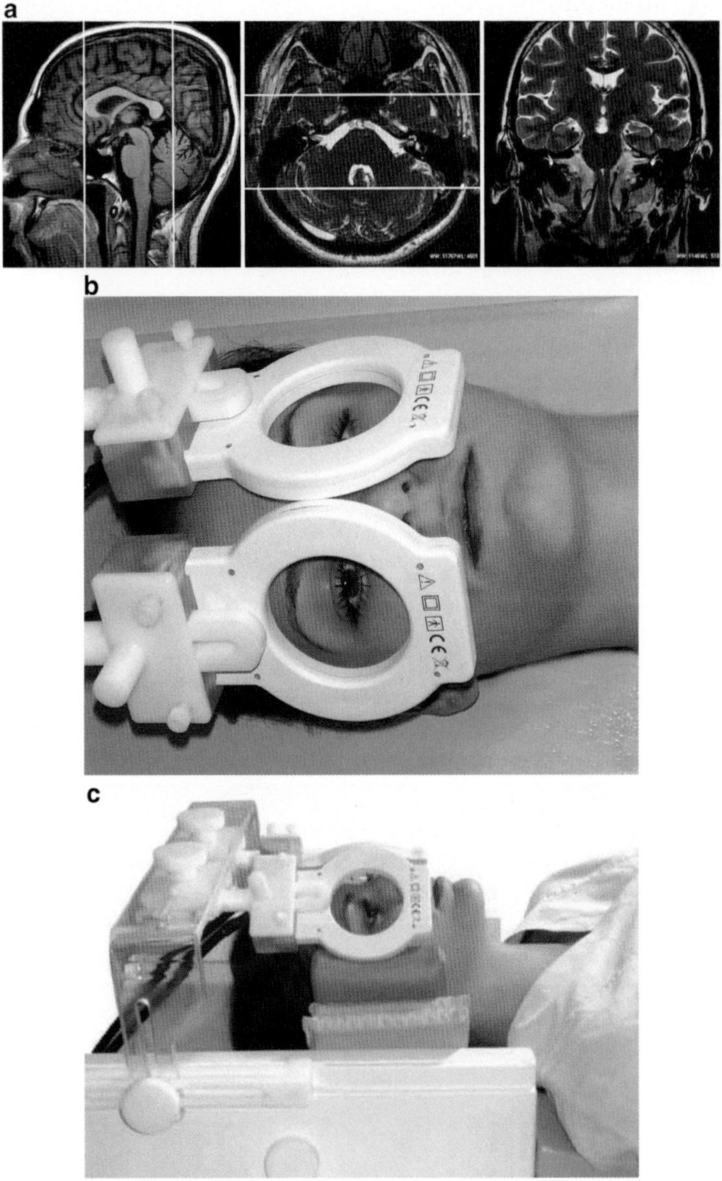

Figure 7.9 (a) Thin slice coronal prescription for trigeminal nerves is shown. (b) Orbital patient positioning using the loop coils. (c) Orbital patient positioning using the loop coils.

Table 7.19 Sample protocols for routine orbital imaging.

Sequences	Comments	Slice order
Three plane localizer	Acquire 9–11 slices in each plane	
Sagittal T2	Prescribe as a localizer to cover the whole brain	R-L
Axial T2 fat sat	Parallel to optical nerves with 2–3 mm slice thickness	S-I
Axial T1	Parallel to optical nerves with 2–3 mm slice thickness	S-I
Coronal T2 or STIR	Plan from axial view to include optic chiasm and globes	A-P
Sagittal T2	Prescribe two different sagittal slice groups, each group should be parallel to each optic nerve	R-L
Post injection	***Scan at least two planes post contrast***	
Axial T1	Same as axial slice prescription as above	S-I
Axial T1 fat sat	Same as axial slice prescription as above	S-I
Coronal T1 fat sat	Choose the middle sagittal slice and prescribe slices parallel to brain stem	A-P

Sample Imaging Protocols

Depending on the patient referral whether it is for orbital globes, optic nerves, or thyroid ophthalmology, different protocols shall be used. Below, a commonly used general protocol you can use for orbital scanning is given as a sample protocol (Table 7.19).

Tips and Tricks

- High resolution coronal T1-w is the best sequence for muscle volume measurements for patients with thyroid ophthalmopathy.
- If you are scanning mainly for globes, use a T1 Fat sat imaging and repeat it postcontrast.
- For MS or trauma patients, you can add Coronal STIR sequence in addition to Coronal T2.
- Always keep the FOV smaller to cover orbits only, increasing the FOV will have negative effect on fat sat imaging, although will decrease the resolution.

Sample Imaging Parameters for 1.5 T

See Table 7.20

Table 7.20 Imaging parameters for an eight channel brain coil is shown.

	T2FS	T1	T1FS	STIR	T2	T1	T2
Planes	Axial	Axial	Axial	Coronal	Coronal	Coronal	Sagittal
Sequence type	FRFSE	FSE	FSE	FSE-IR	FRFSE	FSE	FRFSE
TE	85	MinFull	MinFull	40	120	MinFull	85
TR	4,240	620	480	6,000	3,080	740	3,110
ETL	24	2	3	12	22	3	24
BW	20.83	20.83	16.67	20.83	31.2	20.83	20.83
Slice thickness	3	3	3	3	3	3	3
Slice spacing	0.3	0.3	0.3	0.3	0.3	0.3	0.3
FOV	16	16	16	16	16	16	12
Matrix	320 × 256	288 × 256	288 × 224	288 × 224	288 × 288	352 × 224	288 × 224
NEX/NSA	4	3	3	3	4	2	4
Freq Direction	A-P	A-P	A-P	S-I	S-I	S-I	S-I
SAT band/zip	S-I	S-I	S-I	S-I	S-I	S-I	S-I
TI/FA				140–160			

Graphical Prescription

Graphical prescriptions for orbital imaging are shown in Figs. 7.10–7.12.

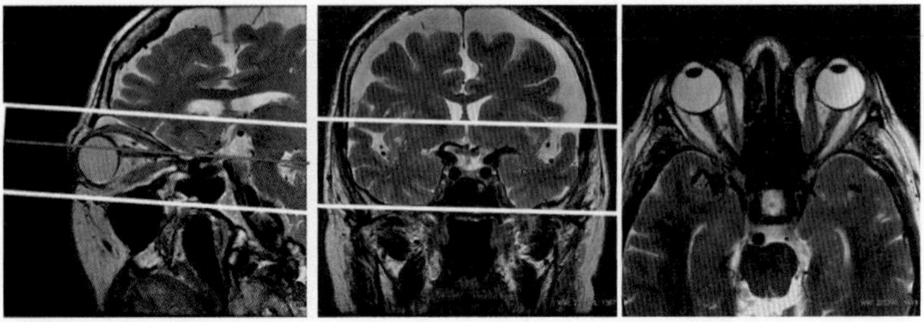

Figure 7.10 Axial slice prescription from sagittal and coronal images is shown.

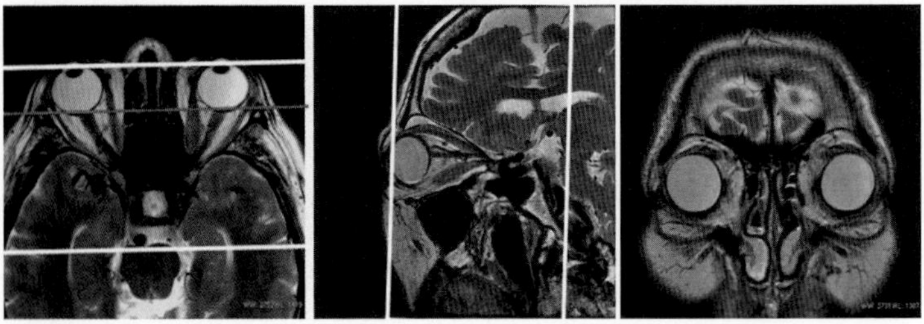

Figure 7.11 Coronal slice prescription from sagittal and axial images is shown.

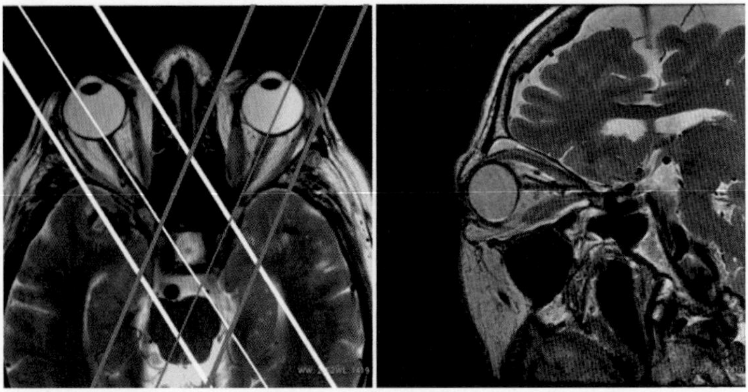

Figure 7.12 Oblique sagittal slice prescriptions from axial images are shown.

Internal Acoustic Canal (IAC)

Patient Preparation and Positioning

It is same as brain (please refer to Head Imaging).

Sample Imaging Protocols

Patients referred for IAC MRI exam usually suffer from tinnitus, hearing loss, or acoustic neurinoma. In general, the sample protocol below would be appropriate for these clinical requests. However, depending on the patient condition and clinical history, you might add additional sequences to this protocol.

- If the 3D sequences are not supported by your system, they might be replaced by 2D sequences.
- Balanced GRE sequences (Fiesta, CISS) provide unique tissue contrast known as T2/T1 for excellent delineation of nerves and fluid. However, tissue with closer T1 and T2 time will not be visualized on these sequences due to this division! Therefore, it should be carefully used for brain tissue–related lesions, which may not be even seen on these sequences (Table 7.21)!

Table 7.21 A routine IAC protocol.

Sequences	Comments	Slice order
Three plane localizer	Acquire 5–7 slices in each plane	
Axial T2	For general routine brain imaging	S-I
Axial 3D fiesta	Cover only IAC with a slice thickness of 1–2 mm	S-I
Axial 3D T1 FS	Cover only IAC with a slice thickness of 1–2 mm	S-I
Coronal 3D fiesta	Plan from axial images to cover only IAC with a slice thickness of 1–2 mm	A-P
Injection	***Contrast injection is recommended if there is no contraindication***	
Axial 3D T1 FS	Same as above	S-I
Coronal 3D T1FS	Plan from axial images to cover only IAC with a slice thickness of 1–2 mm	A-P

Sample Imaging Parameters for 1.5 T

See Table 7.22

Graphical Prescription

Graphical prescriptions for IAC imaging are shown in Figs. 7.13 and 7.14.

Table 7.22 Imaging parameters for an eight channel brain coil is shown.

	3D fiesta	3D T1FS	3D fiesta	T2	T1	T2
Planes	Axial	Axial	Coronal	Axial	Axial	Coronal
Sequence type	Balanced GRE	SPGR	Balanced GRE	FRFSE	FSE	FRFSE
TE	Min	MinFull	Min	120	MinFull	120
TR	Auto	Auto	Auto	3,080	660	3,080
ETL				22	3	22
BW	83	15	83	31.2	31.2	31.2
Slice thickness	1.2	1.6	1.2	2.5	2.5	2.5
Slice spacing	−0.6	−0.8	−0.6	0.5	0.5	0.5
FOV	22	18	22	18	18	18
Matrix	384 × 384	256 × 256	384 × 384	288 × 288	288 × 256	288 × 288
NEX/NSA	4	1	4	6	3	6
Freq Direction	A-P	A-P	S-I	A-P	A-P	S-I
SAT band/zip	Zip2	Zip2	Zip2		S-I	
TI/FA	FA: 65	Auto/FA:13	FA: 65			

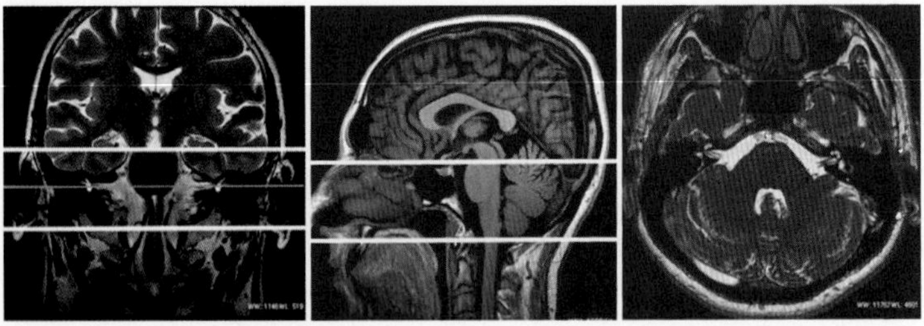

Figure 7.13 Axial slice prescription from coronal and sagittal images is shown.

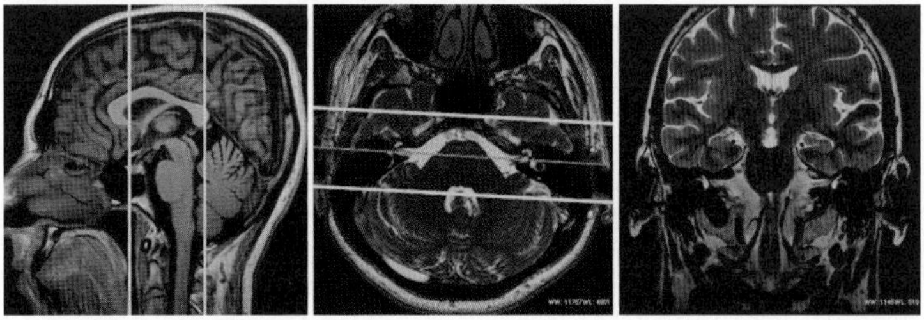

Figure 7.14 Coronal slice prescription from sagittal and axial images is shown.

Pituitary Gland (Hypophysis)

Pituitary gland MRI should be done with thinner slices and preferably with dynamic contrast injection to catch microadenomas (assuming there is no contraindication for contrast injection). Due to the potential effects of hormonal changes on the hypophysis MR imaging, the scan should be performed 7–10 days from initiation of menstruation period for female patients (general recommendation but not necessary).

The decision to include dynamic imaging for patients with pituitary macroadenoma and/or tumor has to be made by the radiologist. If you want to perform the dynamic scanning, you need to scan at least one precontrast phase and then acquire 3–5 more phases/repetitions from initiation of the injection of contrast agent. T1 Fat sat is helpful to delineate the enhancement patterns in patients with macroadenoma before and after operation.

Sample Imaging Protocols

See Table 7.23

Sample Imaging Parameters for 1.5 T

See Table 7.24

Graphical Prescription

Graphical prescriptions for hypophysis imaging are shown in Figs. 7.15 and 7.16.

Table 7.23 A standard pituitary dynamic MRI protocol is given.

Sequences	Comments	Slice order
Three plane localizer	Acquire 5–7 slices in each plane	
Sagittal T1	Parallel to brain midline, covering the pituitary gland with a slice thickness of 2–3 mm	R-L
Coronal T2	Plan from sag images to cover only pituitary gland with 2–3 mm slice thickness, preferably in parallel to pituitary stalk	A-P
Coronal T1	Plan from sag images to cover only hypophysis with a 2-mm slice thickness, preferably in parallel to pituitary stalk	A-P
Dynamic coronal T1	Prescribe 3–5 slices only for pituitary gland. Acquire 1 precontrast and 4–5 postcontrast phases	A-P
Coronal T1	Same as above	A-P
Sagittal T1	Same as above	R-L

Table 7.24 Imaging parameters for an eight channel brain coil is shown.

	T1	T2	T1	Dynamic
Plan	Sagittal	Coronal	Coronal	Coronal
Sequence type	FSE	FRFSE	FSE	FSE
TE	MinFull	113	MinFull	MinFull
TR	560	3,300	560	400
ETL	3	23	3	3
BW	20.8	20	20	10.4
Slice thickness	3	2	2	3
Slice spacing	0.3	0.2	0.2	0.3
FOV	16	16	22	20 × 17
Matrix	224 × 224	352 × 320	288 × 224	224 × 224
NEX/NSA	5	6	6	1
Freq Direction	S-I	S-I	S-I	S-I
SAT band/zip	Oblique inferiorly/zip 512		Oblique inferiorly	O. inferiorly/Z512

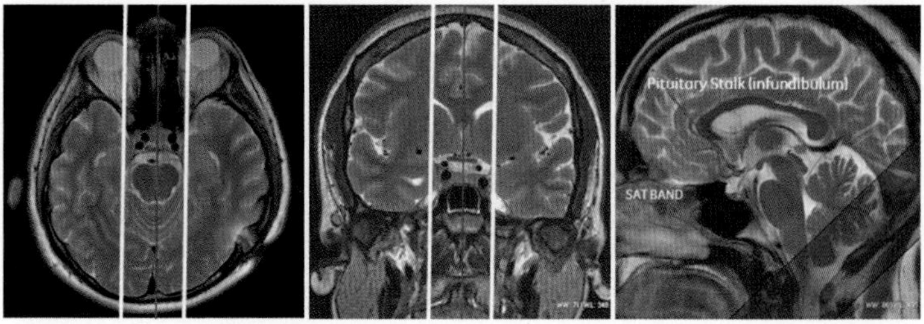

Figure 7.15 **Sagittal slice prescription from axial and coronal images is shown. Please notice the additional saturation band placement inferoposteriorly.**

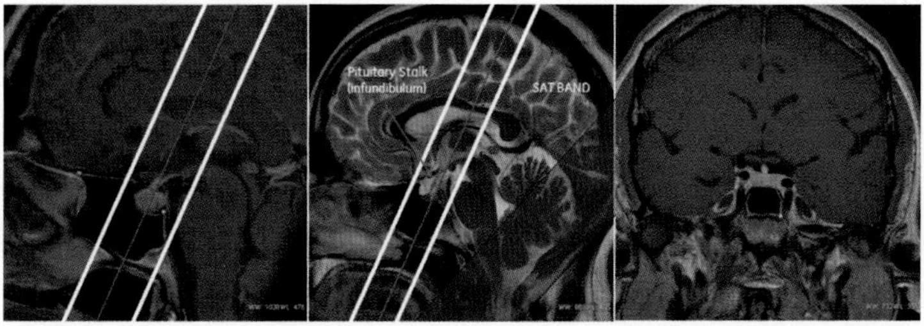

Figure 7.16 **Coronal slice prescription from sagittal images is shown. Please notice the additional saturation band placement inferoposteriorly.**

Cerebro Spinal Fluid (CSF) Flow Measurement

CSF flow measurements were done more frequently in the past and still there is a strong interest in different regions. Therefore, we decided to include CSF flow measurement protocol in this chapter as well.

Like other flow measurements, CSF flow measurement is done using a GRE PC imaging. As we mentioned in Chap. 4, PC imaging is used because of a simple physical rule in MRI: *flowing spins in the blood, body fluids such as*

CSF cause a phase change (proportional to absolute flow) compared to nearby stationary (nonmoving) spins. From this phase change, we can measure absolute flow in MRI quite easily. However, as an MR operator, we need to ensure that we place the slice perpendicular to the direction of flow and choose an appropriate velocity encoding for accurate results. Velocity encoding (venc) here is the key to reduce the user-dependent errors and related underestimation of absolute flow and velocity measurements. Let's explain a bit more on the role of venc for flow measurements:

Any MR image would consist of a magnitude and phase image. For any routine imaging, we simply discard the phase image since magnitude image gives as the majority of information. However, in flow measurements, we keep the phase image in addition to magnitude image. In this case, magnitude imaging is kept as an anatomical landmark but phase image would be critical. A phase image would have a phase range from −180° to +180°. As we mentioned above, if there is no flowing spins, we expect to have a 0 (zero) phase in that pixel. If we have flowing spins in the pixel, we will have a phase value proportional to the amount of velocity in the pixel. For example, if we choose a venc of 100 cm/s, we will have a phase value of 180° in that pixel assuming that the spins are moving at a velocity of 100 cm/s. If we have spins moving at 50 cm/s, then our phase image will give us 90° instead of 180° assuming that we use the same venc. However, if we rescan the same location using a venc of 50 cm/s, then I will end up with a phase value of 180° simply because I set up my dynamic range to map 50 cm/s to 180°. As an MR operator, it is our responsibility to choose the proper venc, so that we can map the maximum velocity in the region of interest to a 180°.

The velocity of CSF fluid in aqueduct (of Sylvius) can range from 2 to 9 cm/s (in normal healthy individuals) and, therefore, choosing a venc of 10 cm/s is usually a good choice. However, if you choose a very low venc value such as 5 cm/s in this case, then you will be getting flow aliasing artifact and would get incorrect results. This problem is easily visible when you look at the resulting phase images. You will see some darker spots (in systolic phases) or white spots (in diastolic phases) in the middle of aqueduct canal for CSF. This problem can be corrected by scanning with a higher venc choice. Notice that we did not mention much on positive or negative flow in the above discussion. The positive or negative phase simply indicates the direction of flow in respect to the chosen flow direction. Some of you might also be confused about the term flow and velocity. We usually measure flow and use the term flow since it is closely connected to velocity. Flow simply means the velocity (cm/s) of the blood within the vessel multiplied by the area (cm2) of the vessel. The units of flow will be mL/s.

Table 7.25 Sample CSF flow protocol.

Sequences	Comments	Slice order
Three plane localizer	Acquire 5 slices in each plane	
Sagittal 3D fiesta/ CISS/or T1	Parallel to brain midline, covering optic chiasm with a slice thickness of 1–3 mm	R-L
2D cine PC for flow measurement	A single slice perpendicular to cerebral aqueduct (of sylvius) with a slice thickness of 5–7 mm and venc of 10 cm/s	S-I
Sagittal 2D PCA for flow visualization	A single slice exactly on the brain midslice with a slice thickness of 5–7 mm and venc of 10 cm/s	R-L

Table 7.26 Imaging parameters for an eight channel brain coil is shown.

	3D fiesta	T1 flair	2D flow	2D flow
Plane	Sagittal	Sagittal	Oblique axial	Sagittal
Sequence type	Balanced GRE	FSE	Cine PC	Cine PC
TE	Min	24	Min	Min
TR	Auto	2,500	Auto	Auto
ETL		7		
BW	83.33	31.2	15.63	15.63
Slice thickness	1.0	3	7	7
Slice spacing	0.0	0.3	0	0
FOV	22	22	16	20
Matrix	384 × 384	288 × 224	256 × 256	256 × 256
NEX/NSA	3	2	8	8
Freq Direction	S-I	S-I	A-P	S-I
VPS/VENC			8/10	8/10
TI/N.phases/FA	FA: 65	TI: 760	20/20	20/20

All the flow measurements should be done with cardiac ECG or PG gating devices and acquire 15–30 phases. Resulting PC image has to be processed with dedicated software for the absolute flow quantification.

Sample Imaging Protocols

See Table 7.25

Sample Imaging Parameters for 1.5 T

See Table 7.26

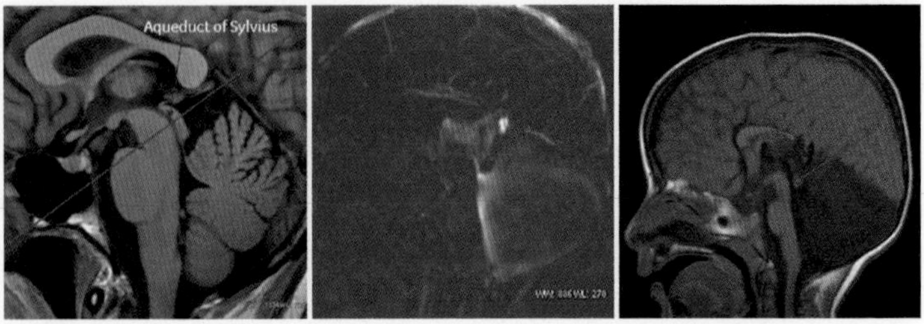

Figure 7.17 Oblique axial slice prescription of 2D cine PC slice from sagittal image. Please notice that oblique slice angle is adjusted to make it perpendicular to aqueduct.

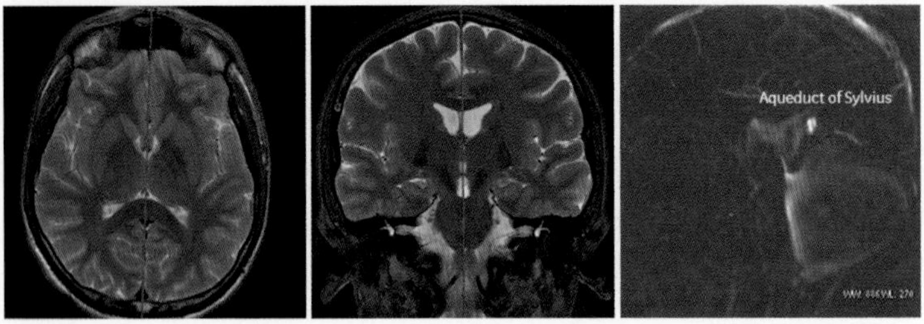

Figure 7.18 Oblique sagittal slice prescription from axial and coronal images is shown.

Graphical Prescription

Graphical prescriptions for CSF flow imaging are shown in Figs. 7.17 and 7.18.

Neck Imaging

Neck imaging is a challenge for MRI due to inhomogeneous anatomical structure of the neck and involuntary patient motion. In this section, we would like to share our experience on how to optimize the neck imaging and improve the MRI image quality for everyday scanning.

In neck imaging, swallowing, gross patient motion, and deep breathing are the main sources of motion-related artifacts. A better attention to patient comfort, utilizing faster sequences (for shorter scan time) reduces the motion-related artifacts resulting from voluntary and involuntary patient motion. Moreover, potential dielectric artifacts can also degrade image quality and may cause regional signal drops in the neck imaging. Even though better understanding dielectric artifacts and developing efficient hardware/software reduces those artifacts greatly, we also recommend using dielectric pads for older 3 T scanners. The sample dielectric pads and how to place them are shown below for your convenience.

Patient Preparation and Positioning

Patient Preparation: The patient consent form should be given to the patient with a detailed explanation on the content. The form should be carefully read, all questions must be answered with clear answers such as "YES" or "NO," and additional clarifications should be written. It must be signed by the patient or legal guardians and confirmed by MR personnel. If there are any surgical implants, radiologist on duty has to make a decision based on implant type and MR compatibility. *If there is any suspicion or lack of information on the implant, do not take any risk with the patient safety and do not scan the patient.* If the form is complete with all the information, the patient should change to MR gown and remove any clothing with any metal. Before the MR exam, explain the nature and duration of the MR exam they will undergo. Also explain that patient motion will make a negative effect on image's quality. Make a habit of informing the patient before every sequence and communicate often to comfort the patient. It is always a good practice to remove the jewelry as well. As the last line of patient safety, it is also a good practice to scan patient with a handheld metal detector before taking the patient to MR room.

Patient Positioning: The neck coil should be centered on the coil. Patient should be in supine position and larynx being centered on the coil center. For better patient comfort and easier breathing, leg support pads should be placed under patient knees. Patient protection headsets and/or immobilization pads should be placed around the head to reduce the noise and gross patient motion. After handing the patient alarm to patient and testing it, you are ready to start the exam. After landmarking the center of the brain coil or just below the eyes using laser marker lights or touch sensors, you can send the patient in and start the exam (Figs. 7.19–7.21).

Let's take a look at the most frequently used protocols and graphical prescriptions for neck imaging:

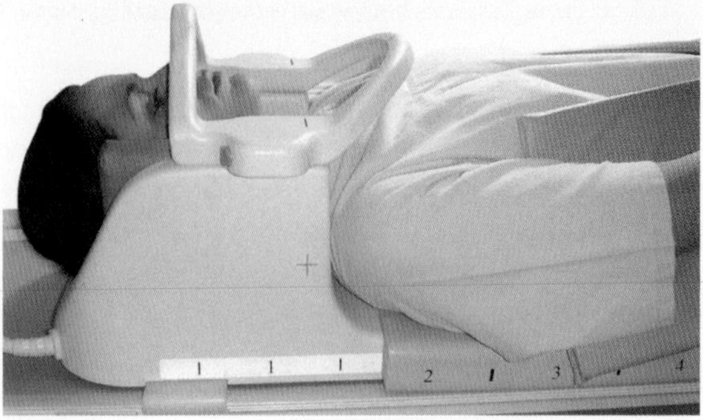

Figure 7.19 Patient positioning on an eight channel spine (CTL) coil.

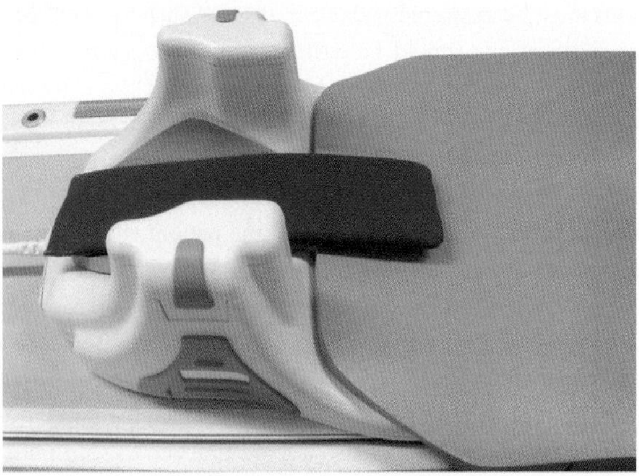

Figure 7.20 A sample dielectric pad and its proper placement on a spine coil on 3.0 T scanner.

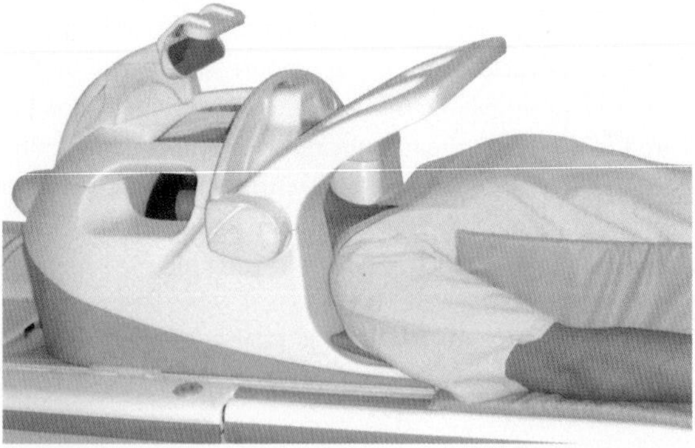

Figure 7.21 Patient positioning on an eight channel neurovascular coil.

Routine Cervical Imaging

Sample Imaging Protocols

A sample routine cervical spine imaging protocol is given in Table 7.27.

Sample Imaging Parameters for 1.5 T

See Table 7.28

Table 7.27 A typical standard cervical spine protocol.

Sequences	Comments	Slice order
Three plane localizer	Acquire 5 slices in each plane	
Sagittal T2	Plan 3 mm sagittal slices over coronal image where you can see the spinal cord to cover the whole spinal canal	R-L
Sagittal T1	Same as above	R-L
Axial T2*GRE/MERGE	Plan 3 mm oblique axial slices from sagittal plane. The slices should be crossing vertebral junctions	S-I

Table 7.28 Imaging parameters for an eight channel spine coil is shown.

	T2	T1	T2*	T1 flair	T2*GRE	T2	T1
Plane	Sagittal	Sagittal	Axial	Sagittal	Axial	Axial	Axial
Sequence type	FRFSE	FSE	GRE	FSE	MERGE	FRFSE	FSE
TE	85	MinFull	13.3	24	MinFull	130	MinFull
TR	3,140	640	509	2,250	500	3,500	720
ETL	27	3	4	7	Auto	25	3
BW	41.67	31.2	31.2	31.2	31.25	31.2	31.2
Slice thickness	3	3	3.0	3	3.5	3.5	3.5
Slice spacing	0.5	0.5	0.5	0.5	0.5	1.5	1.5
FOV	24	24	17	24	19	14	14
Matrix	352 × 256	320 × 224	288 × 224	288 × 224	320 × 192	256 × 256	256 × 256
NEX/NSA	4	4	2	4	2	4	2
Freq Direction	A-P	A-P	R-L	A-P	R-L	A-P	A-P
SAT band	A	A	A	A		R-L	R-L
TI/FA			FA: 30	TI: 750			

Sample Imaging Parameters for 3.0 T

See Table 7.29

Graphical Prescription

Graphical prescriptions for cervical spine imaging are shown in Figs. 7.22 and 7.23.

Table 7.29 Imaging parameters for an eight channel spine coil is shown.

	T2	T1	T2*	T1 flair	STIR	T2	T1
Plane	Sagittal	Sagittal	Axial	Sagittal	Sagittal	Axial	Axial
Sequence type	FRFSE	FSE-XL	MERGE	FSE	FSE-IR	FRFSE	FSE-XL
TE	110	MinFull	MinFull	MinFull	42	102	Minfull
TR	4,000	685	575	2,500	3,400	3,000	900
ETL	24	3		7	12	21	3
BW	31.25	41.7	31.25	62.5	31.25	50.0	41.7
Slice thickness	3.0	3.0	3.0	3.0	3	3.5	3.5
Slice spacing	0.5	0.5	0.5	0.5	0.5	1.5	1.5
FOV	26	26	20	26	24	20	20
Matrix	512 × 256	512 × 224	320 × 224	384 × 224	320 × 224	384 × 256	320 × 256
NEX/NSA	4	4	2	2	4	4	3
Freq Direction	A-P	A-P	R-L	A-P	A-P	A-P	R-L
SAT band			R-L			R-L	
TI/FA			FA: 20	TI: 860	FA: 145		

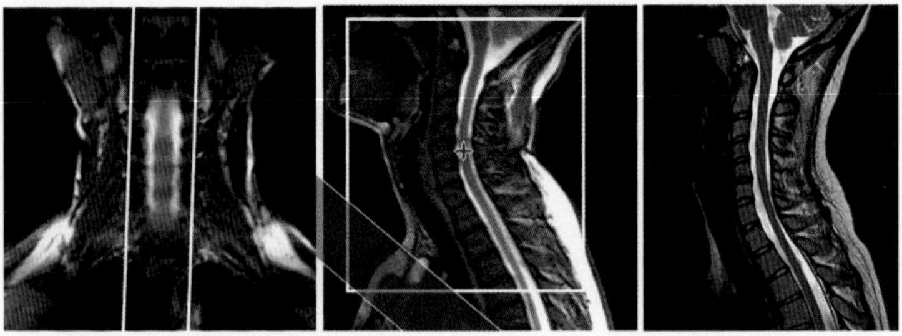

Figure 7.22 Sagittal slice prescription from coronal slices with saturation band is shown.

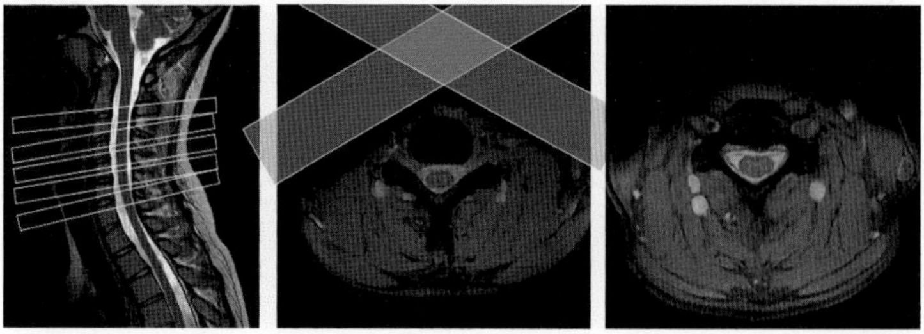

Figure 7.23 Axial slice prescription from sagittal and axial localizer slices with placement of saturation bands is shown.

Table 7.30 Cervical trauma protocol.

Sequences	Comments	Slice order
Three plane localizer	Acquire 5 slices in each plane	
Sagittal T2	Plan 3 mm sagittal slices over coronal image where you can see the spinal cord to cover the whole spinal canal	R-L
Sagittal T1	Same as above	R-L
Sagittal STIR	Same as above	R-L
Sagittal T2*GRE	MERGE or MEDIC type (multiecho recalled gradient echo) sequences are recommended	R-L
Axial T2*GRE	Plan from the sagittal images a continuous block of 3 mm slices from cervical C1 to C7	S-I
Axial T2FS	Plan from the sagittal images a continuous block of 3 mm slices from cervical C1 to C7	S-I
Axial T1	Plan from the sagittal images a continuous block of 3 mm slices from cervical C1 to C7	S-I

Cervical Trauma

Sample Imaging Protocols

The sample protocol for cervical trauma patients can be used (Table 7.30).

Sample Imaging Parameters for 1.5 T

See Table 7.31

Graphical Prescription

Sagittal planning for trauma patients is same as cervical spine imaging. Axial planning is shown in Fig. 7.24.

Table 7.31 Imaging parameters for an eight channel spine coil is shown.

	T2	T1	T2*	STIR	T2*GRE	T2FS	T1
Plan	Sagittal	Sagittal	Sagittal	Sagittal	Axial	Axial	Axial
Sequence type	FRFSE	FSE	MERGE	FSE-IR	MERGE	FRFSE	FSE
TE	85	MinFull	Auto	42	MinFull	102	MinFull
TR	3,140	640	440	3,400	500	3,460	720
ETL	27	3	6	12	Auto	25	3
BW	41.67	31.2	62.5	31.25	31.25	31.25	31.25
Slice thickness	3.0	3	3.0	3.0	3.5	4.0	4.0
Slice spacing	1.0	1.0	1.0	1.0	0.5	0.5	0.5
FOV	24	24	24	24	19	16	16
Matrix	352 × 256	320 × 224	320 × 192	288 × 224	320 × 192	256 × 256	256 × 256
NEX/NSA	4	4	2	4	2	2	2
Freq Direction	A-P	A-P	A-P	A-P	R-L	A-P	A-P
SAT band	A	A	A	A		R-L	R-L
TI/FA				TI: 145			

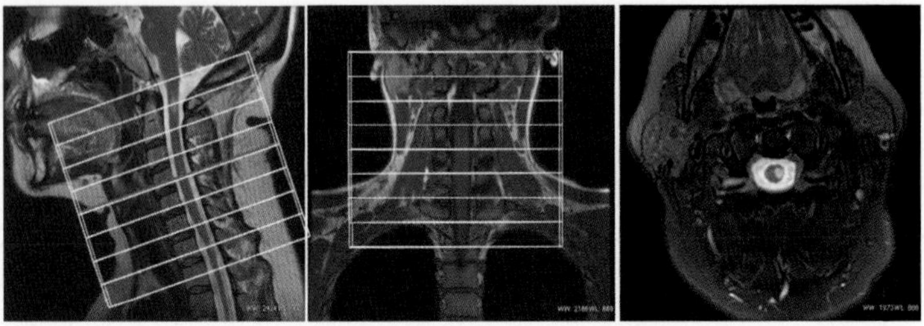

Figure 7.24 Axial slice prescription from sagittal and coronal slices is shown.

Cervical Metastases

Sample Imaging Protocols

The sample protocol for cervical metastases patients is given in Table 7.32.

Sample Imaging Parameters for 1.5 T

See Table 7.33

Table 7.32 A sample protocol for cervical metastases.

Sequences	Comments	Slice order
Three plane localizer	Acquire 5 slices in each plane	
Sagittal T2	Plan 3 mm sagittal slices over coronal image where you can see the spinal cord to cover the whole spinal canal	R-L
Sagittal T1	Same as above	R-L
Sagittal STIR	Same as above	R-L
Axial T2 fat sat	Plan from the sagittal images a continuous block of 4 mm slices from cervical C1 to T1	S-I
Axial T1 fat sat	Same as above	S-I
Coronal T1	Plan from the sagittal images a continuous block of 4 mm slices covering vertebral column	A-P
Postinjection	*Scan at least two planes for postcontrast*	
Axial T1 fat sat	Same as above	S-I
Coronal T1	Same as above	A-P

Table 7.33 Imaging parameters for a eight channel spine coil is shown.

	T2	T1	STIR	T2FS	T1	T1
Plane	Sagittal	Sagittal	Sagittal	Axial	Axial	Coronal
Sequence type	FRFSE	FSE	FSE-IR	FRFSE	FSE	FSE
TE	85	MinFull	42	102	MinFull	MinFull
TR	3,140	640	3,400	3,460	720	760
ETL	27	3	12	25	3	3
BW	41.67	31.2	31.25	31.2	31.2	41.67
Slice thickness	4	4	4	5	5	4
Slice spacing	0.5	0.5	0.5	1.5	1.5	1.0
FOV	24	24	24	14	15	22
Matrix	352 × 224	320 × 224	288 × 224	256 × 256	256 × 256	352 × 256
NEX/NSA	4	4	4	2	2	2
Freq Direction	A-P	A-P	A-P	A-P	A-P	S-I
SAT band	A	A	A		R-L	S-I
TI/b value/FA			TI: 145			

Graphical Prescription

Sagittal planning for metastases patients is same as routine cervical spine imaging. Axial planning is shown in Fig. 7.25 and coronal planning is shown below.

Cervical Scoliosis

Sample Imaging Protocols

The spinal structure of cervical scoliosis patients is quite different than the normal patients. Therefore, it is recommended to image at least two or three different planes/orientations. For better graphical prescription, three-plane localizer or scout imaging should be acquired with larger slice spacing and 5–10 slices. In addition, actual scanning should start with coronal plane, so that the following sagittal and axial images can be prescribed more accurately.

The sample protocol for cervical scoliosis patients is given in Table 7.34.

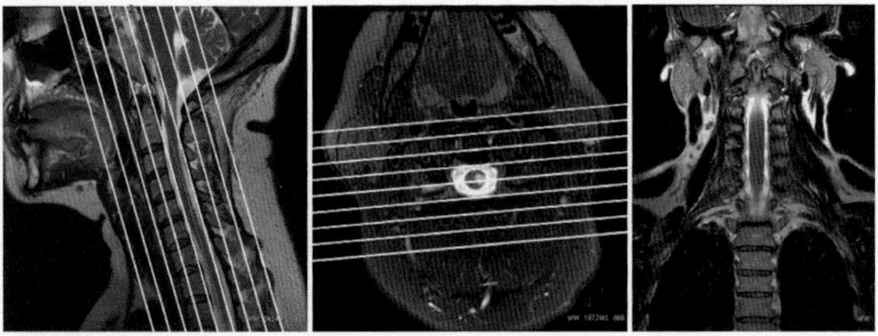

Figure 7.25 Coronal slice prescription from sagittal and axial slices is shown.

Table 7.34 A sample cervical scoliosis protocol is given.

Sequences	Comments	Slice order
Three plane localizer	Acquire 5–10 slices in each plane	
Coronal T2	Plan from the sagittal images a straight coronal images with 3 mm thickness	A-P
Sagittal T2	Plan 3 mm sagittal slices over coronal image where you can see the spinal cord to cover the whole spinal canal	R-L
Sagittal T1	Same as above	R-L
Axial T2*GRE	Plan from the sagittal images a continuous block of 4 mm slices from cervical C1 to T1	S-I
Axial T2	Plan from the sagittal images a continuous block of 4 mm slices from cervical C1 to T1	S-I

Sample Imaging Parameters for 1.5 T

The imaging parameters for kinematic neck exam are same as routine c-spine exam. Please refer to the c-spine parameter table given before.

Graphical Prescription

Graphical prescriptions for cervical scoliosis imaging are shown in Figs. 7.26–7.28.

Cervical Myelography

Sample Imaging Protocols

Even though cervical myelography request is quite uncommon, in some cases you may prescribe cervical myelography for better visualization of spinal cord

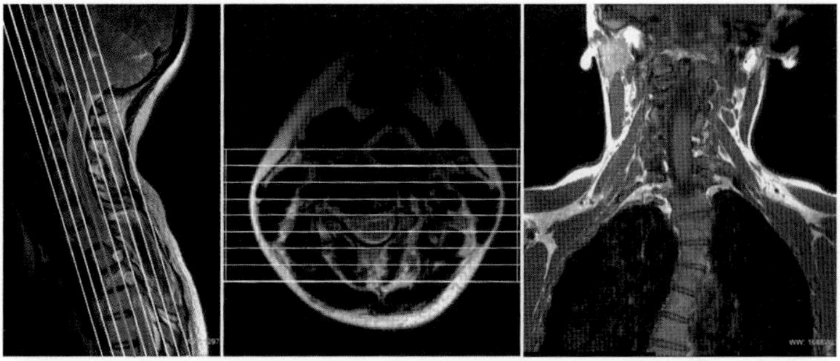

Figure 7.26 Coronal slice prescription from sagittal and axial slices is shown.

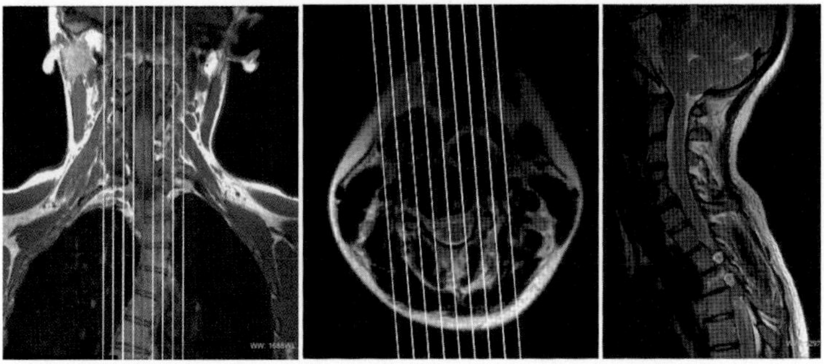

Figure 7.27 Sagittal slice prescription from coronal and axial slices is shown.

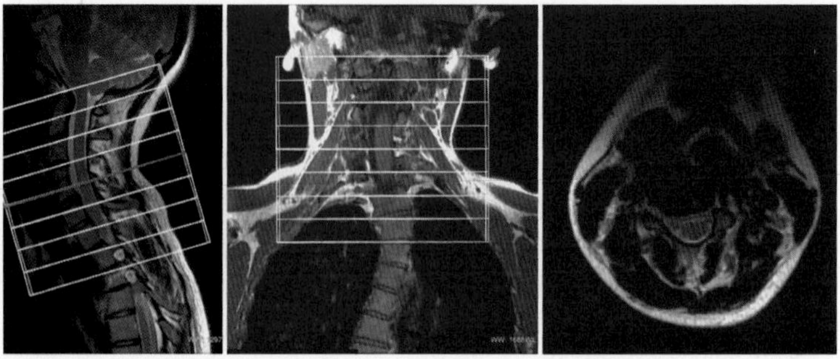

Figure 7.28 Axial slice prescription from sagittal and coronal slices is shown.

Table 7.35 Cervical myelo protocols.

Sequences	Comments	Slice order
Three plane localizer	Acquire 5 slices in each plane	
Sagittal T2	Plan 3 mm sagittal slices over coronal image where you can see the spinal cord to cover the whole spinal canal	R-L
Sagittal T1	Same as above	R-L
Axial T2*GRE/MERGE	Plan 3 mm oblique axial slices from sagittal plane. The slices should be crossing vertebral junctions	S-I
Coronal SSFSE Heavy T2	Plan from the sagittal images parallel to spinal to cord to cover vertebra	A-P
Radial SSFSE myelo	Plan from axial and check from sagittal as radial prescription	
Coronal 3D fiesta	Plan from the sagittal images parallel to spinal to cord to be limited to spinal cord only	A-P

and/or canale. For patient's referent for myelography, additional myelography sequences are prescribed using radial SSFSE/HASTE sequence and 3D Fiesta/TrueFISP sequence (Table 7.35).

Sample Imaging Parameters for 1.5 T

See Table 7.36

Graphical Prescription

Routine sequence planning for metastases patients is same as routine cervical spine imaging. Myelography sequences planning are shown in Figs. 7.29 and 7.30.

Table 7.36 Imaging parameters for an eight channel spine coil is shown.

	T2	T1	T2*	Heavy T2 thick slab	T2 radial	3D fiesta/ CISS	3D cosmic
Plan	Sagittal	Sagittal	Axial	Coronal	Radial	Coronal	Coronal
Sequence type	FRFSE	FSE	MERGE	SSFSE	SSFSE	Balance	Balance
TE	85	MinFull	Auto	Min	Min	Min	Min
TR	3,140	640	500	Min	Min	Auto	Auto
ETL	27	3	Auto	264	264		
BW	41.67	31.2	31.25	31.25	31.25	83.33	50.0
Slice thickness	4	4	3.5	20	20–25	1.6	1.6
Slice spacing	0.5	0.5	0.5	−15		−0.8	0.8
FOV	24	24	19	24	24	26	26
Matrix	352 × 224	320 × 224	320 × 192	320 × 224	320 × 224	320 × 320	352 × 352
NEX/NSA	4	4	2	0.75	0.75	2	2
Freq Direction	A-P	A-P	R-L	S-I	S-I	R-L	R-L
SAT band	A	A	A				
TI/FA			FA: 20			FA: 65	

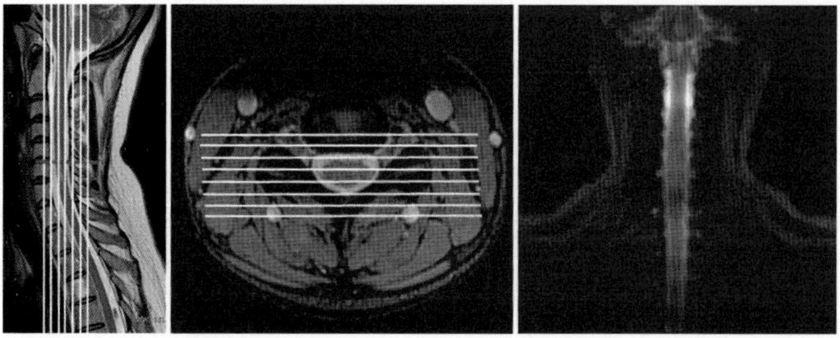

Figure 7.29 Coronal SSFSE thick slab prescription from sagittal and axial slices is shown.

Kinematic Cervical Exams

The purpose of kinematic spinal exams is to better visualize the cord compression under different positions. This way, it may be possible to better diagnose the problems. For kinematic exams, even though there are specific tools available for extension and flexion, these tools are not commonly available in most

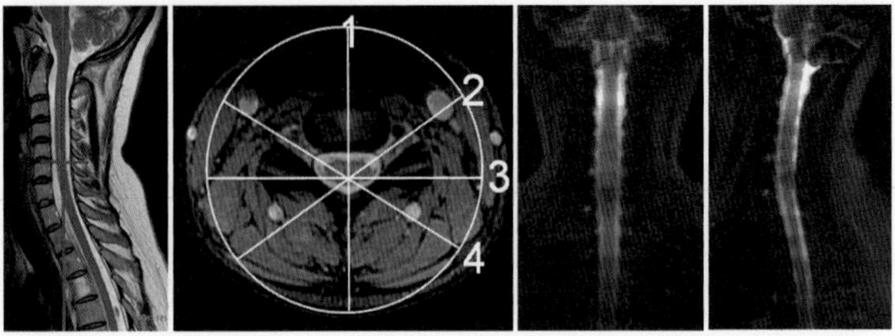

Figure 7.30 SSFSE thick slab radial prescription from sagittal and axial slices is shown.

Table 7.37 A sample kinematic cervical protocols.

Sequences	Comments	Slice order
Three plane or scout	Acquire 5 slices in each plane	
Sagittal T2	Normal position	R-L
Sagittal T2	Hyperextansion	R-L
Sagittal T2	Hyperflexion	R-L
Sagittal T1	Normal position	R-L
Axial T2*GRE	Normal position covering from C2 to C7	S-I

sites. Therefore, each site has its own way of creating kinematic exams, which may cause inconsistency. In your site, if you do not have any MR compatible kinematic tools, you should spend an additional 10 min with each patient to instruct them exactly what they are supposed to do.

For kinematic exams, a sagittal T2 sequence is applied in normal, hyperflexion, and hyperextension position. After that, routine c-spine imaging protocol is applied.

Sample Imaging Protocols

A sample kinematic exam protocol is given in Table 7.37.

Sample Imaging Parameters for 1.5 T

The imaging parameters for kinematic neck exam are same as routine c-spine exam. Please refer to the c-spine parameter table given before.

Graphical Prescription

The graphical plannings are same as routine c-spine imaging.

Nasopharynx and Maxillofacial

Patient Preparation and Positioning

Patient Preparation: Same as neck imaging patient preparation.

Patient Positioning: An eight channel brain or neurovascular coil will be appropriate for these exams in general. The patient cheekbones should be at the center of the coil for best image quality (Figs. 7.31 and 7.32).

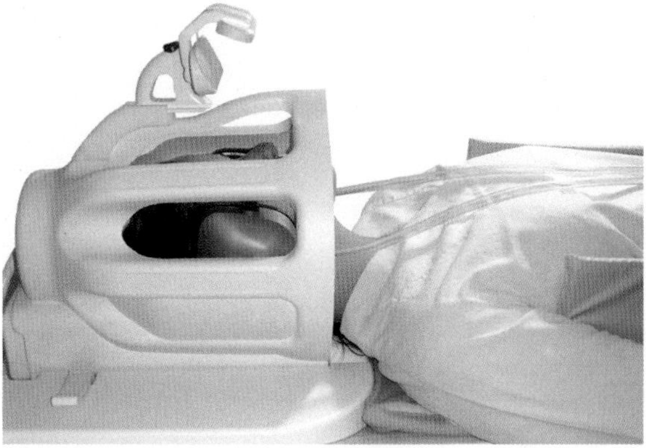

Figure 7.31 Patient positioning on an eight CH brain coil for nasopharynx or maxillofacial MRI.

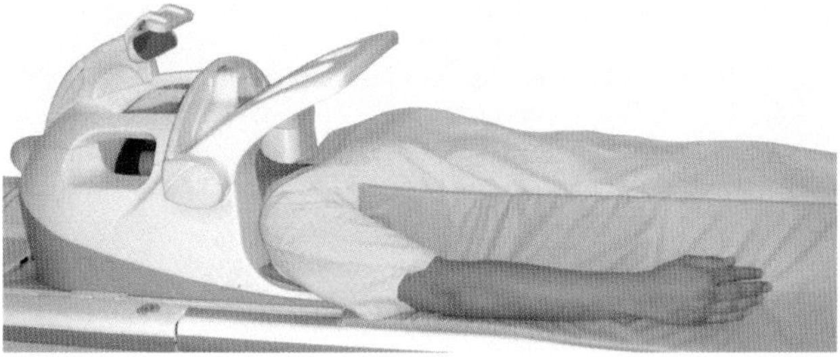

Figure 7.32 Patient positioning on an eight CH neurovascular coil for nasopharynx or maxillofacial MRI.

Sample Imaging Protocols

For nasopharynx exams, depending on the patient teeth filings and sinus cavity, chemical fat sat may not work perfectly. To eliminate any fat sat–related artifacts, we recommend STIR or the recently developed Dixon-based techniques. Dixon method is a 2D or 3D echo technique used to separate fat and water using their inherent resonant frequency differences. The recent interest in Dixon-based methods resulted in a very much improved and stable sequence, which can be used for whole body imaging. Again, we urge our readers to utilize the recently developed techniques to improve their image quality if their system has the capability.

The sample protocol for nasopharynx and maxillofacial MRI is given in Table 7.38.

Sample Imaging Parameters for 1.5 T

See Table 7.39

Graphical Prescription

Graphical prescription details are shown in Figs. 7.33–7.35.

Table 7.38 The sample protocol for nasopharynx and maxillofacial MRI.

Sequences	Comments	Slice order
Three plane localizer	Acquire 5 slices in each plane	
Sagittal STIR	Plan 4–5 mm sagittal slices over coronal image	R-L
Axial T2	The coverage is specific to the lesion or anatomical location	S-I
Axial T1	The coverage is specific to the lesion or anatomical location	S-I
Coronal T2 or T2 fat sat/STIR	Plan from sagittal and axial images and cover the region of interest	A-P
Postcontrast	*If the contrast injection is decided*	
Axial T1	Same as above	S-I
Axial T1 fat sat	Same as above	S-I
Coronal T1 fat sat	Plan same as coronal T2	A-P
Sagittal T1	Similar to STIR prescription as above	R-L

Table 7.39 Imaging parameters for an eight channel neurovascular coil is shown.

	STIR	T2	T1	T2	T1	STIR	T1FS
Plan	Sagittal	Axial	Axial	Coronal	Coronal	Coronal	Axial
Sequence type	FSE-IR	FRFSE	FSE	FRFSE	FSE	FSE-IR	FSE
TE	35	85	MinFull	85	MinFull	35	MinFull
TR	4,925	5,520	620	3,360	760	4,925	780
ETL	12	15	3	18	3	12	3
BW	41.67	31.25	31.25	41.67	41.67	41.67	20.83
Slice thickness	5	5.0	5.0	4.0	4.0	4.0	5.0
Slice spacing	1.0	1.0	1.0	1.0	1.0	1.0	1.0
FOV	26	22	22	24	24	24	22
Matrix	288 × 224	352 × 352	352 × 352	352 × 352	352 × 352	288 × 224	288 × 224
NEX/NSA	2	2	2	2	2	2	2
Freq Direction	S-I	A-P	A-P	S-I	S-I	S-I	A-P
TI/FA	145					145	

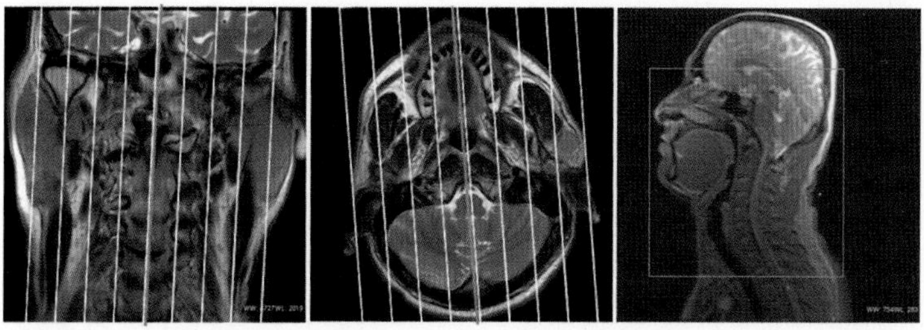

Figure 7.33 Sagittal slice prescription from coronal and axial slices is shown.

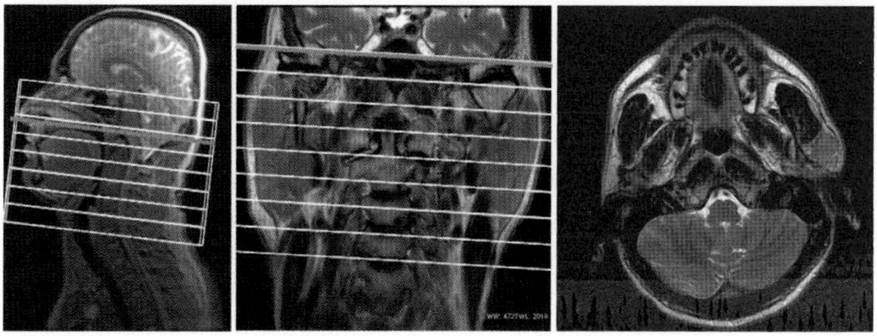

Figure 7.34 Axial slice prescription from sagittal and coronal slices is shown.

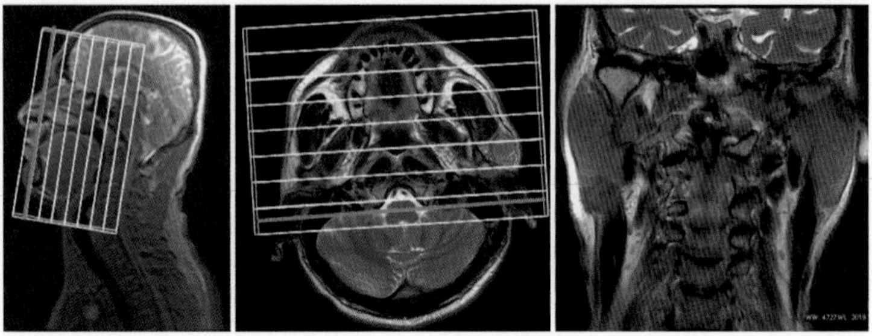

Figure 7.35 Coronal slice prescription from sagittal and axial slices is shown.

Parotid Glands

Patient Preparation and Positioning

Patient Preparation: Same as nasopharynx exam above.

Patient Positioning: Same as nasopharynx exam above.

Sample Imaging Protocols

Sagittal image acquisition is usually not needed for parotid glands if dedicated loop coils are not used. If your radiologist prefer, you can also do a T1 perfusion imaging to see the contrast uptake curves. In this case, you acquire a few phases' precontrast and continue with postcontrast exams for 4–5 min. For perfusion exams, it is recommended to inject single dose contrast agent at 4–5 cc/s injection rate.

Diffusion sequences are also applicable for parotid glands with multiple b values for differential diagnosis.

The sample protocols for the patient referred to MRI for parotid glands exam are shown in Table 7.40.

Sample Imaging Parameters for 1.5 T

See Table 7.41

Graphical Prescription

Graphical prescription details are shown in Figs. 7.36 and 7.37.

Table 7.40 The sample protocol for parotid glands.

Sequences	Comments	Slice order
Three plane localizer	Acquire 5 slices in each plane	
Coronal STIR	Plan 4–5 mm coronal slices over axial and sagittal images	A-P
Coronal T2	Plan same as coronal STIR	A-P
Axial T2	The coverage is specific to the lesion location	S-I
Axial T1	The coverage is specific to the lesion location	S-I
T1 perfusion	*Choose a 2D or 3D T1 sequence and continuously acquire multiphases around 4–5 min starting 10 s before the injection*! (*only dedicated to lesion area*)	S-I
Axial T1	Same as precontrast axial T1	S-I
Axial T1 fat sat	Copy from axial precontrast sequences	S-I
Coronal T1 fat sat	Copy from coronal sequences	A-P

Table 7.41 Imaging parameters for an eight channel neurovascular coil is shown.

	STIR	T2	T2	T2FS	T1	T1	Diff	Perfusion
Plan	Coronal	Coronal	Axial	Axial	Axial	Coronal	Axial	Axial
Sequence type	FSE-IR	FRFSE	FRFSE	FRFSE	FSE	FSE	EPI	SPGR
TE	35	85	85	85	MinFull	MinFull	62.5	Min
TR	5,125	3,180	3,120	3,460	640	720	4,000	Auto
ETL	12	18	18	16	3	3		
BW	41.67	41.67	41.7	31.25	41.67	41.67	250	35.71
Slice thickness	4.0	4.0	4.0	4.0	4.0	4.0	4.0	6
Slice spacing	1.0	1.0	1.0	1.0	1.0	1.0	1.0	−3.0
FOV	20	22	22	22	22	22	22	24
Matrix	256 × 224	352 × 352	288 × 256	224 × 224	288 × 256	352 × 256	128 × 128	224 × 128
NEX/NSA	2	4	4	4	2	4	4	1
Freq Direction	S-I	S-I	A-P	A-P	A-P	S-I	R-L	A-P
Options	FC, Z512							Zip2, Zip512
TI/FA	145			Zip512				TI: Auto/ FA: 12

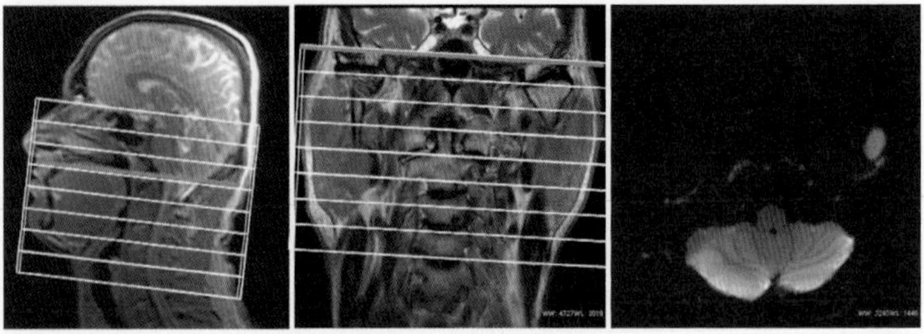

Figure 7.36 Axial slice prescription from sagittal and coronal images is shown.

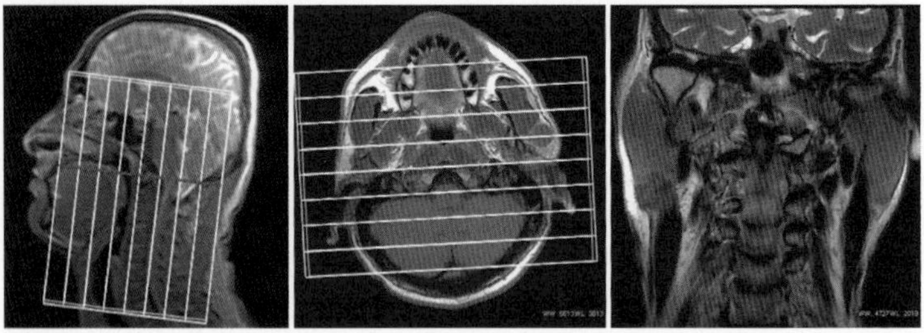

Figure 7.37 Coronal slice prescription from sagittal and axial images is shown.

Soft Tissue Neck

Sample Imaging Protocols

Similar to nasopharynx or maxillofacial MRI, chemical fat saturation may fail for neck soft tissue imaging due to special anatomical structure of the neck. To eliminate any fat sat–related artifacts, we recommend to start imaging with STIR or the recently developed Dixon-based techniques. With STIR-like sequences, traumatic tissue damage, metastases can be visualized in better contrast and help us to prescribe the following sequences specifically for the region of interest.

The sample protocols for the patient referred to MRI for neck soft tissue exam are shown in Table 7.42.

Sample Imaging Parameters for 1.5 T

See Table 7.43

Table 7.42 The sample protocol for soft tissue neck imaging.

Sequences	Comments	Slice order
Three plane localizer	Acquire 5 slices in each plane	
Sagittal STIR	Plan 4–5 mm sagittal slices over axial and coronal images and cover complete neck region	R-L
Axial T2	The coverage is specific to the lesion location	S-I
Axial T1	The coverage is specific to the lesion location	S-I
Coronal T2	Plan from sagittal STIR to cover the complete neck region	A-P
Postinjection	*Inject if needed and scan at least two different planes*	
Axial T1	Same as above	S-I
Axial T1 fat sat	Same as above	S-I
Coronal T1 fat sat	Same as above coronal T2	A-P
Sagittal T1	Same as STIR with 4–5 mm slice thickness	R-L

Table 7.43 Imaging parameters for an eight channel neurovascular coil is shown.

	STIR	T2	T1	T2	T1	STIR	T1FS
Plan	Sagittal	Axial	Axial	Coronal	Coronal	Coronal	Axial
Sequence type	FSE-IR	FRFSE	FSE	FRFSE	FSE	FSE-IR	FSE
TE	35	85	MinFull	85	MinFull	35	MinFull
TR	4,925	5,520	620	3,360	760	4,925	780
ETL	12	15	3	18	3	12	3
BW	41.67	31.25	31.25	41.67	41.67	41.67	20.83
Slice thickness	5	6	6	4	4	4	6
Slice spacing	1.5	1.5	1.5	1	1	1	1.5
FOV	26	22	22	24	24	24	22
Matrix	288 × 224	352 × 352	352 × 20	352 × 352	352 × 352	288 × 224	288 × 224
NEX/NSA	2	2	2	2	2	2	2
Freq Direction	S-I	A-P	A-P	S-I	S-I	S-I	A-P
TI	145					145	

Graphical Prescription

Graphical prescription details are shown in Figs. 7.38–7.40.

Brachial Plexus

Patient preparation and positioning is same as routine neck imaging (Figs. 7.41 and 7.42).

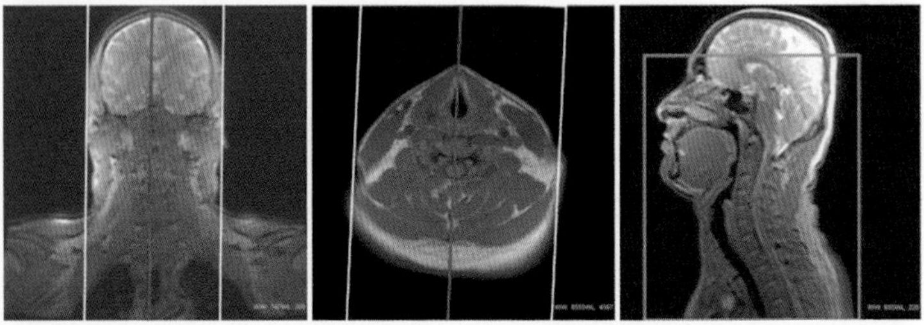

Figure 7.38 Sagittal slice prescription from coronal and axial images is shown.

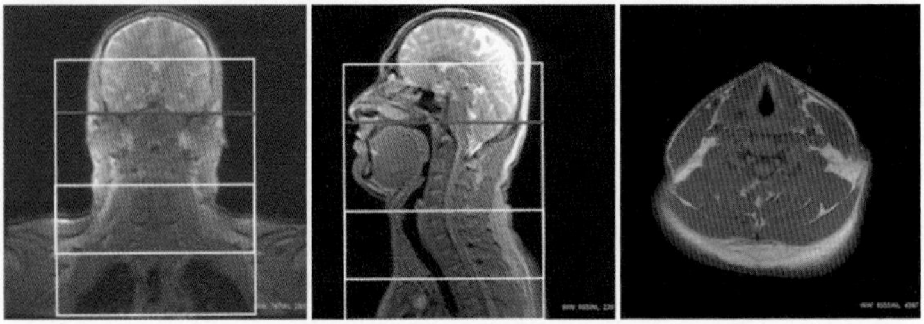

Figure 7.39 Axial slice prescription from coronal and sagittal images is shown.

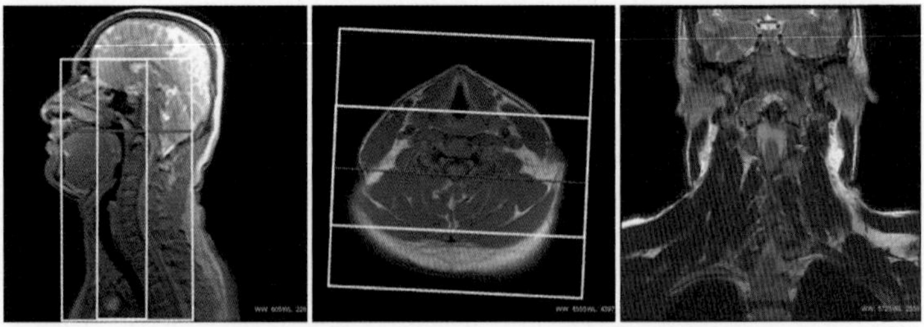

Figure 7.40 Coronal slice prescription from sagittal and axial images is shown.

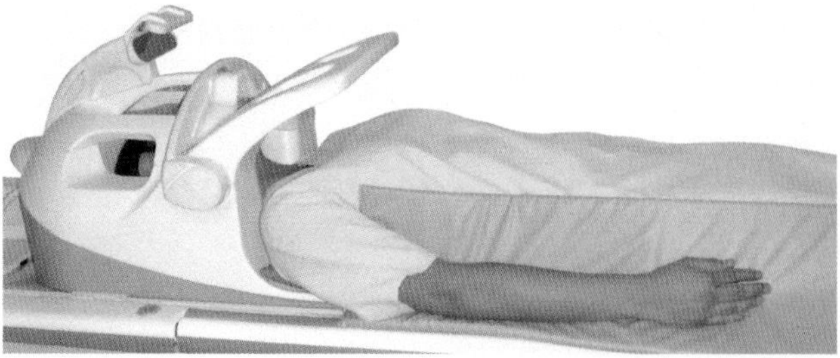

Figure 7.41 Patient positioning on an eight CH neurovascular coil for brachial plexus is shown.

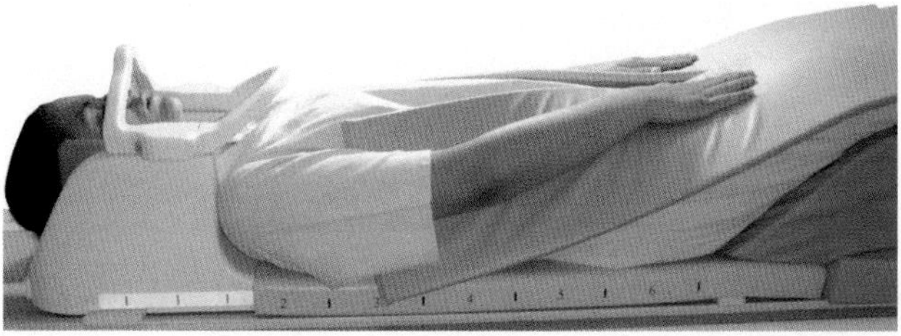

Figure 7.42 Patient positioning on an eight CH spine (CTL) coil for brachial plexus is shown.

Sample Imaging Protocols

The sample protocols for the patient referred to MRI for brachial plexus exam is shown in Table 7.44.

Sample Imaging Parameters for 1.5 T

See Table 7.45

Graphical Prescription

Graphical prescription details are shown in Figs. 7.43–7.45.

Table 7.44 A standard brachial plexus protocol.

Sequences	Comments	Slice order
Three plane localizer	Acquire 5 slices in each plane	
Coronal STIR	Plan from sagittal and axial slices with 3–4 mm slice thickness	A-P
Coronal T2	Copy from coronal STIR sequence	A-P
Coronal T1	Copy from coronal STIR sequence	A-P
Axial T2	Plan from coronal and sagittal images from C3 to aortic arch or axillary region using 4 mm slice thickness	S-I
Axial T1	Copy from axial T2	S-I
Sagittal T2	Plan from coronal STIR with a 3-mm slice thickness	R-L
Postinjection	*If you decide to inject*	
Axial 3DT1 FS	Same axial plan coverage as precontrast sequence. You can use LAVA.VIBE type sequences as well	S-I
Coronal T1	Same as above	A-P

Table 7.45 Imaging parameters for an eight channel neurovascular coil is shown.

	T1	T2	STIR	T2	T1	T2
Plan	Coronal	Coronal	Coronal	Axial	Axial	Sagittal
Sequence type	FSE	FRFSE	FSE-IR	FRFSE	FSE	FRFSE
TE	MinFull	85	38	100	MinFull	85
TR	540	3,600	5,000	5,180	500	4,200
ETL	3	18	12	17	3	24
BW	41.7	41.7	41.7	41.7	41.7	41.7
Slice thickness	4	4	4	4	4	5
Slice spacing	0.4	0.4	0.4	0.4	0.4	0.5
FOV	28	28	28	28	28	24
Matrix	352 × 352	352 × 352	320 × 224	352 × 320	352 × 320	352 × 352
NEX/NSA	2	2	2	2	2	4
Freq Direction	S-I	S-I	S-I	R-L	R-L	S-I
SAT band						I
TI			145			

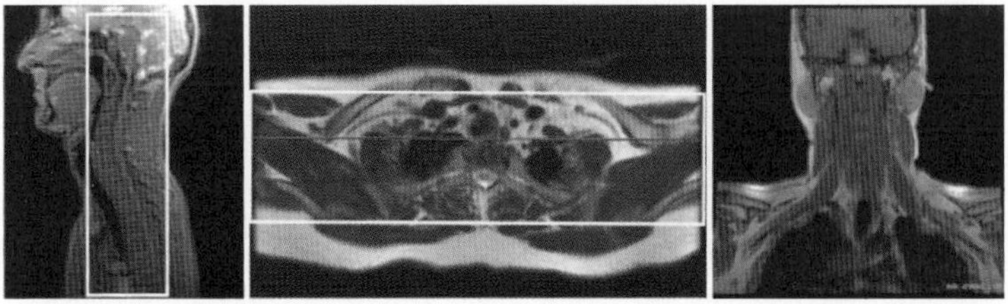

Figure 7.43 Coronal slice prescription from sagittal and axial images is shown.

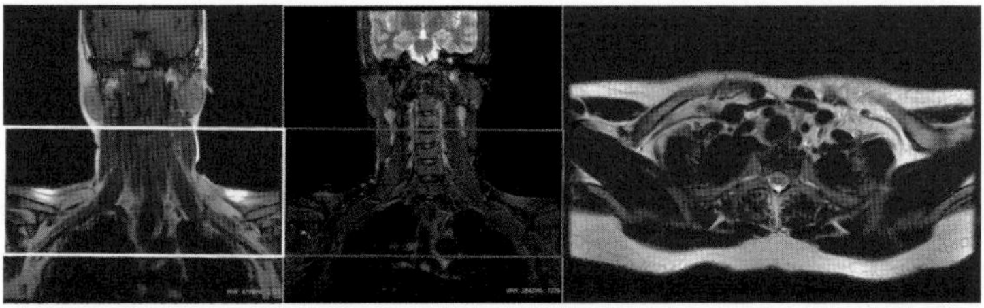

Figure 7.44 Axial slice prescription from coronal images is shown.

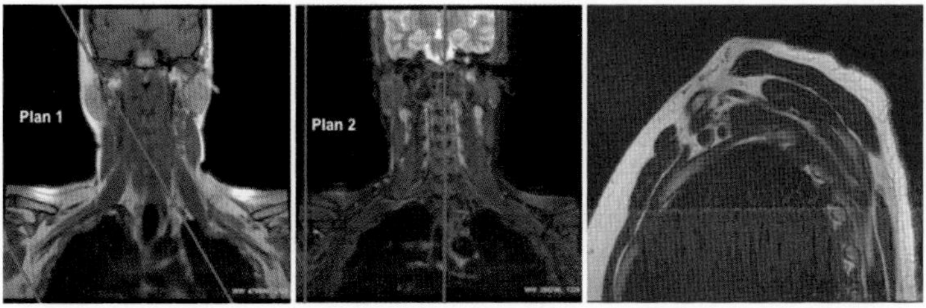

Figure 7.45 Sagittal slice prescription from coronal images is shown.

Thoracic Spine Imaging

Patient Preparation: The patient consent form should be given to the patient with a detailed explanation on the content. The form should be carefully read, all questions must be answered with clear answers such as "YES" or "NO," and additional clarifications should be written. It must be signed by the patient or legal guardians and confirmed by MR personnel. If there are any surgical implants, radiologist on duty has to make a decision based on implant type and MR compatibility. *If there is any suspicion or lack of information on the implant, do not take any risk with the patient safety and do not scan the patient.* If the form is complete with all the information, the patient should change to MR gown and remove any clothing with any metal. Please ensure that female patients remove the bra as well.

Before the MR exam, explain the nature and duration of the MR exam they will undergo. Also explain that patient motion will make a negative effect on image's quality. Make a habit of informing the patient before every sequence and communicate often to comfort the patient. It is always a good practice to remove the jewelry as well. As the last line of patient safety, it is also a good practice to scan patient with a handheld metal detector before taking the patient to MR room.

Patient Positioning: The spine coil should be centered on the table. For better patient comfort and easier breathing, leg support pads should be placed under patient knees. Patient should lie down on the coil in supine position as shown below. The center of sternum should align with the center of the coil. Additional pads should be placed around patient arms to avoid patient skin contact with the MR bore directly. Patient protection headsets and/or patient pads should be placed around the head to reduce the noise and gross patient motion. After handing the patient alarm to patient and testing it, you are ready to start the exam (Fig. 7.46).

In thoracic spine exam, one thing you will notice is increased flow-related artifacts in sagittal and axial planes. This is due to the fact that CSF flows faster in the narrow thoracic and, therefore, causes significantly more flow artifacts. These artifacts are usually magnified in sagittal plane where we use thinner slices with minimal slice spacing or no gap. They will be much less pronounced in axial plane due to thicker slices and larger slice gap. To reduce these artifacts significantly, you can apply gating devices and/or increase slice spacing up to 50%. The new motion insensitive sequences such as PROPELLER and BLADE also do a great job eliminating these artifacts.

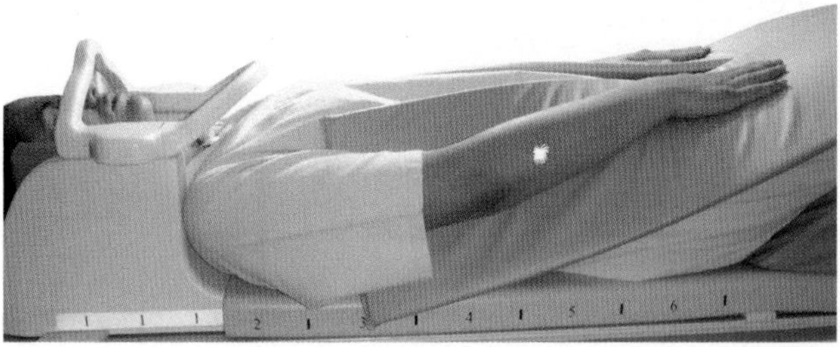

Figure 7.46 Patient positioning on an eight CH spine (CTL) coil for thoracic exam is shown.

Table 7.46 A sample standard thoracic spine protocol.

Sequences	Comments	Slice order
Three plane localizer	Acquire 5 slices in each plane with maximum FOV	
Sagittal FSPGR	Prescribe this sequence to count vertabra for accurate planning (counter)	R-L
Sagittal T2	Plan from coronal and sagittal counter with 3 mm slice thickness to cover the entire thoracic spine	R-L
Sagittal T1	Copy from sagittal T2	R-L
Axial T2	Acquire whole thoracic spine with one or two slice group	S-I

Standard Thoracic Spine

Sample Imaging Protocols

The sample protocols for the patient referred to MRI for routine thoracic spine are shown in Table 7.46.

Sample Imaging Parameters for 1.5 T

See Table 7.47

Graphical Prescription

Graphical prescription details are shown in Figs. 7.47 and 7.48.

Table 7.47 Imaging parameters for an eight channel spine (CTL) coil is shown.

	T2	T1	T2*	STIR	T1 flair	T2	T1
Plan	Sagittal	Sagittal	Sagittal	Sagittal	Sagittal	Axial	Axial
Sequence type	FRFSE	FSE	GRE	FSE-IR	FSE	FRFSE	FSE
TE	106	10	15	30	24	102	MinFull
TR	3,600	640	400	3,400	2,250	6,300	680
ETL	29	3	6	12	7	25	3
BW	41.7	41.7	62	25	31.25	41.7	41.7
Slice thickness	3	3	3	3	3	5	5
Slice spacing	1	1	1	1	1	2.5	2.5
FOV	30	30	30	30	30	20	20
Matrix	416 × 256	416 × 224	352 × 224	288 × 224	512 × 224	384 × 320	352 × 224
NEX/NSA	4	4	2	2	4	2	2
Freq Direction	A-P	A-P	A-P	A-P	A-P	A-P	A-P
SAT band	A	A	A	A	A	R/L	R/L
TI/FA			15	145	860		

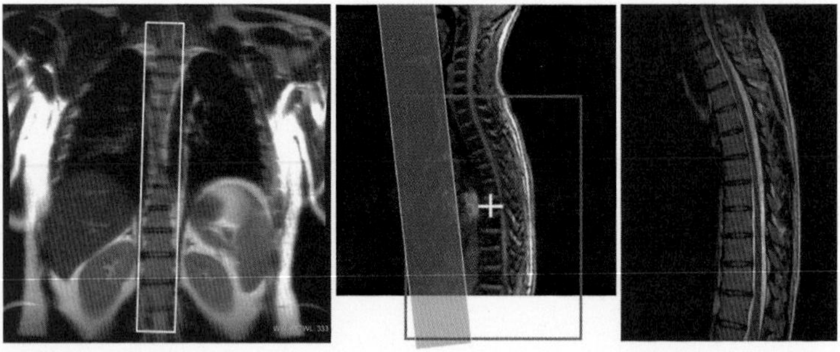

Figure 7.47 Sagittal slice prescription from coronal localizer and sagittal gradient echo counting localizer images is shown.

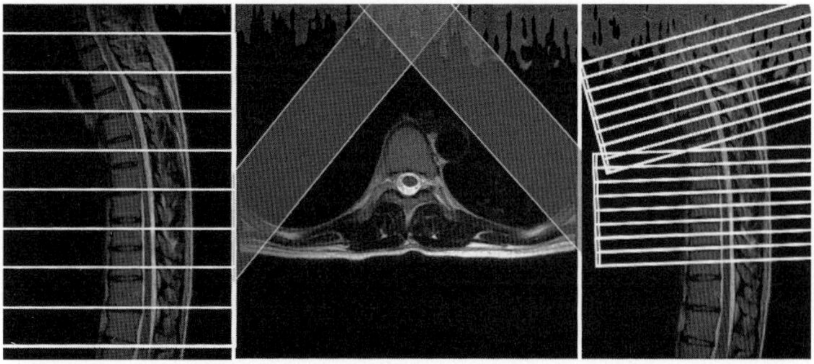

Figure 7.48 Either consecutive or multiangle multigroup axial slice prescription from sagittal slices can be prescribed as shown above. Please also make a note of the placement of saturation bands for more efficient ghosting reduction.

Table 7.48 A sample thoracic trauma protocol

Sequences	Comments	Slice order
Three plane localizer	Acquire 5 slices in each plane	
Sagittal FSPGR	Prescribe this sequence to count vertabra for accurate planning (counter)	R-L
Sagittal T2	Plan from coronal and sagittal counter with 3 mm slice thickness to cover the entire thoracic spine	R-L
Sagittal T1	Same as above	R-L
Sagittal STIR	Same as above	R-L
Coronal T2*GRE	Plan from axial localizer images with 3–4 mm slice thickness. You can use MERGE or MEDIC sequences if applicable	A-P
Axial T2	Acquire slices for region of interest only	S-I
Axial T1	Acquire slices for region of interest only	S-I

Thoracic Trauma

Sample Imaging Protocols

The sample protocols for the patient referred to MRI for thoracic trauma exam are shown in Table 7.48.

Table 7.49 Imaging parameters for an eight channel spine (CTL) coil is shown.

	T2	T1	T2*	STIR	T1 flair	T2	T1
Plan	Sagittal	Sagittal	Coronal	Sagittal	Sagittal	Axial	Axial
Sequence type	FRFSE	FSE	GRE	FSE-IR	FSE	FRFSE	FSE
TE	106	10	15	35	24	102	MinFull
TR	3,600	640	400	3,400	2,250	6,300	680
ETL	22–29	3	6	12	7	22–29	3
BW	41.7	41.7	62	25	31.25	41.7	41.7
Slice thickness	3	3	4	3	3	5	5
Slice spacing	1	1	1	1	1	2.5	2.5
FOV	30	30	33	30	30	20	20
Matrix	352 × 256	352 × 224	352 × 224	288 × 224	512 × 224	384 × 320	352 × 224
NEX/NSA	4	4	2	2	4	2	2
Freq Direction	A-P	A-P	R-L	A-P	A-P	A-P	A-P
SAT band	A	A	R-L	A	A	R/L	R/L
TI/b value/FA			15	145	860		

Sample Imaging Parameters for 1.5 T

See Table 7.49

Graphical Prescription

Sagittal and axial planning for trauma is same as routine thoracic imaging as shown above. The coronal trauma prescription is shown in Fig. 7.49.

Thoracic Metastases

Sample Imaging Protocols

The sample protocols for the patient referred to MRI for thoracic metastases exam is shown in Table 7.50.

Please note that if you start your exam with sagittal fat saturated T2 protocol, there is no additional need to prescribe STIR sequence.

Sample Imaging Parameters for 1.5 T

You can use the same imaging parameters as above.

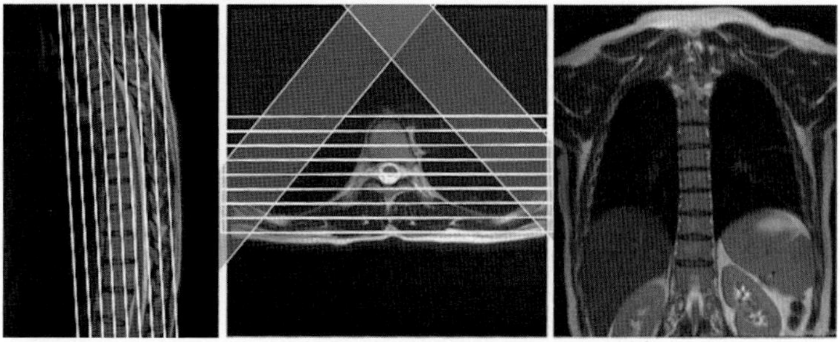

Figure 7.49 Coronal slice prescription from sagittal and axial images with two saturation bands is shown.

Table 7.50 A sample thoracic metastasis protocol.

Sequences	Comments	Slice order
Three plane	Acquire 5 slices in each plane	
Sagittal FSPGR	Prescribe this sequence to count vertabra for accurate planning (counter)	R-L
Sagittal T2	Plan from coronal slices with 3 mm slice thickness to cover the entire thoracic spine	R-L
Sagittal STIR	Same as above. You can use T2 fat sat instead of STIR as well	R-L
Sagittal T1	Same as above	R-L
Axial T2 fat sat	Acquire consecutively for whole thoracic vertabras	S-I
Axial T1	Acquire consecutively for whole thoracic vertabras	S-I
Postinjection	*If you decide to inject, scan at least in two planes*	
Axial T1	Same as above	S-I
Sagittal T1 fat sat	Copy from sagittal T1	R-L
Coronal T1 fat sat	Plan from sagittal slices with 4 mm slice thickness to cover the whole vertebras	A-P

Graphical Prescription

Sagittal and axial planning for trauma is same as routine thoracic imaging as shown above. The coronal thoracic metastases protocol is same as thoracic trauma as shown above.

Table 7.51 A sample thoracic scoliosis protocol.

Sequences	Comments	Slice order
Three plane localizer	Acquire 5–10 slices in each plane	
Coronal T2/ T1	Plan from sagittal slices with 4–5 mm slice thickness to cover the whole vertebras	A-P
Sagittal T2	Plan from coronal and axial images with 3 mm slice thickness to cover the entire spinal canal	R-L
Sagittal T1	Copy from sagittal T2	R-L
Axial T2	Acquire with 5–7 mm slice thickness for whole thoracic vertabras either in one or two consecutive slice group	S-I

Thoracic Scoliosis

The spinal structure of thoracic scoliosis patients is quite different than the normal patients. Therefore, it is recommended to image at least two or three different planes/orientations. For better graphical prescription, localizer or scout imaging should be acquired with larger slice spacing and 5–10 slices. In addition, actual scanning should start with coronal plane, so that the following sagittal and axial images can be prescribed more accurately. If the scoliosis creates more of an S-shaped spine with two very different angulations, then you should plan two different sagittal prescriptions for each orientation.

Sample Imaging Protocols

The sample protocols for thoracic scoliosis patients are given in Table 7.51.

Sample Imaging Parameters for 1.5 T

You can use the same imaging parameters given for routine t-spine imaging.

Graphical Prescription

Graphical prescription details are shown in Figs. 7.50–7.52.

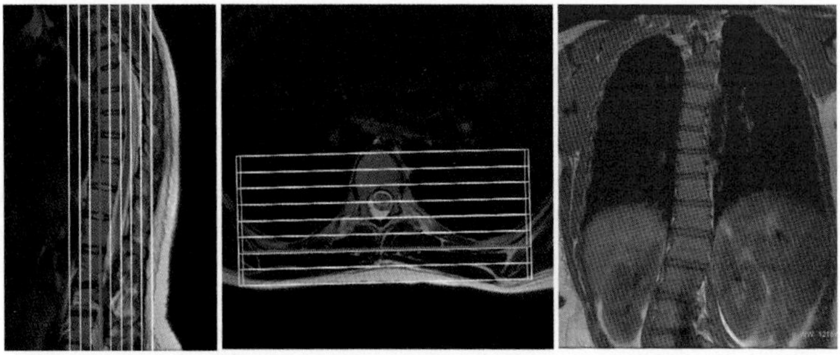

Figure 7.50 Coronal slice prescription from sagittal and axial slices is shown.

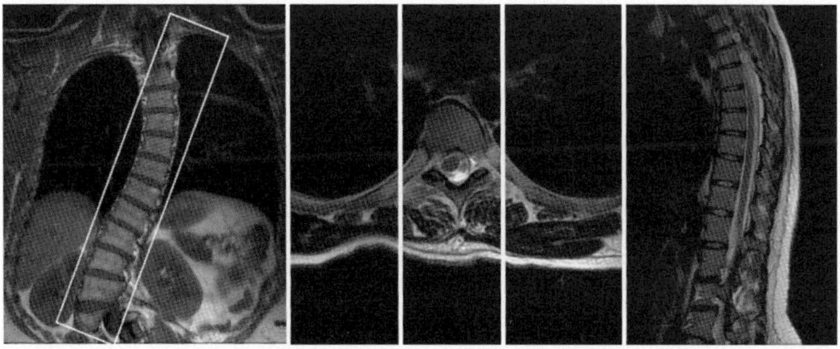

Figure 7.51 Sagittal slice prescription from coronal and axial slices is shown.

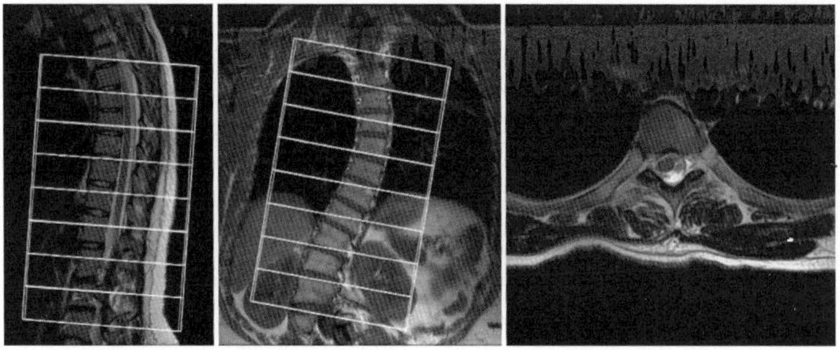

Figure 7.52 Axial slice prescription from sagittal and coronal images is shown.

Lumbar Imaging

Lumbar spine imaging is one of the most frequent MR examinations performed currently. We recommend the following protocols to make sure that lumbar exams are performed as short and simple as possible.

Patient Preparation: The patient consent form should be given to the patient with a detailed explanation on the content. The form should be carefully read, all questions must be answered with clear answers such as "YES" or "NO," and additional clarifications should be written. It must be signed by the patient or legal guardians and confirmed by MR personnel. If there are any surgical implants, radiologist on duty has to make a decision based on implant type and MR compatibility. *If there is any suspicion or lack of information on the implant, do not take any risk with the patient safety and do not scan the patient.* If the form is complete with all the information, the patient should change to MR gown and remove any clothing with any metal. Please ensure that female patients remove the bra as well. Before the MR exam, explain the nature and duration of the MR exam they will undergo. Also explain that patient motion will make a negative effect on image's quality. Make a habit of informing the patient before every sequence and communicate often to comfort the patient. It is always a good practice to remove the jewelry as well. As the last line of patient safety, it is also a good practice to scan patient with a handheld metal detector before taking the patient to MR room.

Patient Positioning: The spine coil should be centered on the table. For better patient comfort and easier breathing, leg support pads should be placed under patient knees. Patient should lie down on the coil in supine position as shown below. About 5 cm superior of iliac bones should align with the center of the coil to be used for lumbar exam. The spine coil usually has signs showing the coil coverage in each coil element. Depending on the patient height you may have a different element centered on lumbar on the patient. Therefore, you should also make a mental note where the coil center is and turn on elements before and after the center coil element. Please be aware that if you turn on more coil elements than needed, you may get an artifact called *annefact or peripheral signal artifact*. Therefore, do not turn on or select more coil elements than you need for your region of interest. However, if you have one of the systems turning on coil elements automatically depending on the FOV placed, then you do not have to worry about coil selection. Please check the localizer images for signal loss and artifacts to ensure that right coil mode and coverage are selected.

Additional MR safety pads should be placed around patient arms to avoid skin contact with the magnet bore directly. Patient protection headsets and/or patient pads should be placed around the head to reduce the noise and gross patient motion. After handling the patient alarm to patient and testing it, you are ready to start the exam (Figs. 7.53 and 7.54).

Let us take a detailed look at the most frequently used lumbar protocols and their prescription if you are ready.

Standard Lumbar Spine

Sample Imaging Protocols

A sample routine lumbar spine protocol referred to MRI for nonspecified back and/or leg pain is given in Table 7.52.

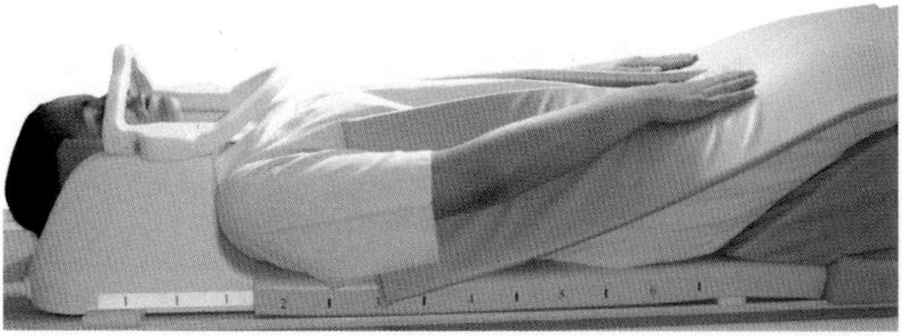

Figure 7.53 Head-first patient positioning on an eight CH spine (CTL) coil for lumbar exam.

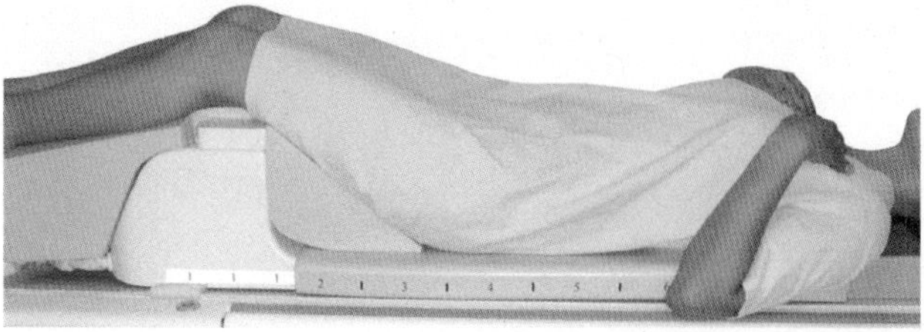

Figure 7.54 Feet-first patient positioning on an eight CH spine (CTL) coil for lumbar exam.

Table 7.52 A sample routine lumbar spine protocol.

Sequences	Comments	Slice order
Three plane localizer	Acquire 5 slices in each plane with maximum FOV	
Sagittal T2	Plan from coronal slices with 3–4 mm slice thickness to cover the entire spinal canal	R-L
Sagittal T1	Copy from sagittal T2	R-L
Axial T2	Acquire from L1-S1 and place the 5 slices for each vertebral disc	S-I

Sample Imaging Parameters for 1.5 T

See Table 7.53

Graphical Prescription

Graphical prescription details are shown in Figs. 7.55 and 7.56.

Table 7.53 Imaging parameters for an eight channel spine (CTL) coil is shown.

	T2	T1	T2*	T1 flair	STIR	T2	T1
Plan	Sagittal	Sagittal	Sagittal	Sagittal	Sagittal	Axial	Axial
Sequence type	FRFSE	FSE	MERGE	FSE	FSE-IR	FRFSE	FSE
TE	102	MinFull	Min	24	42	102	MinFull
TR	4,000	720	400	2,250	3,250	5,260	420
ETL	29	3	4	9	12	27	3
BW	41.67	41.67	62.5	41.67	31.25	41.67	41.67
Slice thickness	4	4	4	4	4	4	4
Slice spacing	1	1	1	1	1	1	1
FOV	30	30	30	30	30	20	20
Matrix	512 × 256	512 × 224	352 × 224	448 × 224	320 × 224	352 × 320	352 × 224
NEX/NSA	4	4	2	4	4	4	4
Freq Direction	A-P	A-P	A-P	A-P	A-P	A-P	A-P
SAT band	A	A	A	A	A	R-L	R-L
TI/b value/FA				800	140		

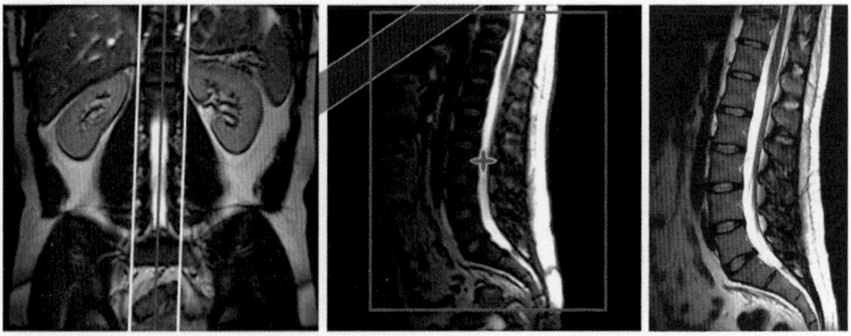

Figure 7.55 Sagittal slice prescription from coronal and sagittal images is shown. Please have a look for center of FOV and placement of saturation band.

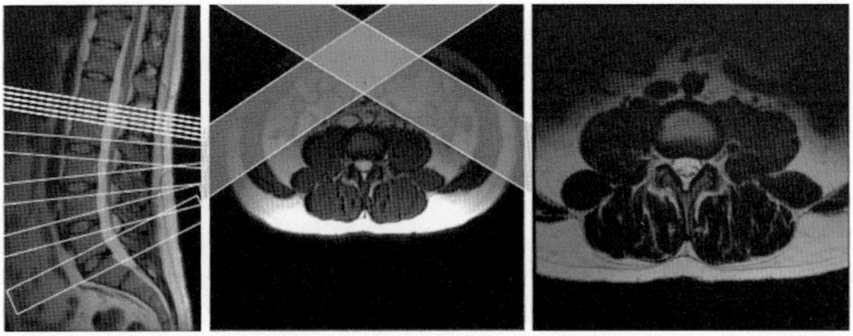

Figure 7.56 Axial slice prescription from sagittal and axial images is shown. Please note that saturation bands are planned from axial views to suppress bowel movements.

Table 7.54 A sample lumbar spine trauma protocol is shown.

Sequences	Comments	Slice order
Three plane localizer	Acquire 5 slices in each plane	
Sagittal T2	Plan from coronal slices with 3 mm slice thickness to cover the entire spinal canal	R-L
Sagittal T1	Copy from sagittal T2	R-L
Sagittal STIR	Copy from previous sagittals	R-L
Coronal T2*GRE	Plan from axial localizer images with 3–4 mm slice thickness. You can use MERGE or MEDIC sequences if applicable	A-P
Axial T2	Acquire slices for region of interest only	S-I
Axial T1	Acquire slices for region of interest only	S-I

Lumbar Trauma

Sample Imaging Protocols

The sample protocols for the patient referred to MRI for thoracic trauma exam is shown in Table 7.54.

Sample Imaging Parameters for 1.5 T

Sample imaging parameters for trauma exam is given above in routine lumbar exam.

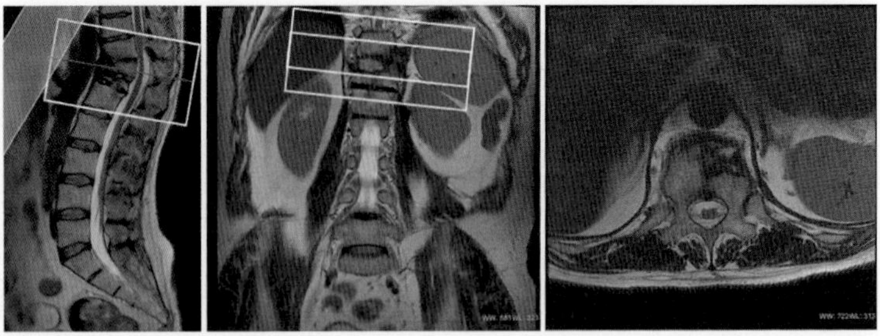

Figure 7.57 Axial slice prescription from sagittal and coronal images is shown.

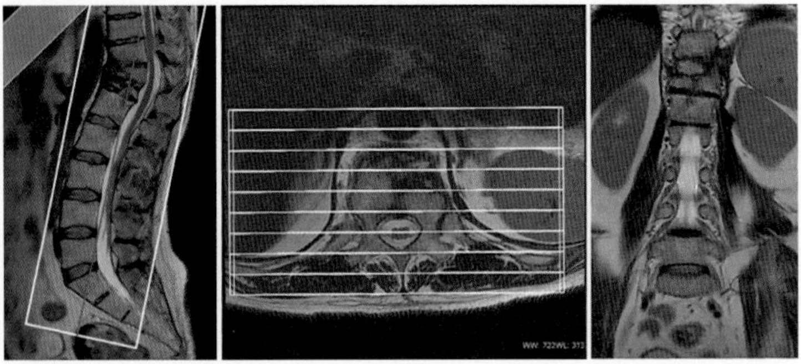

Figure 7.58 Coronal slice prescription from sagittal and axial images is shown.

Graphical Prescription

Sagittal planning for trauma is same as routine lumbar imaging as shown above. The axial coronal trauma prescriptions are shown in Figs. 7.57 and 7.58.

Lumbar Metastases

Sample Imaging Protocols

The sample protocols for the patient referred to MRI for lumbar metastases exam are shown in Table 7.55.

Table 7.55 A sample lumbar metastases protocol.

Sequences	Comments	Slice order
Three plane localizer	Acquire 5 slices in each plane	
Sagittal T2	Plan from coronal slices with 3 mm slice thickness to cover the entire spinal canal	R-L
Sagittal T1	Copy from T2.	R-L
Sagittal STIR	Copy from sagittal T2. You can use T2 fat sat instead of STIR as well	R-L
Axial T2 fat sat	Acquire consecutively for L1-S3	S-I
Axial T1	Copy from axial T2 fat sat	S-I
Postinjection	*If you decide to inject, scan at least in two planes*	
Axial T1 fat sat	Copy from previous axials	S-I
Coronal T1 fat sat	Plan from sagittal slices with 4 mm slice thickness to cover all lumbosacral vertebras	A-P
Sagittal T1 fat sat	Copy from previous sagittal T1	R-L

Graphical Prescription

Sagittal and axial planning for trauma is same as routine Lumbar imaging as shown above. The coronal Lumbar metastases protocol is same as Lumbar trauma as shown above.

Lumbar Scoliosis

The spinal structure of Lumbar scoliosis patients is quite different than the normal patients. Therefore, it is recommended to image at least two or three different planes/orientations. For better graphical prescription, localizer or scout imaging should be acquired with larger slice spacing and 5–10 slices. In addition, actual scanning should start with coronal plane with a T1, T2, or PD weighting, so that the following sagittal and axial images can be prescribed more accurately. If the scoliosis creates more of an S-shaped spine with two very different angulations, then you should plan two different sagittal prescriptions for each orientation.

Sample Imaging Protocols

The sample protocols for lumbar scoliosis patients are given in Table 7.56.

Table 7.56 A sample lumbar scoliosis protocol.

Sequences	Comments	Slice order
Three plane localizer	Acquire 5–10 slices in each plane	
Coronal T2	Plan from sagittal slices with 4–5 mm slice thickness to cover the whole vertebras	A-P
Sagittal T2	Plan from coronal and axial images with 3 mm slice thickness to cover the entire spinal canal	R-L
Sagittal T1	Copy from sagittal T2	R-L
Axial T2	Acquire with 5–7 mm slice thickness for whole lumbosacral vertabras either in one or two consecutive slice group	S-I

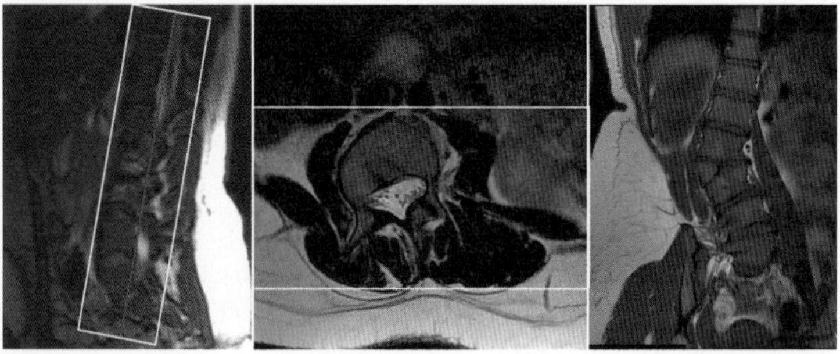

Figure 7.59 Coronal slice prescription from sagittal and axial images is shown.

Sample Imaging Parameters for 1.5 T

Sample imaging parameters for lumbar scoliosis exam can be seen from thoracic scoliosis exam.

Graphical Prescription

Graphical prescription details are shown in Figs. 7.59–7.61.

Lumbar Myelography

Sample Imaging Protocols

Even though lumbar myelography request is not quite common as the lumbar protocols we discussed above, we sometimes prescribe lumbar myelography

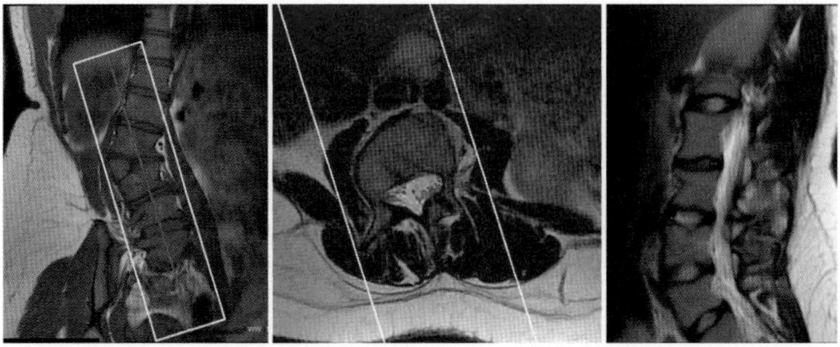

Figure 7.60 Sagittal slice prescription from coronal and axial images is shown.

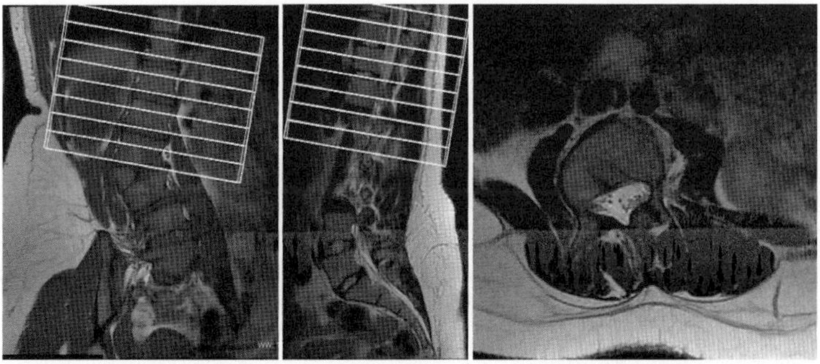

Figure 7.61 Axial slice prescription from coronal and sagittal images is shown.

for better visualization of spinal cord and/or canale. For patients referent for myelography, additional myelography sequences are prescribed using radial SSFSE/HASTE sequence, 3D FRFSE/RESTORE T2 sequence, and 3D Fiesta/TrueFISP sequence. The thin slice and high in-plane resolution capability of these sequences combined with their superb contrast (T2/T1) make lumbar myelography exams much more diagnostic.

The sample protocol for lumbar myelography patients is given in Table 7.57.

Sample Imaging Parameters for 1.5 T

Sample imaging parameters for lumbar myelography exam can be seen from cervical myelography exam.

Table 7.57 A sample for lumbar myelography protocol.

Sequences	Comments	Slice order
Three plane localizer	Acquire 3–5 slices in each plane	
Sagittal T2	Plan 3 mm sagittal slices over coronal image where you can see the spinal cord to cover the whole spinal canal	R-L
Sagittal T1	Same as above	R-L
Axial T2	Plan 3–4 mm oblique axial slices from sagittal images. The slices should be crossing vertebral junctions and cover from L1 to S1	S-I
Coronal SSFSE thickslap	Plan from the sagittal images parallel to spinal to cord to cover vertebra	A-P
Radial SSFSE myelo	Plan from axial and check from sagittal as radial prescription	S-I
Coronal 3D fiesta	Plan from the sagittal images parallel to spinal to cord to be limited to spinal cord only	S-I

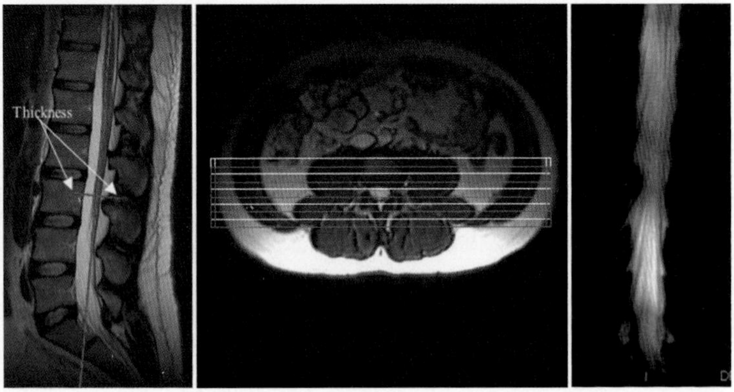

Figure 7.62 Coronal SSFSE thick slice prescription from sagittal and axial slices is shown.

Graphical Prescription

Graphical prescription details are shown in Figs. 7.62–7.64.

Lumbar Kinematic Protokolleri

The purpose of kinematic spinal exams is to better visualize the cord compression under different positions. This way, it may be possible to better diagnose the problems. For kinematic exams, even though there are specific tools

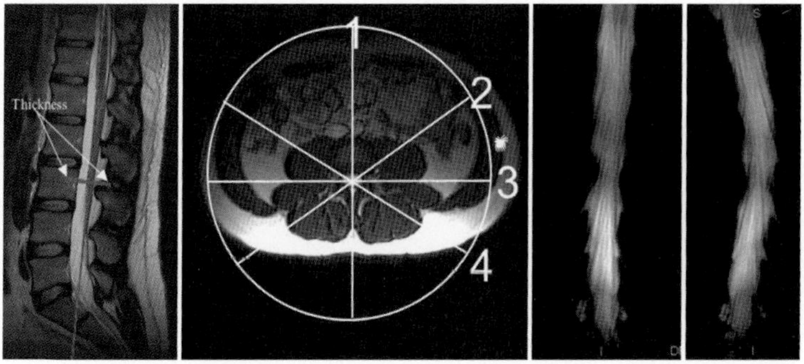

Figure 7.63 Radial planning from sagittal and axial slices is shown.

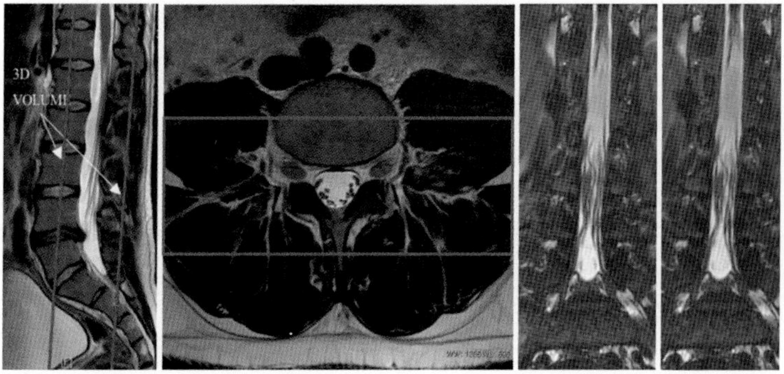

Figure 7.64 3D coronal fiesta/true FISP/b-FFE sequence slice prescription from sagittal and axial images is shown.

available for extension and flexion, these tools are not commonly available in most sites. Therefore, each site has its own way of creating kinematic exams, which may cause inconsistency. In your site, if you do not have any MR compatible kinematic tools, you should spend an additional 10 min with each patient to instruct them exactly what they are supposed to do.

For kinematic exams, a sagittal T2 sequence is applied in normal, hyperflexion, and hyperextension position. After that, routine lumbar spine imaging protocol is applied.

Sample Imaging Protocols

A sample kinematic exam protocol is given in Table 7.58.

Sample Imaging Parameters for 1.5 T

Sample imaging parameters for lumbar kinematic exam are same as routine lumbar spine exam.

Graphical Prescription

All graphical planning for kinematic exam is same as routine lumbar imaging as shown above.

Table 7.58 A sample lumbar kinematic protocol.

Sequences	Comments	Slice order
Three plane	Acquire 5 slices in each plane	
Sagittal T2	Normal position	R-L
Sagittal T2	Hyperextansion	R-L
Sagittal T2	Hyperflexion	R-L
Sagittal T1	Neutral position	R-L
Axial T2	Neutral position covering from L1 to S1 with 3 mm	S-I

Chapter 8

Musculoskeletal Imaging: MRI Protocols, Imaging Parameters, and Graphical Prescriptions

Musculoskeletal system is the locomotor system that gives us ability to move using muscular and skeletal systems. Musculoskeletal system has various structures such as; bone, muscle, cartilage, tendons, joints, etc. All these structures of musculoskeletal system can be imaged with MRI and therefore is a significant portion of routine clinical MR imaging.

In this chapter, musculoskeletal system imaging applications will be covered in the same order for easier organization and follow-up. For each section, we will discuss patient preparation, patient positioning, imaging protocols, graphical prescriptions, and sample imaging parameters.

Temporomandibular Joint (TMJ)

Temporomandibular joints (TMJ) joint imaging can be done with a number of different coils depending on the availability at your site. Even though today high-density coils with eight channel of above can give you good quality, the TMJ imaging dedicated coils do produce a very nice image quality. The TMJ dedicated coils usually has a holder device to fix them in the desired position and can be used for bilateral joint imaging with small loop coils as shown in the figure below. These loop coils are practically surface coils and can have different diameters. The coil shown in this book is two 3 in. diameter coil. These coils will get relatively uniform signal within the 3 in. in diameter and 3 in. in depth. Therefore, they provide high signal for the TMJ joints. If you

M. Elmaoğlu and A. Çelik, *MRI Handbook: MR Physics, Patient Positioning, and Protocols*, DOI 10.1007/978-1-4614-1096-6_8,

have one of the new multichannel brain coils but not the loop coils, you can still follow the guidance in the book to acquire very nice TMJ images.

Quite often TMJ imaging can be done in dynamic imaging or so-called kinematic imaging. Kinematic imaging requires imaging TMJ joint while the mouth is closed and opened at different levels, so that the joint and disc position can be imaged dynamically. To keep mouth open at different levels without motion is possible by using kinematic devices from different companies. However, if you do not have any special hardware for this type of exam, you can still do the kinematic exam by explaining the patient the procedure and give instructions during the scan accordingly. The kinematic exam starts with the mouth shut. Then, we repeat the scan while the patient opens his/her mouth 1–2 cm in each time until we reach the maximum opening.

A step-by-step approach to TMJ MR imaging is given below.

Patient Preparation and Positioning

Patient Preparation: The patient consent form should be given to the patient with a detailed explanation on the content. The form should be carefully read, all questions must be answered with clear answers such as "YES" or "NO," and additional clarifications should be written. It must be signed by the patient or legal guardians and confirmed by MR personnel. If there are any surgical implants, radiologist on duty has to make a decision based on implant type and MR compatibility. *If there is any suspicion or lack of information on the implant, do not take any risk with the patient safety and do not scan the patient.* If the form is complete with all the information, the patient should change to MR gown and remove any clothing with any metal. It is always a good practice to remove the jewelry as well. As the last line of patient safety, it is also a good practice to scan patient with a handheld metal detector before taking the patient to MRI room.

Patient Positioning: The TMJ coil shown in Figs. 8.1 and 8.2 has two pieces firmly fixed in a holder. The holder enables you to position the coil in the desired location and can be fixed in this location, so that it does not move during the scan. When you position the coil, ask the patient to open and close the mouth while you feel exactly where the TMJ joint is with your hand. The loop coil center should be placed directly at the TMJ joint. The coils should be as close to the face as possible without disturbing the patient. If you do not have the TMJ dedicated coils, you can use general purpose brain coil for imaging.

Please make sure that you give the patient alarm/buzzer to patient's hand and test it before sending in. The landmarking should be on the center of loop coils using laser lights or touch sensor. It is always recommended to let the patient know how long the scan is going to take and also keep communicating frequently to make them as comfortable as possible in the MR bore (Fig. 8.2). Let's take a look at the most frequently used protocols and graphical prescriptions for TMJ imaging:

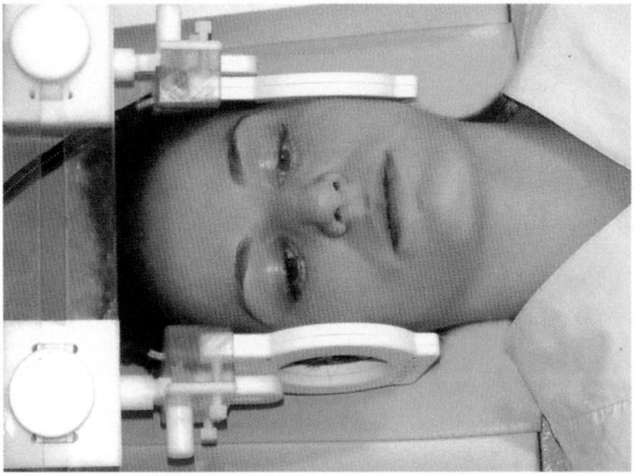

Figure 8.1 A sample patient positioning in a TMJ dedicated loop coils.

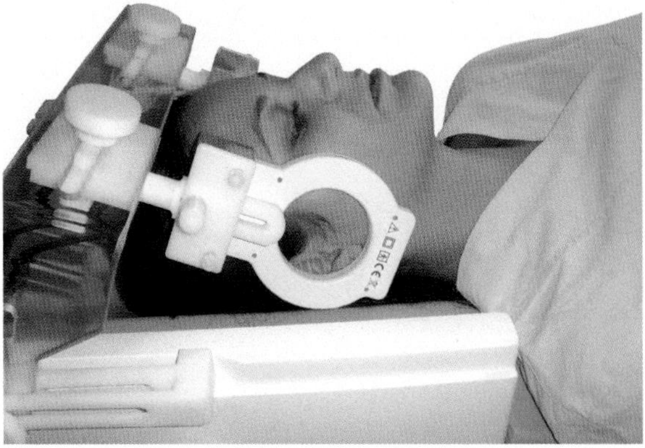

Figure 8.2 A sample patient positioning in a TMJ dedicated loop coils.

Table 8.1 A standard TMJ imaging protocol.

Sequences	Comments	Slice order
Three plane localizer	Acquire 5–7 slices in each plane	
Axial FGRE	Prescribe a fast sequence with 3 mm slice only for the joint	S-I
Sagittal T1	Prescribe two groups of sagittal slices for each joint with 2–3 mm slice thickness	R-L
Sagittal T2 GRE*	Prescribe two groups of sagittal slices for each joint with 2–3 mm slice thickness	R-L
Sagittal PD or hybrid PD fat sat	Prescribe two groups of sagittal slices for each joint with 2–3 mm slice thickness	R-L
Kinematic sagittal	Prescribe a single sagittal slice for each joint and repeat it at five different positions	R-L
Mouth open fully	*While the mouth is opened fully with a hardware*	
Sagittal PD	Prescribe two groups of sagittal slices for each joint with 2–3 mm slice thickness	R-L
Sagittal T2 GRE*	Prescribe two groups of sagittal slices for each joint with 2–3 mm slice thickness	R-L

Sample Imaging Protocols

In addition to the sample protocol above, a coronal T2 and/or Hybrid PD Fat Sat sequence can be prescribed as well for better visualization of degenerated tissue and effusion (Table 8.1).

Kinematic Imaging: For kinematic exams, we usually use a T2* sequence such as FGRE or SPGR to image the joint at different mouth opening levels. The main purpose with the kinematic exams is to visualize the position of the disk dynamically. The kinematic exam starts with the mouth shut. Then, we repeat the scan while the patient opens his/her mouth 1–2 cm in each time until we reach the maximum opening.

Sample Imaging Parameters for 1.5 T

See Table 8.2

Graphical Prescription

The graphical prescriptions for axial, sagittal, and coronal imaging are given in Figs. 8.3–8.5.

Table 8.2 A sample of TMJ imaging parameters is given for a dedicated TMJ coil.

	T2*	T1	T2*	PD	Kinematic	T2*	PD fat sat
Plan	Axial	Sagittal	Sagittal	Sagittal	Sagittal	Coronal	Sagittal
Sequence type	SPGR	FSE	GRE	FSE	SPGR	GRE	FSE
TE	MinFull	MinFull	15	24	MinFull	14	35
TR	100	600	450	1,800	Auto	500	2,250
ETL		2		7			8–9
BW	31.2	20.83	8.93	16.6	13.89	8.93	17.86
Slice thickness	3	3	3	3	4	3	3
Slice spacing	0.3	0.3	0.3	0.3	0	0.3	0.3
FOV	20	10	10	10	12	18	12
Matrix	224 × 224	288 × 224	288 × 224	288 × 224	256 × 192	288 × 256	256 × 224
NEX/NSA	2	4	3	4	2	2	4
Freq direction	A-P	S-I	S-I	S-I	S-I	S-I	S-I
FA/Zip	15		20		25	25	Zip512

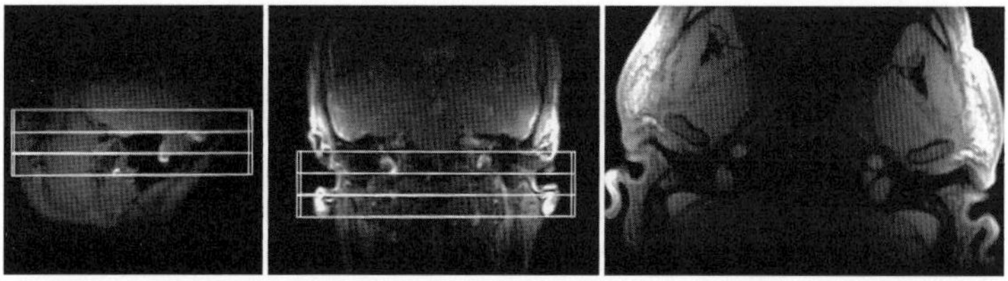

Figure 8.3 Axial slice prescription from sagittal and coronal localizer images is shown.

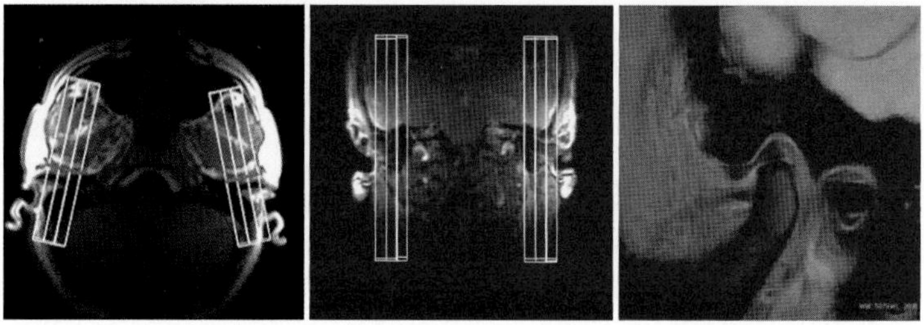

Figure 8.4 Oblique sagittal slice prescription from axial and coronal images is shown.

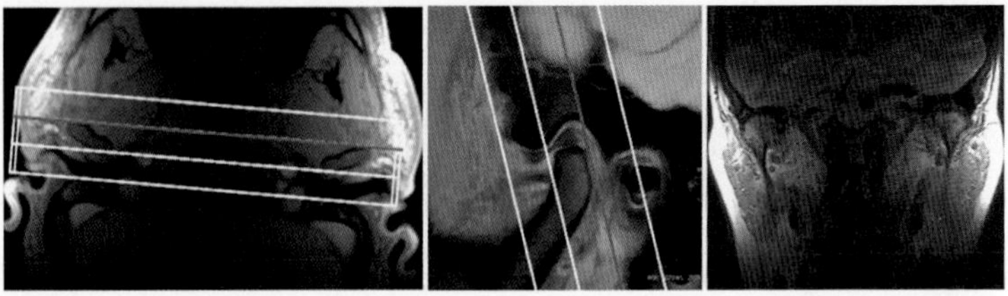

Figure 8.5 Coronal slice prescription from axial and sagittal images is shown.

Shoulder

Shoulder imaging is one of the most common MSK imaging procedure. Appropriate patient positioning and correct graphical prescriptions are key points to obtain diagnosable image quality in shoulder imaging.

For shoulder imaging, dedicated multichannel phased array coils should be preferred. However, general purpose flexible coils or other available surface coils can be used if your site does not have one of the dedicated shoulder coils.

Patient Preparation and Positioning

Patient Preparation: The patient consent form should be given to the patient with a detailed explanation on the content. The form should be carefully read, all questions must be answered with clear answers such as "YES" or "NO," and additional clarifications should be written. It must be signed by the patient and confirmed by MR personnel. If there is any surgical implant, radiologist on duty has to make a decision based on implant type and MR compatibility. *If there is any suspicion or lack of information on the implant, do not take any risk with the patient safety and do not scan the patient.* If the form is complete with all the information, the patient should change to MR gown and remove any clothing with any metal. It is always a good practice to remove the jewelry as well. As the last line of patient safety, it is also a good practice to scan patient with a handheld metal detector before taking the patient to MR room (Fig. 8.6).

Patient Positioning: The shoulder coil is placed on the shoulder to be imaged and fixed with additional straps. The patient lies down on supine position and shoulder coil is placed if there is a coil holder or positioning pad on the table. Additional pads should be placed under the patient arm to make humerus almost parallel to the table. The palm of the hand should be pointing upward as well for best patient position (anatomical position or external rotation).

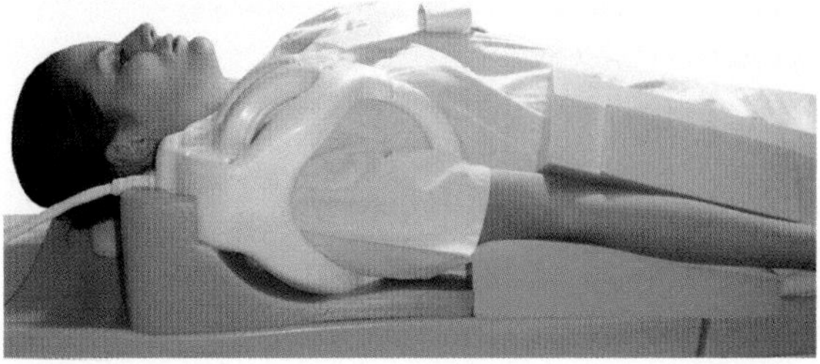

Figure 8.6 A sample patient positioning for a dedicated phase array shoulder coil. Please note that the patient arm is in external rotation (palm point upward in this position).

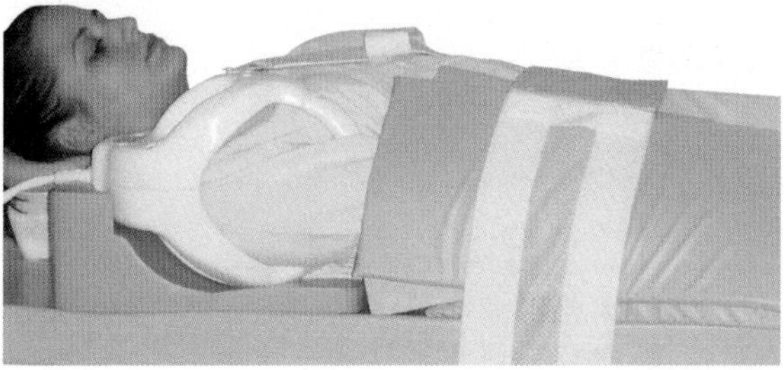

Figure 8.7 A sample patient positioning for a dedicated shoulder coil. Please note that the additional MR safety pads and immobilization straps are placed for motion reduction and patient protection.

However, if the patient is unable to stay in this position due to injury or pain, you can position the arm in a comfortable way. To reduce gross patient motion artifacts, an additional strap should be placed over the patient at the elbow level or a bit more inferior as shown in Fig. 8.7. A proper patient positioning in a multichannel coil is shown in the figure below for your information.

Please make sure that you placed the MR safety pads on both sides of the patient in order to protect patient from potential RF burn. This is particularly important for obese patients where they might touch the magnet easily.

Additionally, you should give the alarm bell to patient and ask them to test it before sending patient in. After landmarking the center of coil using laser lights or touch sensors, you can send the patient in and start the exam. It is always recommended to let the patient know how long the scan is going to take and also keep communicating frequently to make them as comfortable as possible in the MR bore.

Table 8.3 A routine shoulder imaging protocol.

Sequences	Comments	Slice order
Three plane or scout	Acquire 5 slices in each plane	
Axial GRE	Prescribe a straight axial with 3–4 mm slice only for joint	S-I
Oblique coronal PD fat sat	Prescribe parallel to supraspinatus muscle or tendon	A-P
Oblique coronal T1	Same as coronal PD fat sat	A-P
Sagittal PD fat sat	Prescribe perpendicular to the coronal slice orientation from coronal images	R-L
Additions		
Axial PD fat sat	This sequence can be prescribed instead of axial GRE for trauma patients	S-I
Coronal STIR	Prescribe this sequence for trauma patient and/or fat sat issues	A-P
Sagittal T2	Prescribe this sequence instead of PD fat sat if there are fat sat issues	R-L

Sample Imaging Protocols

A sample shoulder imaging protocol for a patient referred to the MRI for shoulder scan is given in Table 8.3.

Tips and Tricks

Hybrid PD Sequence: For MSK imaging PD weighted protocols in this book, you will notice that the parameters are slightly different. Usually, tissues like disk, labrum, cartilage, and fluid are isointense in a standard PD weighted images and hypointense in T2 weighted images (when TE is longer than 50 ms). Therefore, for better differential diagnosis, additional sequences are generally required. However, longer TE provides better signal differences in pathologic changes such as edema (in traumatic cases), tears, cartilage damage, or other tumoral developments but doesn't help to differentiate the superficial cartilage and bone. The hybrid sequence has intermediate contrast weighting and provides better differentiation for bone-normal and abnormal cartilage tissues and fluid. To provide this weighting, we usually recommend slightly longer

Table 8.4 A sample shoulder imaging parameter is given for a multichannel shoulder coil.

	T2*	PD fat sat	T1	PD fat sat	T2	PD fat sat	T1
Plan	Axial	Coronal	Coronal	Sagittal	Sagittal	Axial	Axial
Sequence type	MERGE	FRFSE	FSE	FRFSE	FRFSE	FRFSE	FSE
TE	MinFull	40	MinFull	37.5	85	40	MinFull
TR	513	2,420	560	2,560	3,040	2,480	740
ETL		9	3	9	15	9	2
BW	31.25	20.83	50.0	20.83	31.25	20.83	41.67
Slice thickness	4.0	4.0	4.0	3.0	3.0	4.0	4.0
Slice spacing	1.0	1.0	1.0	1.0	1.0	1	1.0
FOV	17	14–16	14–16	16	16	14–17	14–17
Matrix	288 × 224	256 × 224	352 × 256	320 × 224	352 × 320	320 × 256	384 × 224
NEX/NSA	2	4	3	4	2	3	2
Freq direction	R-L	S-I	S-I	S-I	S-I	R-L	R-L
SAT band/zip		RL/Z512		I	I	I	
TI/FA	25						

TE (around 35–40 ms) and ETL (8–9) for PD sequences in this book to create somewhat a hybrid PD contrast with additional T2 weighting. As a result, fluid, abnormal cartilage, and pathological structures appear hyperintense while normal cartilage remains isointense. This type of sequence provides better contrast between soft tissue (e.g., cartilage, disk, and labrum) and fluid.

Shoulder imaging acquisition should be done as soon as possible. When the acquisition times become longer, patient motion artifacts can degrade image quality significantly.

Sample Imaging Parameters for 1.5 T

A sample imaging sequence parameter for a routine shoulder imaging is given in Table 8.4.

Graphical Prescription

See Figs. 8.8–8.11

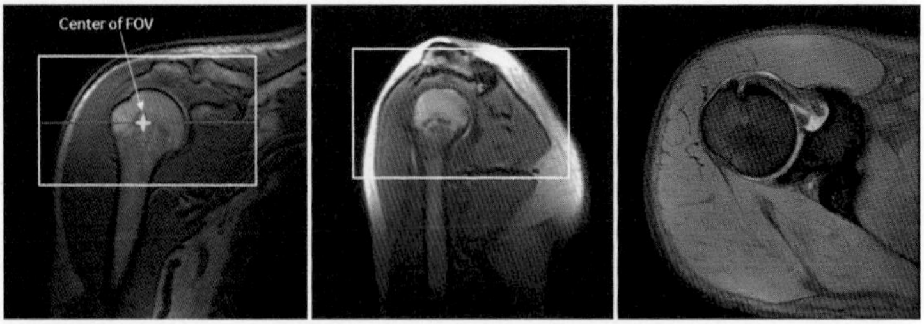

Figure 8.8 Axial slice prescription from sagittal and coronal localizer images is shown.

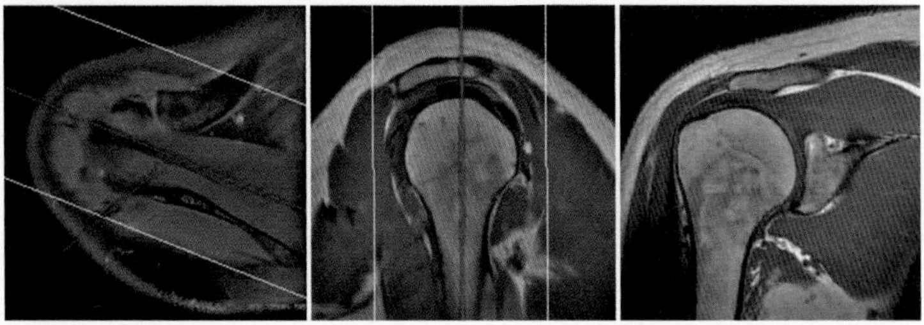

Figure 8.9 Coronal slice prescription from sagittal and axial images is shown using supraspinatus tendon as a reference point for rotator cuff tear.

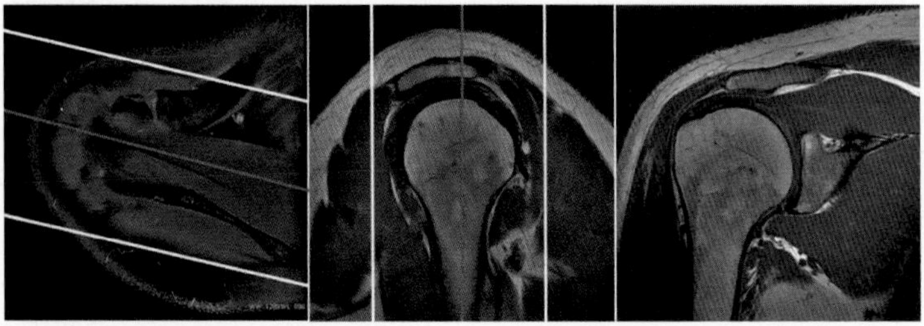

Figure 8.10 Coronal slice prescription from axial and sagittal images is shown using supraspinatus muscle as a reference point.

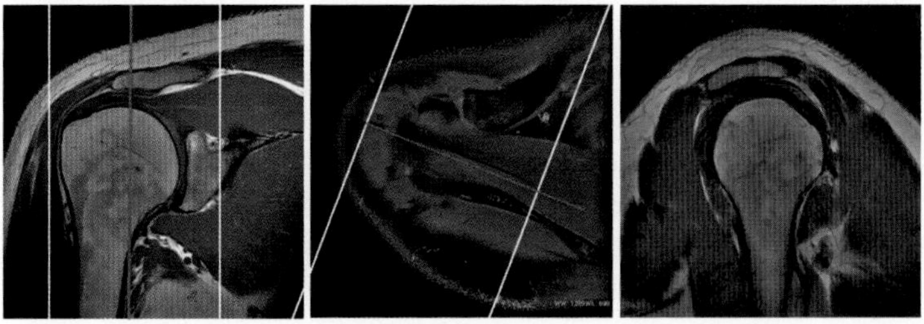

Figure 8.11 Sagittal slice prescription from coronal and axial images is shown.

Elbow Imaging

Elbow imaging can be done with several different coils. If you have a general flexible coil available at your site, you can put the patient feet first on supine position and let the arms at the side. Then you can wrap the coil around the elbow. This is the most comfortable position for the patient. However, if you do not have any working flexible coils, you can use one of the smaller diameter coils such as knee, foot, or loop coils to scan the patient head first on prone position. This is also called superman position. Somewhat contrary to the position name, it is a *super uncomfortable* position for the patient though.

If you have to scan a patient in a cast and cannot be placed straight, you can also use other coils such as shoulder coil for an efficient scan.

Patient Preparation: The patient consent form should be given to the patient with a detailed explanation on the content. The form should be filled and signed by the patient with the help of MR personnel. If there are any surgical implants, radiologist on duty has to make a decision based on implant type and MR compatibility. *If there is any suspicion or lack of information on the implant, do not take any risk with the patient safety and do not scan the patient.* If the form is complete with all the information, the patient should change to MR gown and remove any clothing with any metal. It is always a good practice to remove the jewelry as well. As the last line of patient safety, it is also a good practice to scan patient with a handheld metal detector before taking the patient to MR room.

Patient Positioning: If you do have a flexible coil, you can position the patient supine, feet first or head first and you can wrap the coil around the elbow of interest. Quite similar to shoulder imaging patient preparation, place additional pads under the patient's arm to make humerus almost parallel to the table.

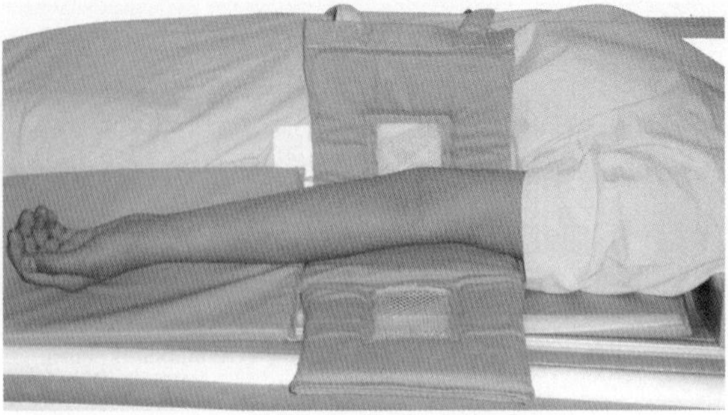

Figure 8.12 A sample patient positioning for elbow in a general purpose flexible coil. Please note that the patient palm point upward in this position (external rotation).

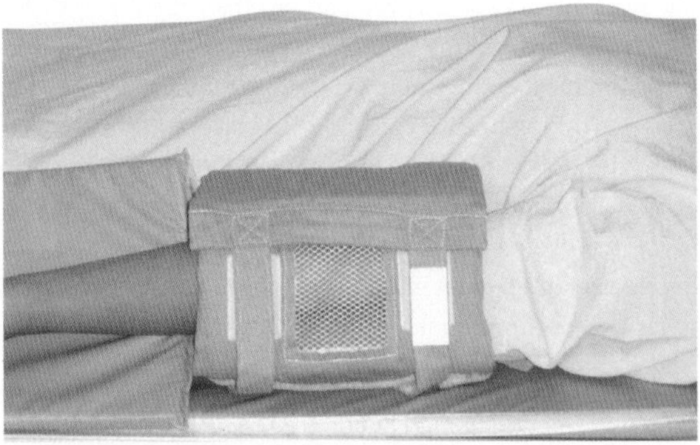

Figure 8.13 A sample patient positioning for elbow in a general purpose flexible coil.

The palm of the hand should be pointing upward as well for best patient position as shown in Fig. 8.12. However, if the patient is unable to stay in this position due to injury or pain, you can position the arm in a more comfortable way. To reduce gross patient motion artifacts, immobilization straps should be placed over the patient arm at the elbow level or a bit more inferior.

Please make sure that you give the patient alarm/buzzer to patient's hand and test it. After landmarking the center of coil using laser lights or touch sensors, you can send the patient in and start the exam. It is always recommended to let the patient know how long the scan is going to take and also keep

Table 8.5 A routine elbow imaging protocol.

Sequences	Comments	Slice order
Three plane localizer	Acquire 5 slices in each plane	
Axial GRE	Prescribe a 3–4 mm slice only for the joint	S-I
Coronal PD fat sat	Prescribe 3 mm coronal slices from axial GRE and sagittal localizer images	A-P
Coronal T1	Copy from coronal PD fat sat	A-P
Sagittal PD fat sat	Prescribe from coronal and axial images, perpendicular to the joint	R-L
Additions		
Axial PD fat sat	This sequence can be prescribed for trauma patients	S-I
Coronal STIR	Prescribe this sequence for trauma patient and/or fat sat issues	A-P
Sagittal PD and T2	Prescribe this sequence for instead of PD fat sat if there are fat sat issues	R-L
Sagittal GRE	Prescribe this sequence for bone lesions or cartilage defects	R-L
Axial T1	Prescribe this sequence for trauma patients	S-I

communicating frequently to make them as comfortable as possible in the MR bore (Fig. 8.13).

Sample Imaging Protocols

A sample imaging protocol for elbow scan is given in Table 8.5.

Sample Imaging Parameters for 1.5 T

Elbow imaging parameters can differ depending on the coil availability or selection. An eight channel small diameter coil (e.g., knee) and flexible coil optimized imaging parameters are given in Tables 8.6 and 8.7, respectively.

Graphical Prescription

See Figs. 8.14–8.16

Table 8.6 A sample routine elbow imaging parameter is given for a multichannel coil.

	T2*	PD fat sat	T1	PD fat sat	T2*	STIR	PD fat sat	T1
Plane	Axial	Coronal	Coronal	Sagittal	Sagittal	Coronal	Axial	Axial
Sequence type	MERGE	FSE-XL	FSE	FSE	MERGE	FSE-IR	FSE	FSE
TE	MinFull	40	MinFull	35	MinFull	42	40	MinFull
TR	400	2,480	580	2,920	490	4,000	2,480	740
ETL	3	12	3	12	3	12	9	2
BW	31.25	20.83	31.25	20.83	31.25	20.83	20.83	41.67
Slice thickness	4	3	3	4	4	3	4	4
Slice spacing	0.5	0.5	0.5	0.5	0.5	0.5	0.5	0.5
FOV	15	16	16	16	16	16	15	15
Matrix	288 × 192	256 × 224	352 × 224	288 × 224	288 × 192	224 × 224	288 × 256	352 × 224
NEX/NSA	2	4	2	4	2	2	3	2
Freq direction	R-L	R-L	R-L	A-P	A-P	R-L	R-L	R-L
SAT band/zip		SI/Zip512		S-I		Zip512	S-I	S-I
TI/FA	25				25	TI:145		

Table 8.7 A sample routine elbow imaging parameters is given for a flexible coil.

	T2*	PD fat sat	T1	PD fat sat	T2*	T2	PD fat sat	T1
Plane	Axial	Coronal	Coronal	Sagittal	Sagittal	Coronal	Axial	Axial
Sequence type	MERGE	FSE-XL	FSE	FSE	MERGE	FRFSE	FSE	FSE
TE	MinFull	37	MinFull	37	MinFull	85	40	MinFull
TR	400	2,420	440	2,500	490	3,620	2,600	740
ETL	3	9	3	10	3	18	9	2
BW	31.25	17.86	13.89	20.83	31.25	20.83	15.63	41.67
Slice thickness	4.0	3.0	3.0	4.0	4.0	3.0	4.0	4.0
Slice spacing	0.5	0.5	0.5	0.5	0.5	0.5	0.5	0.5
FOV	15	15	15	16	16	15	15	15
Matrix	288 × 192	256 × 192	256 × 192	256 × 192	288 × 192	256 × 256	256 × 224	320 × 224
NEX/NSA	2	4	4	4	2	4	4	2
Freq direction	R-L	R-L	R-L	A-P	A-P	R-L	R-L	R-L
SAT band/zip		Z512	Z512			Z512		
TI/FA	25				25			

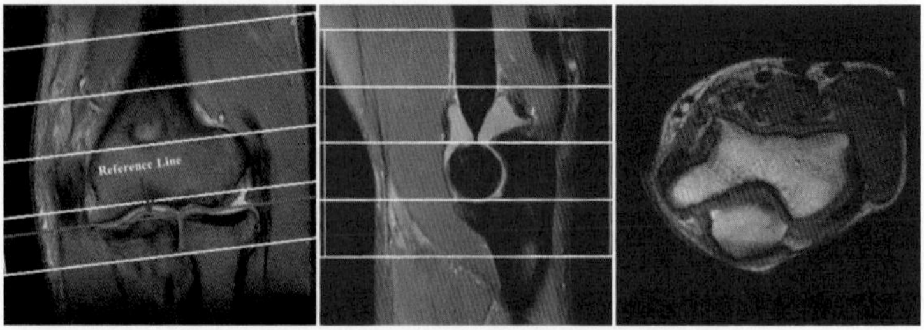

Figure 8.14 Axial planning from coronal and sagittal images is shown.

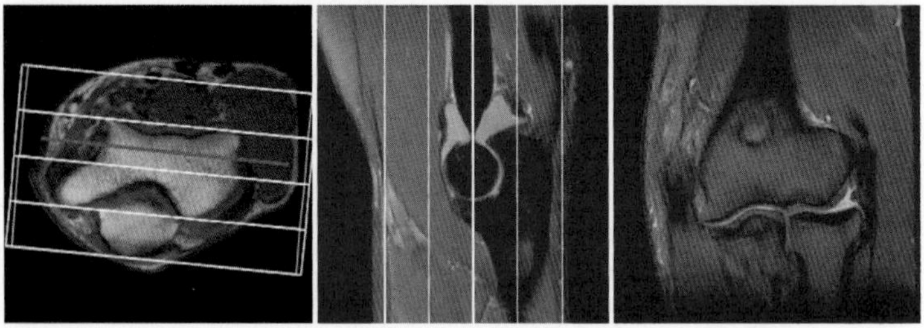

Figure 8.15 Oblique coronal prescription from axial and sagittal images is shown.

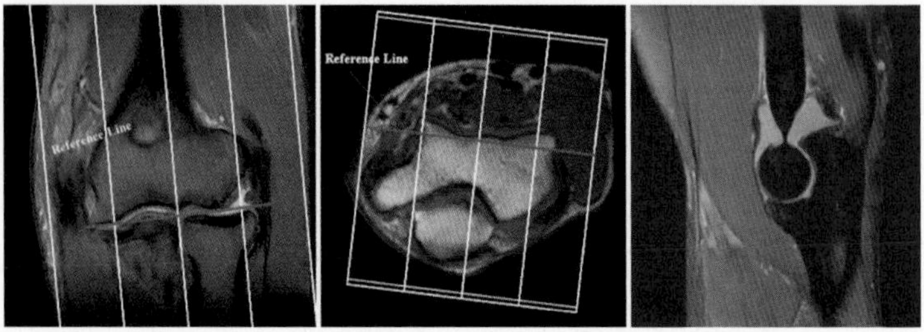

Figure 8.16 Oblique sagittal prescription from coronal and axial images is shown.

Wrist Imaging

Similar to elbow imaging, wrist imaging can be done with several different coils. If you have a dedicated multichannel wrist coil available at your site, you can put the patient feet first on supine position and let the arms at the side. Then you can place the wrist to be imaged in the coil. This is the most comfortable position for the patient. However, if you do not have any dedicated coils, you can use one of the smaller diameter coils such as knee or loop coils to scan the patient head first on prone position. This is also called superman position, but it is a *rather uncomfortable* position for the patient.

Patient Preparation: The patient consent form should be given to the patient with a detailed explanation on the content. The form should be filled and signed by the patient with the help of MR personnel. If there are any surgical implants, radiologist on duty has to make a decision based on implant type and MR compatibility. *If there is any suspicion or lack of information on the implant, do not take any risk with the patient safety and do not scan the patient.* If the form is complete with all the information, the patient should change to MR gown and remove any clothing with any metal. It is always a good practice to remove the jewelry as well. As the last line of patient safety, it is also a good practice to scan patient with a handheld metal detectors before taking the patient to MR room.

Patient Positioning: If you do have a dedicated wrist coil, you can place and fix the coil on the table. Then, you can position the patient supine, feet first (preferred) or head first.

In this position, the coil can be placed straight and patient wrist is centered in the middle of the coil as shown in Figs. 8.17 and 8.18. This is the most comfortable position. However, if you need to choose superman position for clinical needs or coil availability, the patient is positioned prone and head first. Then the arm is extended straight while the palm is pointing down. This position is quite uncomfortable for the patient and arm starts shaking after a short while uncontrollably.

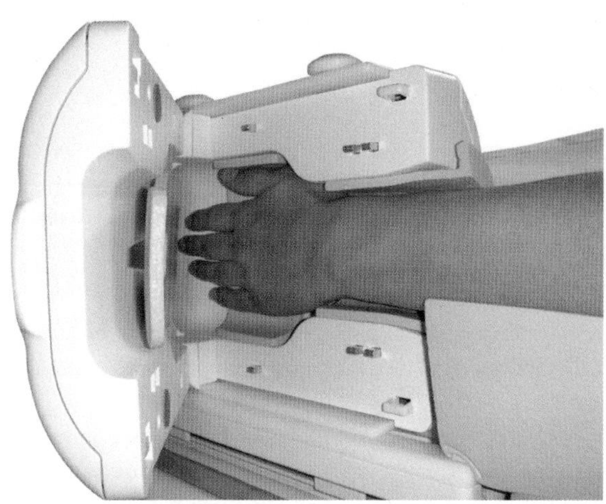

Figure 8.17 A sample of feet first and supine patient positioning for a dedicated multichannel wrist coil is shown. Please note that the coil stands vertical here and wrist is placed sideways in the middle of the coil.

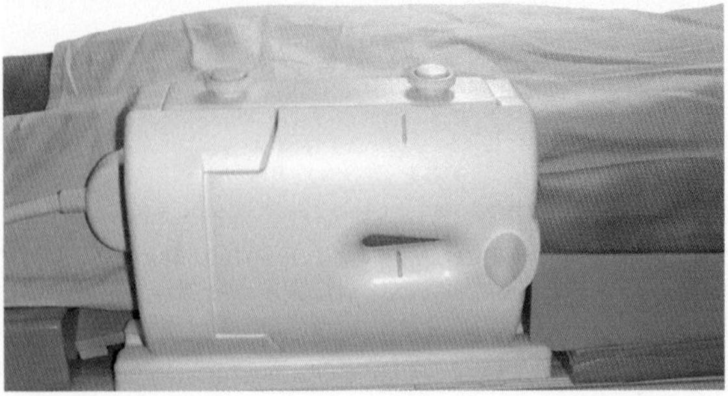

Figure 8.18 A sample of feet first and supine patient positioning for a dedicated multichannel wrist coil is shown. Please note that the coil stands vertical here and wrist is placed sideways in the middle of the coil.

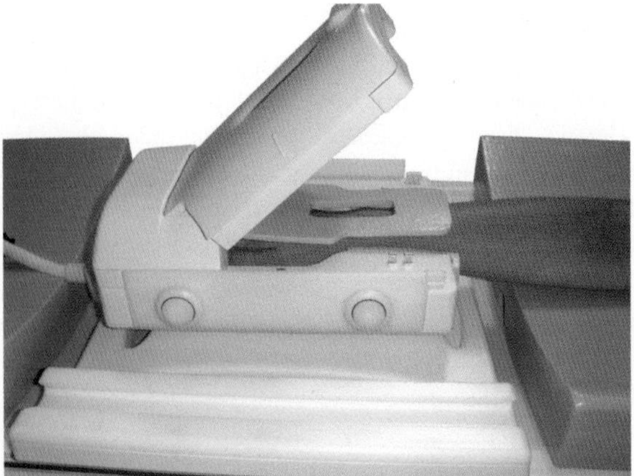

Figure 8.19 A sample head first and prone patient positioning for a dedicated, multichannel wrist coil is shown. Please note that the coil stands horizontal here and wrist is placed in the coil palm on the table.

Therefore, it is quite important to place pads under the patient arm and place a strap over the elbow level to increase patient comfort as well as image quality.

Please make sure that you give the patient alarm/buzzer to patient's hand and test it. After landmarking the center of coil using laser lights or touch sensors, you can send the patient in and start the exam. It is always recommended to let the patient know how long the scan is going to take and also keep communicating frequently to make them as comfortable as possible in the MR bore (Figs. 8.19–8.22).

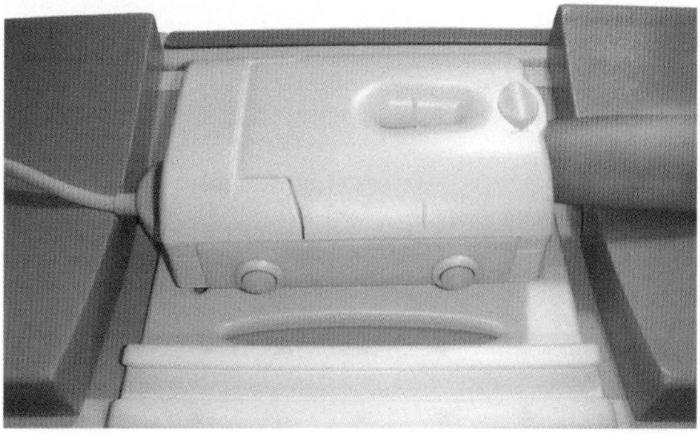

Figure 8.20 A sample head first and prone patient positioning for a dedicated, multichannel wrist coil is shown. Please note that the coil stands horizontal here and wrist is placed in the coil palm on the table.

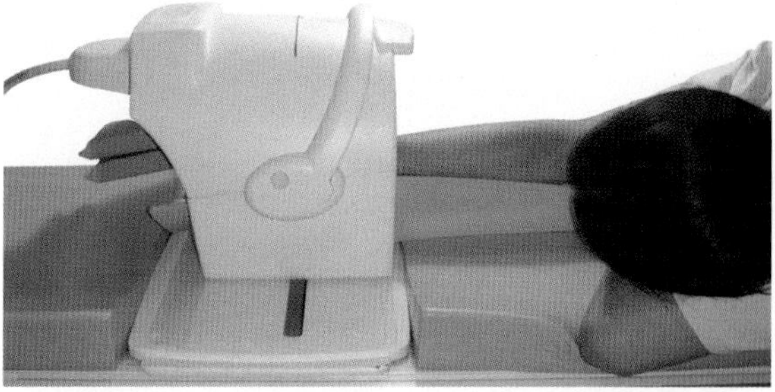

Figure 8.21 A sample head first and prone patient positioning for a multichannel knee coil is shown.

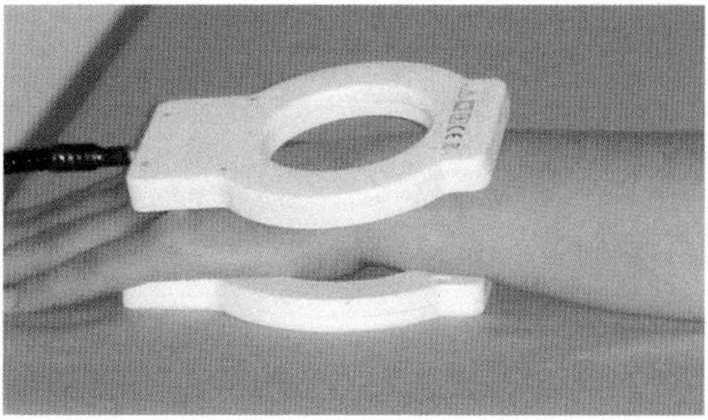

Figure 8.22 A sample head first and prone patient positioning for a dual loop coil (TMJ coil) is shown. Please note that the coil stands horizontal here and wrist is placed in the coil palm on the table.

Table 8.8 A routine wrist imaging protocol is given.

Sequences	Comments	Slice order
Three plane localizer	Acquire 5 slices in each plane	
Axial T1	Prescribe 3 mm slices only for the joint	S-I
Axial PD fat sat	Prescribe 3 mm slices only for the joint	S-I
Coronal PD fat sat	Prescribe 2–3 mm coronal slices from axial and sagittal images	A-P
Coronal T1	Prescribe 2–3 mm coronal slices from axial and sagittal images	A-P
Sagittal T2*GRE	Prescribe from coronal slices perpendicular to the joint	R-L
Additions		
Axial T2	Prescribe this sequence for instead of PD fat sat if there are fat sat issues	S-I
Coronal STIR	Prescribe this sequence for instead of PD fat sat if there are fat sat issues	A-P
Coronal 3DFiesta	Prescribe this sequence 1–2 mm thickness to better visualize triangular fibrocartilage complex (TFC)	A-P

Sample Imaging Protocols

A sample imaging protocol for a routine wrist scan is given in Table 8.8.

A sample imaging protocol for a patient referred to the MRI for a clinical wrist indication such as tumor, trauma, rheumatoid arthritis, or lesion scan is given in Table 8.9.

Sample Imaging Parameters for 1.5 T

Wrist imaging parameters can differ depending on the coil availability or selection. An eight channel dedicated wrist coil and dual loop coil optimized imaging parameters are given in Tables 8.10 and 8.11, respectively.

Tips and Tricks

Please note that the PD sequences in the protocols are hybrid weighted and parameters are different than standard PD. This sequence is applied to most of the MSK protocols in order to improve differential diagnosis and decrease the number of sequence in the protocols.

Table 8.9 A sample wrist imaging protocol for potential indications such as tumor, trauma, rheumatoid arthritis, or lesion is given.

Sequences	Comments	Slice order
Three plane localizer	Acquire 5 slices in each plane	
Axial T1	Prescribe 3 mm slices only for the joint	S-I
Axial STIR	Prescribe 3 mm slices only for the joint	S-I
Coronal STIR	Prescribe 2–3 mm coronal slices from axial images	A-P
Coronal PD fat sat	Prescribe 2–3 mm coronal slices from axial and sagittal images	A-P
Coronal T1		A-P
Sagittal T2*GRE or T2 FSE	Prescribe straight sagittal slices from coronal slices perpendicular to the axial and coronal planes	R-L
Sagittal PD fat sat	Same as sagittal slice prescription as above	R-L
Postcontrast	*Inject contrast agent if required*	
Axial T1 Fat sat	Same as axial slice prescription as above	S-I
Coronal T1 Fat sat	Same as coronal slice prescription as above	A-P
Sagittal T1 Fat sat	Same as sagittal slice prescription as above	R-L

Table 8.10 Part I: A sample routine wrist imaging parameter is given for a dedicated multichannel (eight channel wrist) coil.

	T1	T2	PD fat sat	T1	T2*GRE	PD fat sat	PD fat sat
Plane	Axial	Axial	Axial	Coronal	Coronal	Coronal	Sagittal
Sequence type	FSE	FRFSE	FSE	FSE	Merge	FSE-XL	FSE
TE	MinFull	125	42	MinFull	MinFull	40	37.5
TR	560	4,260	3,220	680	500	2,040	2,560
ETL	3	15	9	3	3	9	9
BW	20.83	31.2	17.86	20.8	31.2	17.86	17.86
Slice thickness	3.0	3.0	3.0	3.0	3.0	3.0	3.0
Slice spacing	0.5	0.5	0.5	0.3	0.3	0.3	0.5
FOV	9×9	9×9	9×9	9×9	9×9	9×9	9×9
Matrix	352×256	352×256	256×256	352×320	256×224	256×256	256×256
NEX/NSA	2	3	4	3	2	4	4
Freq direction	A-P	A-P	A-P	S-I	S-I	S-I	A-P
SAT band/ZIP	S-I	S-I	SI/Z512	S-I	SI/Z512	SI/Z512	SI/Z512
TI/FA					20		

Table 8.11 Part II: A sample routine wrist imaging parameter is given for a dedicated multichannel (eight channel wrist) coil.

	T1FS	STIR	3DT1FS	STIR	T2*GRE	3D Fiesta	T1
Plane	Axial	Axial	Coronal	Coronal	Sagittal	Coronal	Sagittal
Sequence type	FSE	FSE-IR	SPGR	FSE-IR	Merge	Fiesta	FSE
TE	MinFull	35	MinFull	34	MinFull	Min	MinFull
TR	880	4,000	Auto	4,000	500	Auto	560
ETL	3	10		10	3	–	3
BW	20.83	12.5	31.2	12.5	31.2	62.5	25
Slice thickness	4	4	1.4	3	3	1.0	3
Slice spacing	0.4	0.4	−0.7	0.3	0.3	−0.5	0.3
FOV	12	12	12	9	9	9	9
Matrix	320 × 224	256 × 160	256 × 256	256 × 160	256 × 224	320 × 320	352 × 288
NEX/NSA	2	4	2	4	2	4	4
Freq direction	A-P	R-L	S-I	S-I	S-I	S-I	A-P
SAT band/ZIP		Zip512	Zip2	Z512	SI/Z512	Zip2	
TI/FA		TI:145		TI:150	20	65	

Hybrid PD Sequence: For MSK imaging PD weighted protocols in this book, you will notice that the parameters are slightly different. Usually tissues like disk, labrum, cartilage, and fluid are isointense in standard PD weighted images and hypointense in T2 weighted images (when TE is longer than 50 ms). Therefore, for better differential diagnosis, additional sequences are generally required. However, longer TE provides better signal differences in pathologic changes such as edema (in traumatic cases), tears, cartilage damage, or other tumoral developments but doesn't help to differentiate the superficial cartilage and bone. The hybrid sequence has intermediate contrast weighting and provides better differentiation for bone-normal and abnormal cartilage tissues and fluid. To provide this weighting, we usually recommend slightly longer TE (around 35–40 ms) and ETL (8–9) for PD sequences in this book to create somewhat a hybrid PD contrast with additional T2 weighting. As a result, fluid, abnormal cartilage, and pathological structures appear hyperintense while normal cartilage remains isointense. This type of sequence provides better contrast between soft tissue (e.g., cartilage, disk, labrum) and fluid.

Graphical Prescription

See Figs. 8.23–8.25

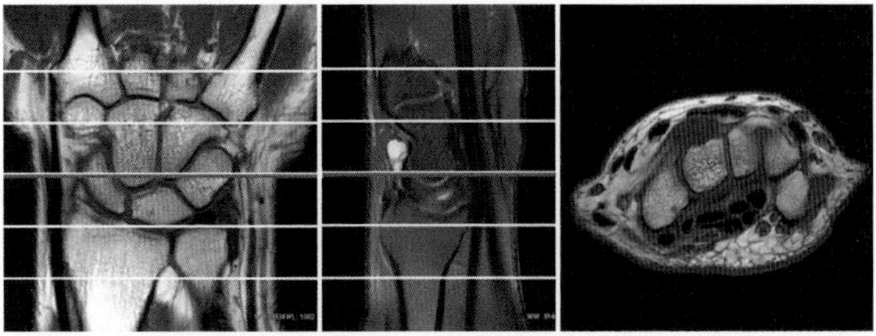

Figure 8.23 Axial planning from coronal and sagittal images is shown.

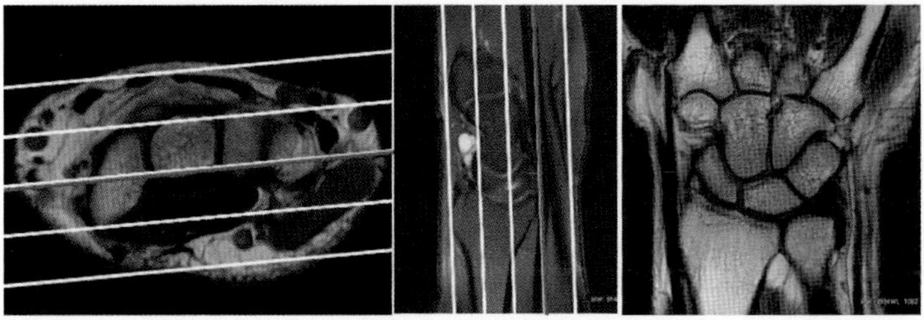

Figure 8.24 Oblique coronal prescription from axial and sagittal images is shown.

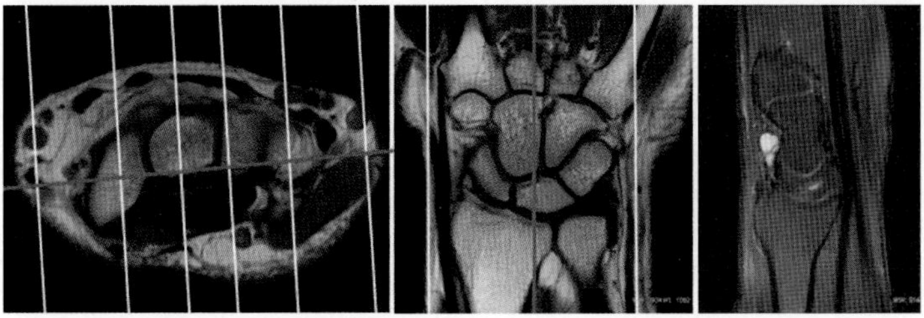

Figure 8.25 Oblique sagittal prescription from axial and coronal images is shown.

Hip Imaging

Bidirectional (anterior-posterior) multichannel coils are usually used for hip MRI. Depending on the vendor, the coil availability may vary for hip scanning. You should choose the most appropriate coil in case of multiple coil availability. It is also a common practice to use a cardiac coil for hip scanning whenever

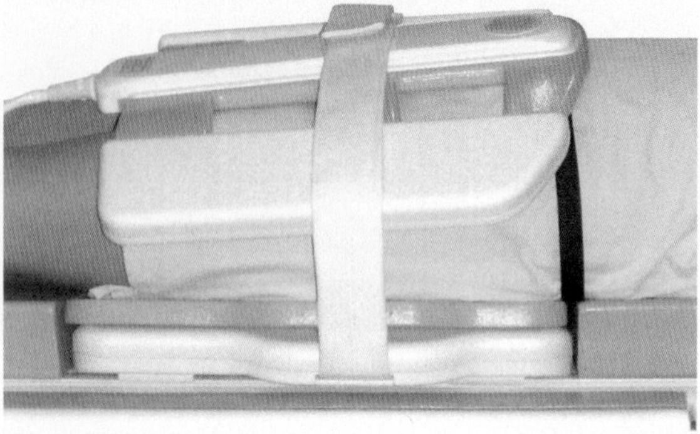

Figure 8.26 A sample for feet first and supine patient positioning in a multichannel cardiac coil is shown. The dark line (black belt) marks the iliac crest.

it is possible. The cardiac coils usually have smaller size and smaller multiple coil elements; therefore, they may provide higher signal than a regular multichannel coil.

Patient Preparation: The patient consent form should be given to the patient with a detailed explanation on the content. The form should be filled and signed by the patient with the help of MR personnel. If there are any surgical implants, radiologist on duty has to make a decision based on implant type and MR compatibility. The official confirmation of radiologist in the form is usually required. *If there is any suspicion or lack of information on the implant, do not take any risk with the patient safety and do not scan the patient.* If the form is complete with all the information, the patient should change to MR gown and remove any clothing with any metal. It is always a good practice to remove the jewelers as well. As the last line of patient safety, it is also a good practice to scan patient with a handheld metal detector before taking the patient to MR room. Finally, have the patient go to the restroom before the exam.

Patient Positioning: Place the coil straight at the center of the MR table. To reduce the breathing artifacts, the coil top should align with iliac crest (superior border of ilium wings) as shown with the dark line in Fig. 8.26. In other words, the abdomen should be left outside the coil coverage as shown in Figs. 8.26 and 8.27. After handling the patient alarm to patient and testing it, you are ready to start the exam.

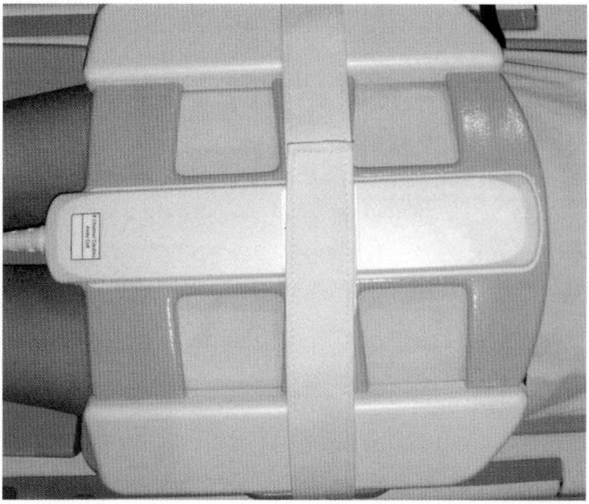

Figure 8.27 A sample for feet first and supine patient positioning in a multichannel cardiac coil is shown. The dark line (black belt) on Fig. 8.25 marks the iliac crest.

Please make sure that you give the patient alarm bell and test it before sending in. After landmarking the center of coil using laser lights or touch sensors, you can send the patient in and start the exam. It is always recommended to let the patient know how long the scan is going to take and also keep communicating frequently to make them as comfortable as possible in the MR bore.

Sample Imaging Protocols

A sample imaging protocol for a patient referred to the MRI for hip scan is given in Tables 8.12 and 8.13.

Sample Imaging Parameters for 1.5 T

See Table 8.14

Graphical Prescription

See Figs. 8.28–8.31

Table 8.12 A routine hip imaging protocol is given.

Sequences	Comments	Slice order
Three plane localizer	Acquire 5 slices in each plane	
Axial T1	Prescribe 3–4 mm slices only for the joint	S-I
Axial PD and T2 fat sat	Prescribe 3–4 mm slices only for the joint	S-I
Coronal PD fat sat	Prescribe 3–4 mm coronal slices from axial images	A-P
Coronal T1	Prescribe 3–4 mm coronal slices from axial images	A-P
Sagittal PD fat sat	Prescribe straight sagittal slices from coronal images	R-L
Additions		
Axial T2*GRE	Prescribe this fast sequence for avascular necrosis (AVN)	S-I
Coronal STIR	Prescribe this sequence for instead of PD fat sat if there are fat sat issues	A-P
Coronal PD fat sat	Prescribe this sequence as oblique coronal for labrum imaging	A-P

Table 8.13 A sample hip imaging protocol for potential indications such as tumor, trauma, rheumatoid arthritis, or infection diseases is given.

Sequences	Comments	Slice order
Three plane localizer	Acquire 5 slices in each plane	
Axial T1	Prescribe 4 mm slices only for the joint	S-I
Axial T2 fat sat	Prescribe 4 mm slices only for the joint	S-I
Coronal STIR	Prescribe 4 mm coronal slices from axial images	A-P
Coronal T1	Prescribe 4 mm coronal slices from axial images	A-P
Postcontrast	*Inject contrast agent if required*	
Axial T1 fat sat	Same as axial slice prescription as above	S-I
Coronal T1 Fat sat	Same as coronal slice prescription as above	A-P

Table 8.14 A sample routine hip imaging parameter is given for a multichannel coil.

	T1	PD andT2 fat sat	T1	PD fat sat	T2 fat sat	STIR	T1 fat sat	Labrum
Plane	Axial	Axial	Coronal	Coronal	Axial	Coronal	Axial	Oblique
Sequence	FSE	FRFSE	FSE	FRFSE	FRFSE	FSE	FSE	FSE
TE/TI	MinFull	40/80	MinFull	68	85	40/TI:145	MinFull	40
TR	720	4,000	560	3,420	4,520	4,300	620	2,840
ETL	3	12	3	19	20	12	3	14
BW	41.67	20.83	41.67	31	41.67	31	41.67	15.63
Slice thickness	4.0	4.0	4.0	4.0	5.0	5.0	4.0	4.0
Slice spacing	1.0	1.0	1.0	1.0	1.5	1.5	1.0	1.0
FOV	40	40	32	32	40	40	40	18
Matrix	416 × 352	352 × 256	416 × 352	320 × 256	416 × 352	320 × 224	320 × 256	256 × 256
NEX/NSA	3	2	2	4	3	3	3	4
Freq direction	R-L	R-L	S-I	S-I	R-L	S-I	R-L	S-I
Parallel imaging	ON	ON	OFF	OFF	ON	OFF	ON	OFF

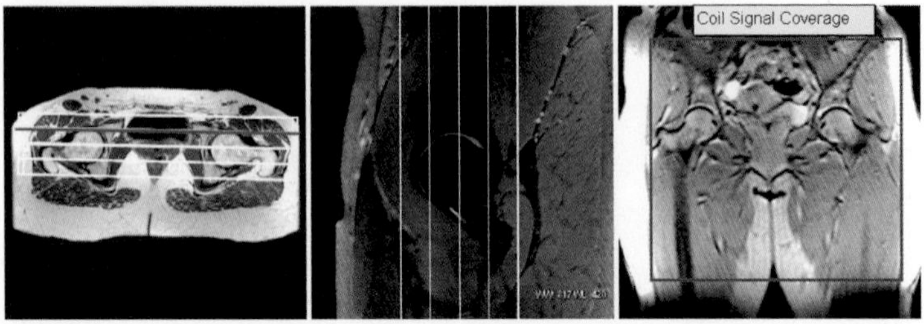

Figure 8.28 Coronal prescription from axial and sagittal images is shown.

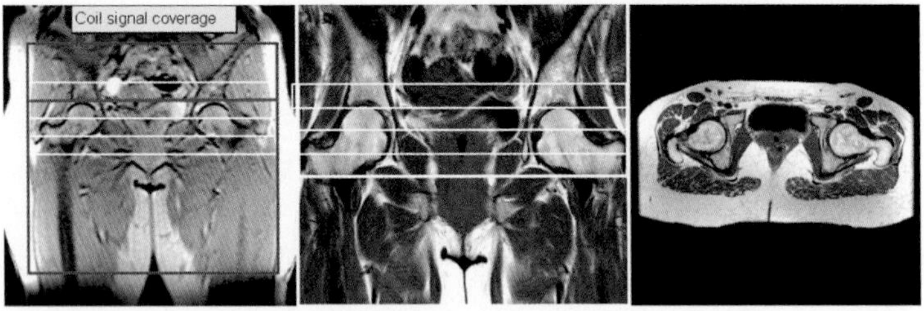

Figure 8.29 Axial planning from coronal images is shown.

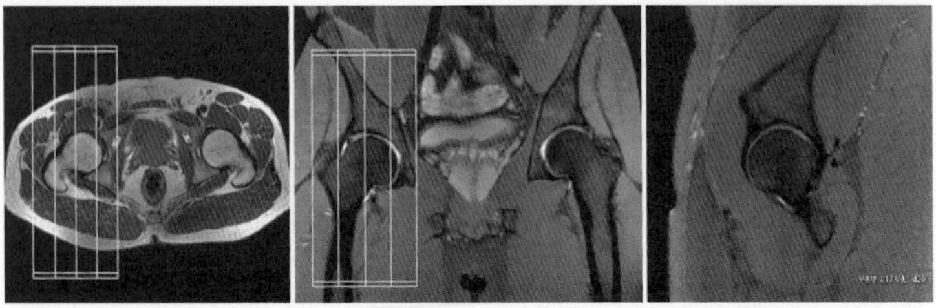

Figure 8.30 Sagittal prescription from axial and coronal images is shown.

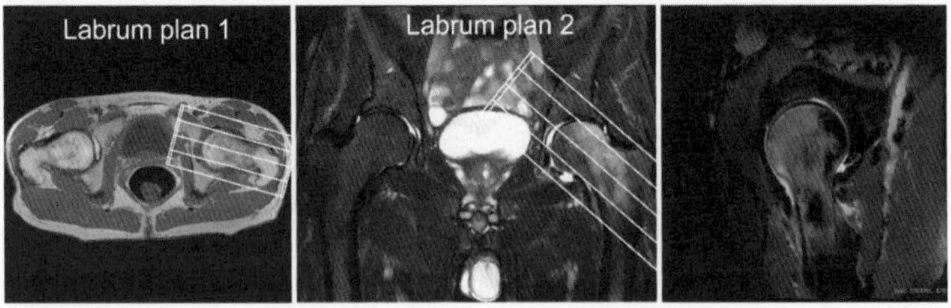

Figure 8.31 Labrum prescriptions from axial and coronal images are shown.

Knee Imaging

Knee joints are usually imaged unilaterally using dedicated coils. The knee and foot coils are usually what we call transmit/receive coils rather than receive only coils. Transmit/receive coils have the design features to be able to transmit the RF pulse directly from a transmitter element in the coil and receives the signal with receiver elements. This way, we can eliminate possible wrap around or aliasing artifacts from the other knee. Most of the MR systems use dedicated single channel (quadrature) transmit receive knee coils. However, most of the recent MR systems come with multichannel (8 or 16) dedicated transmit/receive knee and/or foot coils. The utilization of dedicated multichannel knee coils can make significant improvements in MR image SNR and can be used for either shorter scan time or increased spatial resolution. If you do not have a dedicated knee coil, it is possible to use other available coils. However, the image parameters should be modified to compensate for the SNR loss.

Patient Preparation: The patient consent form should be given to the patient with a detailed explanation on the content. The form should be filled and signed by the patient with the help of MR personnel. If there are any surgical implants, radiologist on duty has to make a decision based on implant type and MR compatibility. *If there is any suspicion or lack of information on the implant, do not take any risk with the patient safety and do not scan the patient.* If the form is complete with all the information, the patient should change to MR gown and remove any clothing with any metal. It is always a good practice to remove the jewelers as well. As the last line of patient safety, it is also a good practice to scan patient with a handheld metal detector before taking the patient to MR room. Finally, have the patient go to the restroom before the exam.

Patient Positioning: Place the knee coil straight at the center of the MR table. When you place the patient's knee in the coil, insert a small pad under the knee joint to slightly bend the knee (about 15°). The patella should be aligned with the center of the coil for good positioning. When the coil top is attached and locked, place additional pads between the knee and coil to further immobilize the knee. These pads can significantly reduce the motion artifacts. The other knee should be placed as further ways from the coil as possible to prevent any wrapping or aliasing, especially with receive-only coil.

Please make sure that you give the patient alarm bell to patient and ask them to test it before sending in. After landmarking the center of coil using laser lights or touch sensors, you can send the patient in and start the exam.

It is always recommended to let the patient know how long the scan is going to take and also keep communicating frequently to make them as comfortable as possible in the MR bore (Figs. 8.32–8.35).

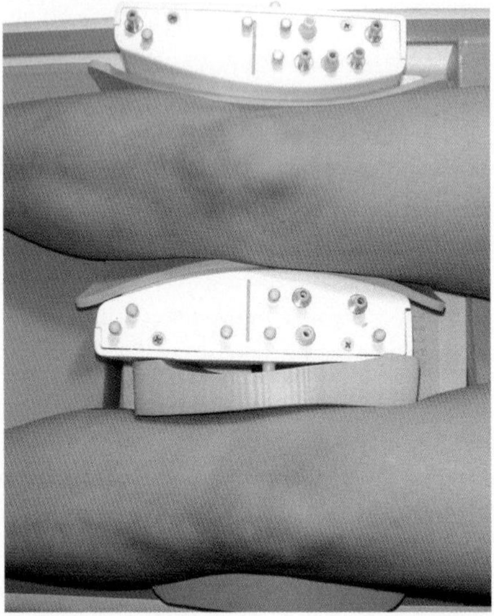

Figure 8.32 A sample for feet first and supine patient positioning in a multichannel transmit/receive knee coil is shown. Please note that this coil design includes a small pad under the knee joint.

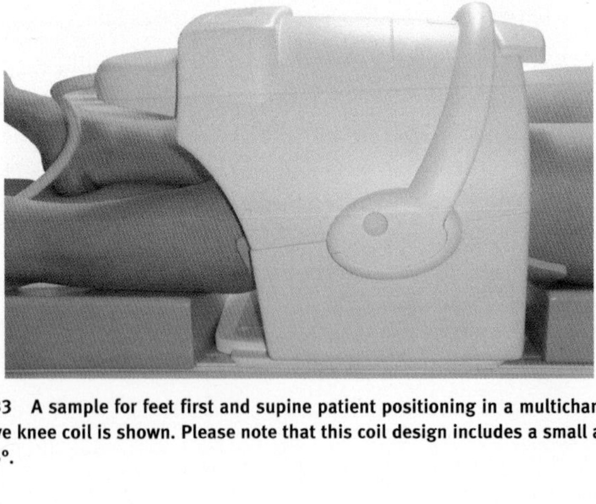

Figure 8.33 A sample for feet first and supine patient positioning in a multichannel transmit/receive knee coil is shown. Please note that this coil design includes a small angulation around 15°.

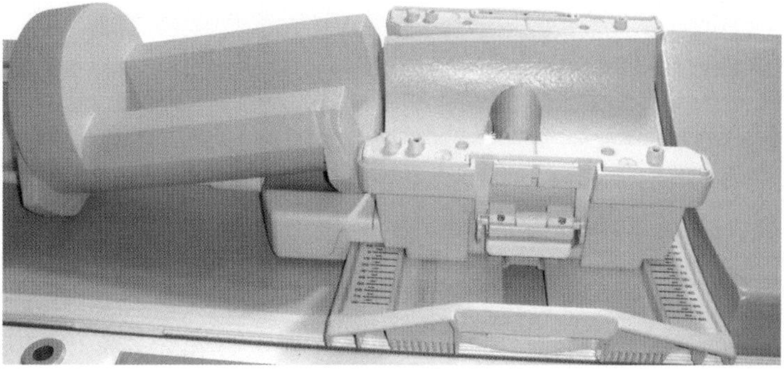

Figure 8.34 A sample single channel transmit/receive knee coil is shown.

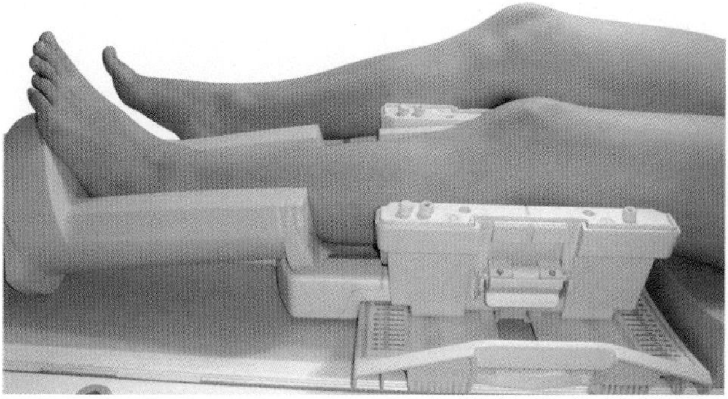

Figure 8.35 A sample feet first and supine patient positioning for a single channel transmit/ receive knee coil is shown.

Tips and Tricks

Please note that the single-channel (quadrature) knee coil shown in Fig. 8.34 has a flat design since it is also used for foot imaging. Therefore, we place the provided small gray pad in the center of coil underneath the knee joint. This pad roughly creates a 10–15° flexion of the knee in order to visualize the anterior cruciate ligament (ACL) better (Fig. 8.35).

Sample Imaging Protocols

A sample imaging protocol for a patient referred to the MRI for knee scan is given in Tables 8.15 and 8.16.

Table 8.15 A routine knee imaging protocol is given.

Sequences	Comments	Slice order
Three plane localizer	Acquire 5 slices in each plane by adding a lateral shift to routine scout image for the knee of interest if it is off center!	
Axial PD fat sat	Prescribe 3–4 mm slices only for the joint covering the patella	S-I
Coronal PD fat sat	Prescribe 3–4 mm coronal slices parallel to posterior horns of bilateral femoral condyles	A-P
Sagittal PD fat sat	Prescribe 3–4 mm sagittal slices perpendicular to coronal prescription (perpendicular to bilateral condyles)	R-L
Sagittal T1	Copy from previous sagittal	R-L
Additions		
Axial T2*GRE	Prescribe this sequence for potential AVN, bone lesions, trauma, and patellar chondromalacia	S-I
Coronal T2*GRE	Prescribe this sequence for potential AVN, bone lesions, trauma, and patella chondromalacia	A-P
Coronal STIR	Prescribe this sequence for instead of PD Fat Sat if there is fat sat issue	A-P
Coronal T1	Prescribe this sequence for trauma or bone lesions	A-P
Sagittal PD	Prescribe this sequence in case of fat sat issues	R-L

Tips and Tricks

Hybrid PD Sequence: For MSK imaging PD weighted protocols in this book, you will notice that the parameters are slightly different. Usually, tissues like disk, labrum, cartilage, and fluid are isointense in a standard PD weighted images and hypointense in T2 weighted images (when TE is longer than 50 ms). Therefore, for better differential diagnosis, additional sequences are generally required. However, longer TE provides better signal differences in pathologic changes such as edema (in traumatic cases), tears, cartilage damage, or other tumoral developments but doesn't help to differentiate the superficial cartilage and bone. The hybrid sequence has intermediate contrast weighting and provides better differentiation for bone-normal and abnormal cartilage tissues and fluid. To provide this weighting, we usually recommend

Table 8.16 A sample knee imaging protocol for potential indications such as tumor, trauma, rheumatoid arthritis, or bone lesion is given.

Sequences	Comments	Slice order
Three plane localizer	Acquire 5 slices in each plane by adding a lateral shift to routine scout image for the knee of interest if it is off center!	
Axial PD fat sat	Prescribe 3–4 mm slices only for the joint covering the patella	S-I
Axial T1 Fat sat	Prescribe 3–4 mm slices only for the joint covering the patella	S-I
Coronal STIR	Prescribe 3–4 mm coronal slices parallel to posterior horns of bilateral femoral condyles	A-P
Sagittal T2	Prescribe 3–4 mm sagittal slices perpendicular to coronal prescription (perpendicular to bilateral condyles)	R-L
Sagittal T1	Copy from previous sagittal	R-L
Postcontrast	*Inject contrast agent if required*	
Axial T1 Fat sat	Prescribe 3–4 mm slices only for the joint covering the patella	S-I
Coronal T1 Fat sat	Copy from previous coronal	A-P
Sagittal T1	Copy from previous sagittal	R-L

slightly longer TE (around 35–40 ms) and ETL (8–9) for PD sequences in this book to create somewhat a hybrid PD contrast with additional T2 weighting. As a result, fluid, abnormal cartilage, and pathological structures appear hyperintense while normal cartilage remains isointense. This type of sequence provides better contrast between soft tissue (e.g., cartilage, disk, and labrum) and fluid.

Sample Imaging Parameters for 1.5 and 3.0 T

See Tables 8.17 and 8.18

Graphical Prescription

See Figs. 8.36–8.38

Table 8.17 A sample routine knee imaging parametersis given for a multichannel coil at 1.5 T.

	PD fat sat	PD fat sat	PD fat sat	T1	T2*GRE	T2	PD
Plane	Axial	Coronal	Sagittal	Sagittal	Coronal	Sagittal	Sagittal
Sequence type	FSE	FSE	FSE	FSE	Merge	FRFSE	FSE
TE	42	42	42	MinFull	MinFull	102	MinFull
TR	2,880	2,420	3,180	560	500	4,340	2,940
ETL	9	9	9	3	3	15	7
BW	25.00	20.83	20.83	20.83	31.2	20.83	62.5
Slice thickness	4	4	4	4	4	4	4
Slice spacing	1	1	1	1	1	1	1
FOV	16	16	15	15	16	16	16
Matrix	352 × 256	320 × 256	320 × 256	384 × 320	288 × 224	384 × 320	352 × 320
NEX/NSA	4	3	3	2	2	2	2
Freq direction	A-P	S-I	A-P	A-P	S-I	A-P	A-P
SAT band/ZIP							
TI/b value/FA					20		

Table 8.18 A sample routine knee imaging parameter is given for a multichannel coil at 3.0 T.

	PD fat sat	PD fat sat	PD fat sat	PD	T2	STIR	T1 fat sat
Plane	Axial	Coronal	Sagittal	Sagittal	Sagittal	Coronal	Axial
Sequence type	FRFSE	FRFSE	FRFSE	FRFSE	FRFSE	FSE-IR	FSE
TE	40	32	30	25	125	42	MinFull
TR	2,300	2,260	2,260	2,260	5,920	3,000	725
ETL	5	5	5	5	25	12	3
BW	31.2	31.2	31.2	41.7	41.7	41.7	31.2
Slice thickness	3	3	3	3	4	3	2
Slice spacing	1	1	1	1	1	0.3	0.2
FOV	16	16	16	16	24	16	16
Matrix	448 × 256	384 × 256	384 × 256	512 × 288	384 × 256	288 × 224	288 × 256
NEX/NSA	2	2	2	2	4	2	2
Freq direction	A-P	S-I	A-P	A-P	S-I	S-I	A-P
SAT band							
TI/b value/FA						150	

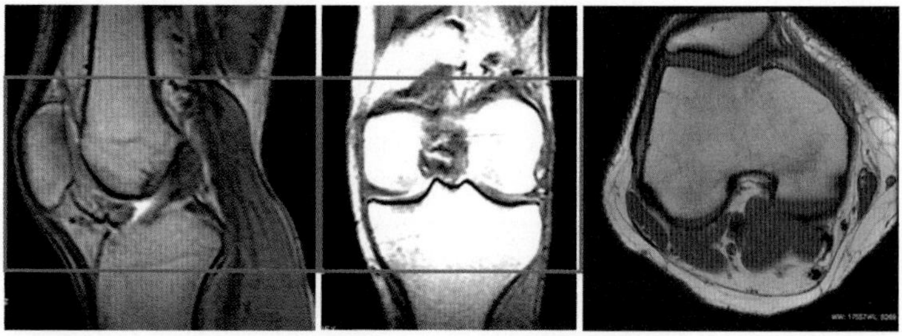

Figure 8.36 Axial planning from sagittal and coronal images is shown.

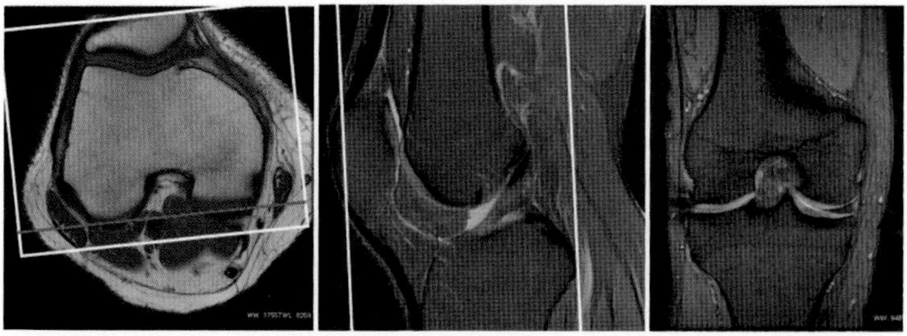

Figure 8.37 Coronal prescription from axial and sagittal images is shown.

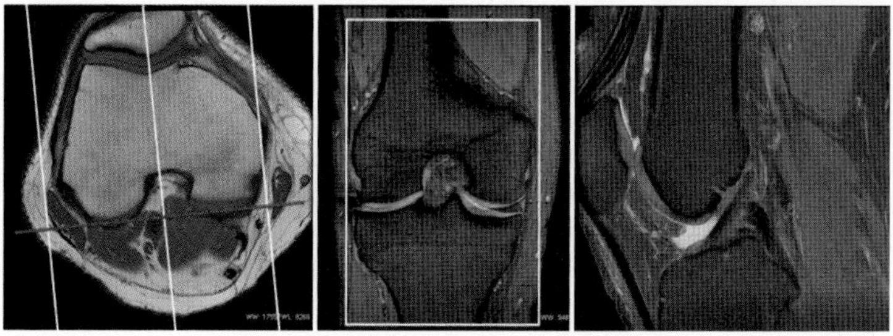

Figure 8.38 Sagittal prescription from axial and coronal images is shown.

Ankle Imaging

Ankle is usually imaged unilaterally using dedicated coils. The ankle coils can be either transmit/receive or receive-only coils. The utilization of dedicated multichannel ankle/foot coils can make significant improvements in SNR, which can be used for either shorter scan time or increased spatial resolution. If you do not have a dedicated coil, it is possible to use other available coils. However, the image parameters should be modified to compensate for the SNR loss. To prevent fat saturation issues, the ankle or more specifically tarsal sinus should be centered in the coil and FOV.

Patient Preparation: The patient consent form should be given to the patient with a detailed explanation on the content. The form should be filled and signed by the patient and MR personnel. If there are any surgical implants, radiologist on duty has to make a decision based on implant type and MR compatibility. *If there is any suspicion or lack of information on the implant, do not take any risk with the patient safety and do not scan the patient*. If the form is complete with all the information, the patient should change to MR gown and remove any clothing with any metal. It is always a good practice to remove the jewelers as well. As the last line of patient safety, it is also a good practice to scan patient with a handheld metal detector before taking the patient to MR room.

Patient Positioning: Place the ankle coil straight at the center of the MR table. When you place the patient's ankle in the coil, you can use patient support pads to immobilize the foot and keep it straight during the scan. The ankle-specific pads can significantly reduce the motion artifacts. The other foot should be placed as further away from the coil as possible to prevent any wrapping or aliasing, especially with receive-only coils.

Please make sure that you give the patient alarm bell to patient and ask to test it before sending patient in. After landmarking the center of coil using laser lights or touch sensors, you can send the patient in and start the exam. It is always recommended to let the patient know how long the scan is going to take and also keep communicating frequently to make them as comfortable as possible in the MR bore (Figs. 8.39 and 8.40).

Sample Imaging Protocols

A sample protocol for a patient referred to the MRI for ankle scan is given in Tables 8.19 and 8.20.

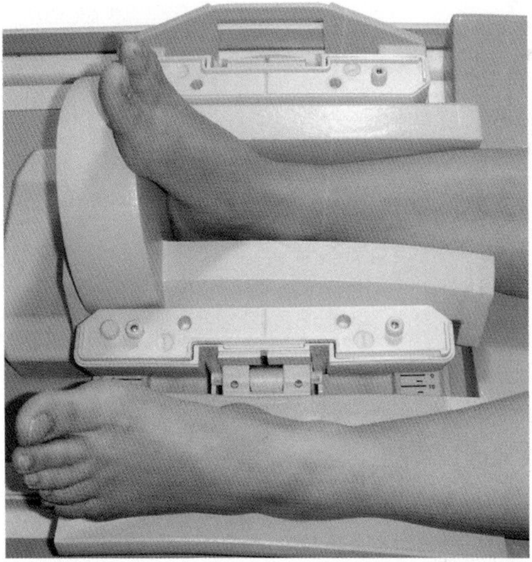

Figure 8.39 A sample feet first and supine patient positioning for a single channel transmit/receive ankle coil is shown.

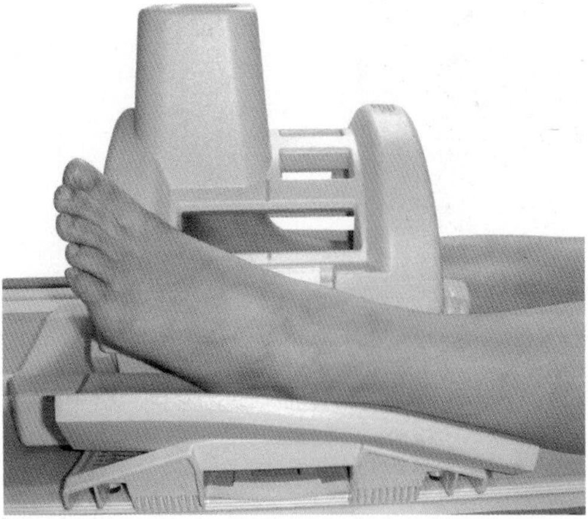

Figure 8.40 A sample feet first and supine patient positioning for a single channel transmit/receive ankle coil is shown.

Table 8.19 A routine ankle imaging protocol is given.

Sequences	Comments	Slice order
Three plane localizer	Acquire 5 slices in each plane by adding a lateral shift	
Sagittal PD fat sat (hybrid)	Prescribe 3–4 mm sagittal slices perpendicular to tibiotalar joint (superior facet) in coronal plane and parallel to foot floor in axial plane. Center of the FOV should be placed at tarsal sinus	R-L
Sagittal T1	Same as sagittal PD fat sat	R-L
Axial PD fat sat (hybrid)	Prescribe 3–4 mm slices only for the joint either straight or parallel to posterior talar articular surface	S-I
Axial T1	Same as axial PD fat sat	S-I
Coronal T2*GRE	Prescribe perpendicular to superior facet surface	A-P
Additions		
Sagittal STIR	Prescribe this sequence for instead of PD fat sat if there are fat sat issues	R-L
Sagittal PD and T2	Prescribe this sequence in case of fat sat issues	R-L
Sagittal T2* GRE	Prescribe this sequence for potential AVN, bone lesions, and trauma	R-L
Coronal PD fat sat (hybrid)	Prescribe this sequence instead of GRE	A-P
Coronal T1	Prescribe this sequence for trauma or bone lesions	A-P

Table 8.20 A sample ankle imaging protocol for potential indications such as tumor, trauma, rheumatoid arthritis, or bone lesion is given.

Sequences	Comments	Slice order
Three plane localizer	Acquire 5 slices in each plane by adding a lateral shift	
Sagittal T1	Prescribe 3–4 mm sagittal slices perpendicular to tibiotalar joint in coronal plane and parallel to foot floor in axial plane. Center of the FOV should be placed at tarsal sinus	R-L
Sagittal STIR	Copy from previous sagittal	R-L
Axial PD fat sat	Prescribe 3–4 mm slices only for the joint either straight or parallel to posterior talar articular surface	S-I
Axial T1 fat sat	Same as axial PD fat sat	S-I
Coronal STIR	Prescribe 3–4 mm slices perpendicular to superior facet joint	A-P
Postcontrast	*Inject contrast agent if required*	
Axial T1 Fat sat	Copy from previous axial	S-I
Coronal T1 Fat sat	Copy from previous coronal	A-P
Sagittal T1	Copy from previous sagittal	R-L

Table 8.21 A sample routine ankle imaging parameters is given for a quadrature coil at 1.5 T.

	T1	STIR	PD fat sat	PD fat sat	T1	T2	T2*GRE
Plane	Sagittal	Sagittal	Sagittal	Axial	Axial	Axial	Coronal
Sequence type	SE	FSE	FSE	FSE	FSE	FSE	GRE
TE	MinFull	35	44	37.6	MinFull	85	13
TR	500	3,900	2,220	3,100	640	3,220	520
ETL		12	9	10	3	18	
BW	15.6	41.67	25	20.8	20.8	31.25	10.4
Slice thickness	4.0	4.0	4.0	4.0	4.0	4.0	4.0
Slice spacing	0.5	0.5	0.5	0.5	0.5	0.5	0.5
FOV	16	16	16	16	16	16	16
Matrix	384 × 320	256 × 256	320 × 224	288 × 224	512 × 320	352 × 320	384 × 256
NEX/NSA	1.5	4	2	2	2	3	2
Freq direction	S-I	S-I	S-I	A-P	A-P	A-P	S-I
SAT band/zip		Zip512					
TI/FA		145					25

Sample Imaging Parameters for 1.5 T

See Table 8.21

Sample Imaging Parameters for 3.0 T

See Table 8.22

Graphical Prescription

See Figs. 8.41–8.44

Table 8.22 A sample routine ankle imaging parameter is given for a quadrature coil at 3.0 T.

	T1	PD fat sat	PD fat sat	T1	T2	T2*GRE	STIR
Plane	Sagittal	Sagittal	Axial	Axial	Axial	Coronal	Coronal
Sequence type	FSE	FSE	FSE	FSE	FSE	GRE	FSE
TE	MinFull	35	30	MinFull	85	MinFull	120
TR	525	2,400	3,100	650	5,050	450	5,700
ETL	3	7	8	3	16		12
BW	31.25	31.25	31.25	41.67	41.67	15.63	25.0
Slice thickness	3.0	3.0	3.0	3.0	3.0	3.0	3.0
Slice spacing	1.0	1.0	1.0	1.0	1.0	1.0	1.0
FOV	15	15	15	15	15	16	16
Matrix	512 × 256	384 × 288	384 × 256	512 × 320	352 × 352	512 × 256	320 × 224
NEX/NSA	2	2	2	1	2	2	2
Freq direction	S-I	S-I	A-P	A-P	A-P	S-I	S-I
TI/FA						FA:20	TI:180

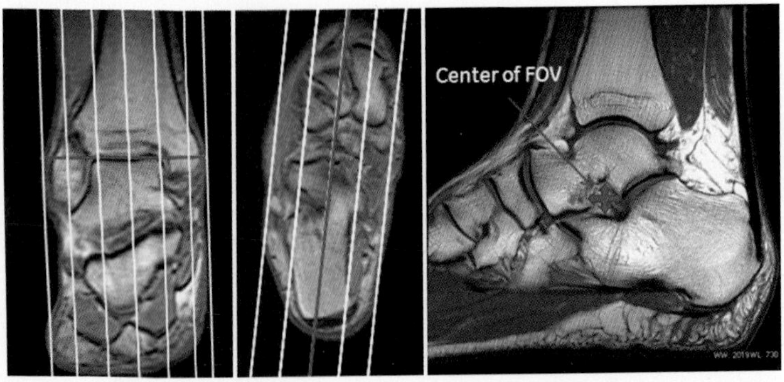

Figure 8.41 Sagittal prescription from coronal and axial images is shown.

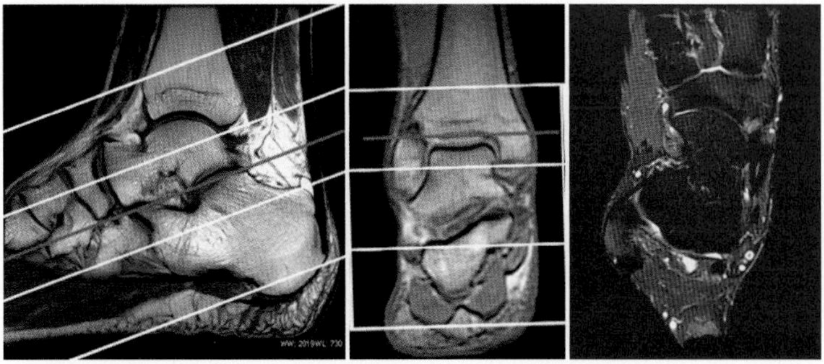

Figure 8.42 Oblique axial planning from sagittal and coronal images is shown.

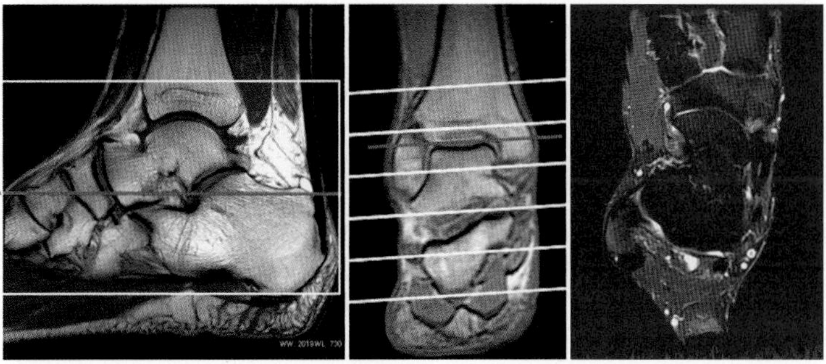

Figure 8.43 Straight axial planning from sagittal and coronal images is shown.

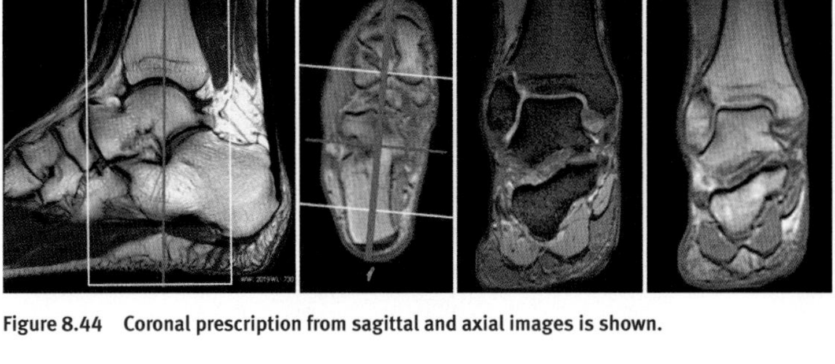

Figure 8.44 Coronal prescription from sagittal and axial images is shown.

Forefoot Imaging (Morton's Neuroma)

Forefoot is usually imaged unilaterally using dedicated coils. The coils can be either transmit/receive or receive-only coils. If you do not have a dedicated coil, it is possible to use other available coils. However, the image parameters should be modified to compensate for the SNR loss. A proper patient positioning and graphical prescription is necessary for an efficient fat sat. Otherwise, the image quality might suffer from improper fat saturation. The anatomy of interest should be centered in the coil and selected FOV should not be larger than anatomy of interest. Forefoot imaging can be performed usually for Morton's neuroma, which is a benign neuroma of intermetatarsal plantar nerve.

Patient Preparation: The patient consent form should be given to the patient with a detailed explanation on the content. The form should be carefully read, all questions must be answered with clear answers such as "YES" or "NO," and additional clarifications should be written. It must be signed by the patient or legal guardians and confirmed by MR personnel. If there are any surgical implants, radiologist on duty has to make a decision based on implant type and MR compatibility. *If there is any suspicion or lack of information on the implant, do not take any risk with the patient safety and do not scan the patient*. If the form is complete with all the information, the patient should change to MR gown and remove any clothing with any metal. It is always a good practice to remove the jewelry as well. As the last line of patient safety, it is also a good practice to scan patient with a handheld metal detector before taking the patient to MRI room.

Patient Positioning: Place the coil straight at the center of the MR table. When you place the patient's foot in the coil, you can use patient support pads to immobilize the foot and to properly position the forefoot in the coil. When the coil top is attached and locked, additional pads should be placed between the coil anterior and foot. The other foot should be placed as further away from the coil as possible to prevent any wrapping or aliasing, especially with receive-only coils.

Please make sure that you give the patient alarm bell and test it. After landmarking the center of coil using laser lights or touch sensors, you can send the patient in and start the exam. It is always recommended to let the patient know how long the scan is going to take and also keep communicating frequently to make them as comfortable as possible in the MR bore (Figs. 8.45–8.47).

Sample Imaging Protocols

A sample imaging protocol for a patient referred to the MRI for a forefoot scan is given in Table 8.23.

Note: Please have a look at the parameters of PD Fat sat (Hybrid).

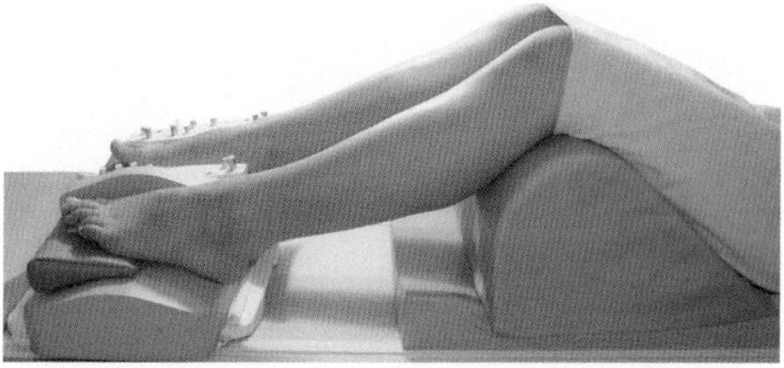

Figure 8.45 A sample feet first and supine patient forefoot positioning for a multichannel transmit/receive coil is shown.

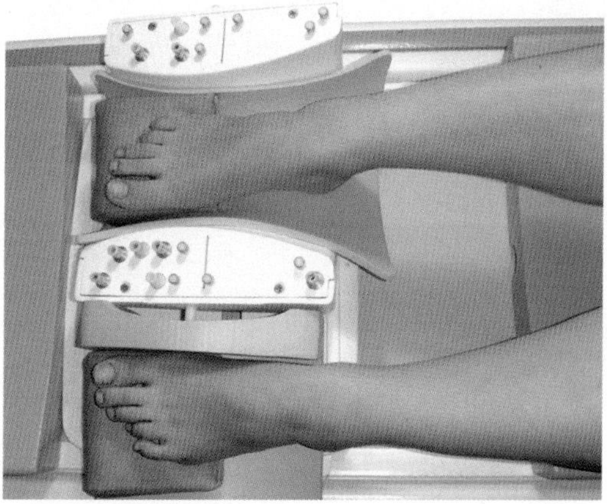

Figure 8.46 A sample feet first and supine patient forefoot positioning for a multichannel transmit/receive coil is shown.

Sample Imaging Parameters for 1.5 T

See Table 8.24

Sample Imaging Parameters for 3.0 T

See Table 8.25

Graphical Prescription

See Figs. 8.48–8.50

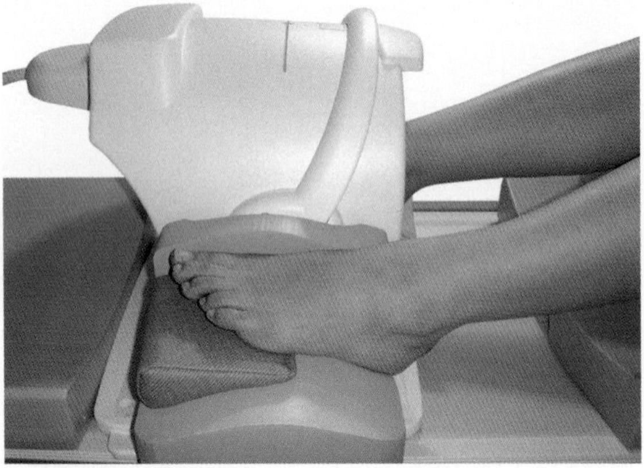

Figure 8.47 A sample feet first and supine patient forefoot positioning for a multichannel transmit/receive coil is shown.

Table 8.23 A routine ankle imaging protocol is given.

Sequences	Comments	Slice order
Three plane localizer	Acquire 5 slices in each plane	
Axial PD fat sat	Prescribe 3–4 mm slices only for the region of interest	S-I
Axial T1	Copy from previous axial (PD fat sat)	S-I
Coronal T2 fat sat	Prescribe 3–4 mm slices perpendicular to metatarsals	A-P
Coronal T1	Same as coronal T2 fat sat	A-P
Sagittal STIR	Prescribe 3–4 mm sagittal slices perpendicular to superior facet in coronal plane and parallel to foot floor in axial plan	R-L
Sagittal T1	Same as sagittal PD fat sat	R-L
Additions		
Coronal T2*GRE	Prescribe this sequence for trauma and bone fractures	A-P
Coronal STIR	Prescribe this sequence for instead of PD fat sat if there is fat sat issue	A-P
Coronal T1 FS	Prescribe this sequence for soft tissue tumors and infections. Can be repeated postcontrast	A-P
Postcontrast	Inject contrast agent if required	
Axial T1 Fat sat	Copy from previous axial	S-I
Coronal T1 Fat sat	Copy from previous coronal	A-P
Sagittal T1	Copy from previous sagittal	A-L

Table 8.24 A sample forefoot imaging parameter is given for a multichannel coil at 1.5 T.

	T1	STIR	PD fat sat	T1	T1	T2 Fat sat	T2*	T1 Fat sat
Plane	Sagittal	Sagittal	Axial	Axial	Coronal	Coronal	Coronal	Coronal
Sequence type	FSE	FSE-IR	FSE	FSE	FSE	FRFSE	GRE	FSE
TE	MinFull	35	40	MinFull	MinFull	85	MinFull	MinFull
TR	700	4,700	3,250	700	550	2,850	650	580
ETL	2	12	9	2	3	12		3
BW	41.67	20.83	31.25	31.25	31.25	20.83	11.90	31.25
Slice thickness	4.0	4.0	4.0	4.0	3.0	3.0	3.0	3.0
Slice spacing	0.5	0.5	0.5	0.5	0.5	0.5	0.5	0.5
FOV	16	16	14	14	14	14	14	14
Matrix	384 × 320	288 × 224	352 × 224	320 × 320	320 × 320	288 × 256	320 × 224	320 × 224
NEX/NSA	2	2	4	2	2	2	2	2
Freq direction	S-I	S-I	R-L	R-L	S-I	S-I	S-I	S-I
TI/FA		145					25	

Table 8.25 A sample forefoot imaging parameters is given for a multi-channel coil at 3.0 T.

	T1	T2 fat sat	T2 fat sat	T1	T1	T2 fat sat	STIR
Plane	Sagittal	Sagittal	Axial	Axial	Coronal	Coronal	Coronal
Sequence type	FSE	FRFSE	FRFSE	FSE	FSE	FRFSE	FSE-IR
TE	MinFull	85	85	MinFull	MinFull	85	120
TR	825	4,150	4,950	700	600	3,000	5,700
ETL	2	15	15	3	3	15	12
BW	62.5	31.25	31.25	62.5	62.5	31.25	25.0
Slice thickness	4	4	4	4	3	3	3
Slice spacing	0.5	0.5	0.5	0.5	0.5	0.5	0.5
FOV	18	18	18	18	18	18	18
Matrix	384 × 256	384 × 256	384 × 256	384 × 256	384 × 256	384 × 256	320 × 224
NEX/NSA	2	2	2	2	2	2	2
Freq direction	S-I	S-I	R-L	R-L	S-I	S-I	S-I
TI/b value/FA							180

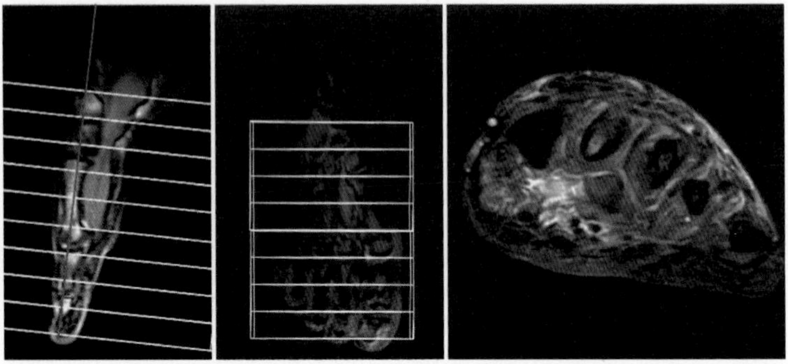

Figure 8.48 Oblique axial planning from sagittal and coronal images is shown.

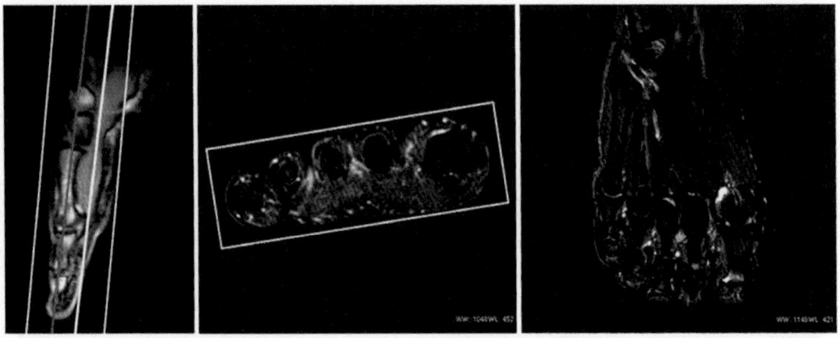

Figure 8.49 Coronal prescription from sagittal and axial images is shown.

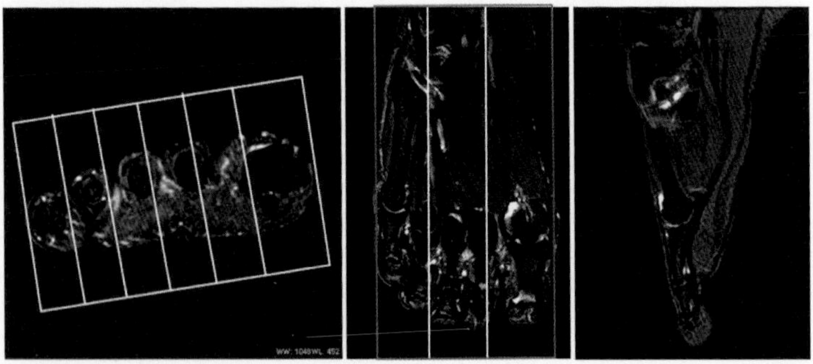

Figure 8.50 Sagittal prescription from axial and coronal images is shown.

Long Bones (Femur, Tibia, Cruris)

Long bones of the body can be imaged bilaterally using multichannel coils. For optimized image quality, it is important to select the best available coil for the region of interest. For example, cardiac coil may be a bit too small for bilateral imaging of femur for good coverage. Instead, a multichannel body/abdomen coil can be used. However, flex coils, knee coil, cardiac coil, etc. can be used to image a specific region of interest.

Patient Preparation: The patient consent form should be given to the patient with a detailed explanation on the content. The form should be carefully read, all questions must be answered with clear answers such as "YES" or "NO," and additional clarifications should be written. It must be signed by the patient or legal guardians and confirmed by MR personnel. If there are any surgical implants, radiologist on duty has to make a decision based on implant type and MR compatibility. *If there is any suspicion or lack of information on the implant, do not take any risk with the patient safety and do not scan the patient.* If the form is complete with all the information, the patient should change to MR gown and remove any clothing with any metal. It is always a good practice to remove the jewelry as well. As the last line of patient safety, it is also a good practice to scan patient with a handheld metal detector before taking the patient to MRI room.

Patient Positioning: Place the coil straight at the center of the MR table. The anatomy of the interest is centered in the coil to receive uniform signal from the entire region of interest. For example, for femur imaging, the coil should cover femur and hips. For humerus imaging, shoulder and elbow should be within the coil coverage. For cruris imaging, knee and foot should be within the coil coverage. For humerus imaging, the patient can be moved to the left or right to place the region of interest as close as possible to isocenter.

Please make sure that you give the patient alarm/buzzer to patient's hand and test it. After landmarking the center of coil using laser lights or touch sensors, you can send the patient in and start the exam. It is always recommended to let the patient know how long the scan is going to take and also keep communicating frequently to make them as comfortable as possible in the MR bore (Figs. 8.51–8.53).

Sample Imaging Protocols

A sample imaging protocol for a patient referred to the MRI for long bone scan is given in Tables 8.26 and 8.27.

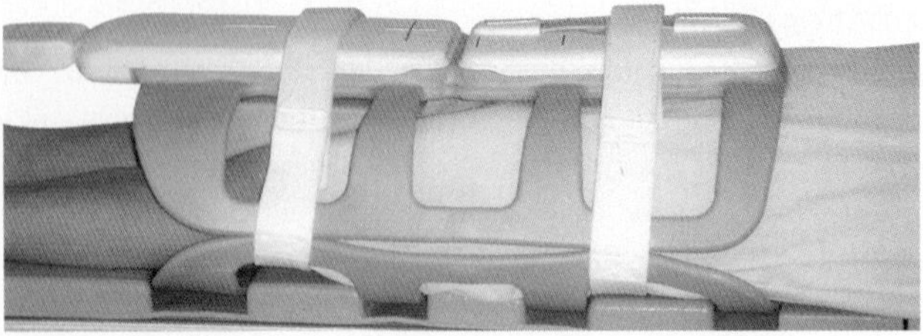

Figure 8.51 A sample of feet first and supine patient femur positioning in a multichannel coil is shown.

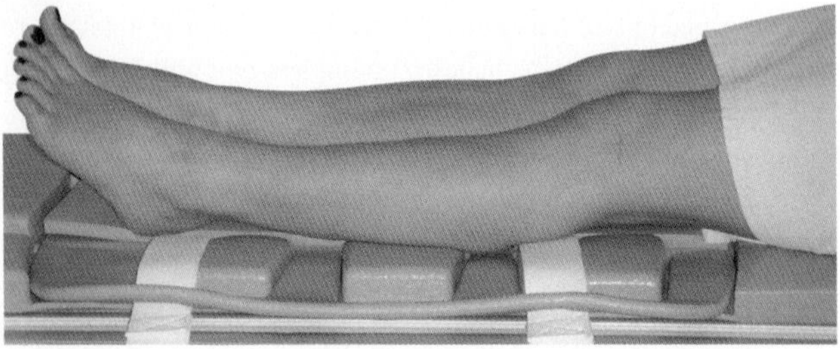

Figure 8.52 A sample feet first and supine patient tibia (cruris) positioning in a multichannel coil is shown. For tibia imaging, knee and foot should be within the coil coverage.

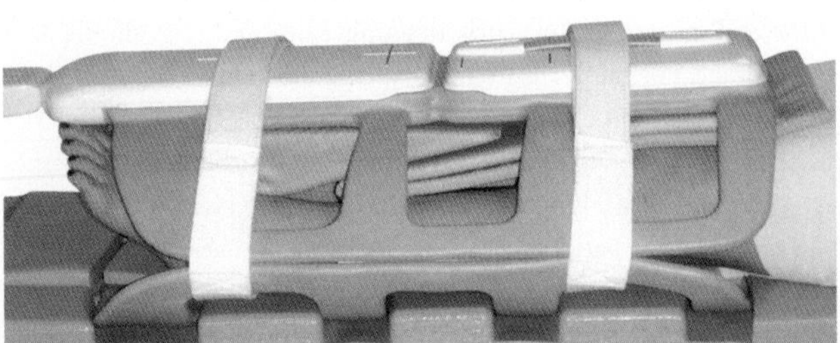

Figure 8.53 A sample feet first and supine patient tibia (cruris) positioning for a multichannel coil is shown. Please look at the positioning of anterior part of the coil which should be parallel to posterior part.

Table 8.26 A routine long bone imaging protocol is given.

Sequences	Comments	Slice order
Three plane localizer	Acquire 5 slices in each plane	
Coronal STIR	Prescribe coronal slices to cover the entire anatomy from sagittal and axial images	A-P
Coronal T1	Copy from coronal STIR sequence	A-P
Axial PD and T2 fat sat	Prescribe straight axial slices only for the region of interest. Slice thickness can be selected by the operator depending on the coverage of interest	S-I
Axial T1	Copy from previous axial	S-I
Sagittal T2	Prescribe sagittal slices perpendicular to coronal prescription	R-L
Additions		
Coronal T2*GRE	Prescribe this sequence for trauma or bone lesions	A-P

Table 8.27 A sample long bone imaging protocol for potential indications such as tumor, trauma, soft tissue, or bone lesion is given.

Sequences	Comments	Slice order
Three plane localizer	Acquire 5 slices in each plane	
Coronal STIR	Prescribe coronal slices to cover the entire region of interest from sagittal and axial images	A-P
Coronal T1	Copy from previous coronal sequence	A-P
Axial PD and T2 fat sat	Prescribe straight axial slices only for the region of interest. Slice thickness can be selected by the operator depending on the coverage of interest	S-I
Axial T1	Copy from previous axial	S-I
Sagittal T2 fat sat	Prescribe sagittal slices perpendicular to coronal prescription	R-L
Postcontrast	*Inject contrast agent if required*	
Axial T1 fat sat	Copy from previous axial	S-I
Coronal T1	Copy from previous coronal. Sagittal plane can be chosen depending on the lesion location, extension, etc.	A-P

Sample Imaging Parameters for 1.5 T

See Table 8.28

Graphical Prescription

See Figs. 8.54–8.56

Table 8.28 A sample long bone imaging parameters is given for a multichannel coil at 1.5 T.

	T1	STIR	PD and T2FS	T1	T2	T2FS	T1FS
Plane	Coronal	Coronal	Axial	Axial	Axial	Coronal	Coronal
Sequence type	FSE	FSE-IR	FRFSE	FSE	FRFSE	FRFSE	FSE
TE	MinFull	42	42/85	MinFull	120	70	MinFull
TR	740	6,220	4,360	760	4,440	3,420	575
ETL	3	12	12	3	20	19	3
BW	41.67	20.83	20.83	41.67	41.67	31.25	41.67
Slice thickness	6.0	6.0	5–8	5–8	5–8	6.0	6.0
Slice spacing	1.0	1.0	2.5	2.5	2.5	1.0	1.0
FOV	44	44	40	40	40	40	44
Matrix	416 × 416	320 × 256	352 × 256	480 × 480	480 × 480	352 × 256	352 × 352
NEX/NSA	2	2	2	2	2	4	2
Freq direction	S-I	S-I	R-L	R-L	R-L	S-I	S-I
Parallel imaging	ON	ON	ON	ON	ON	OFF	OFF

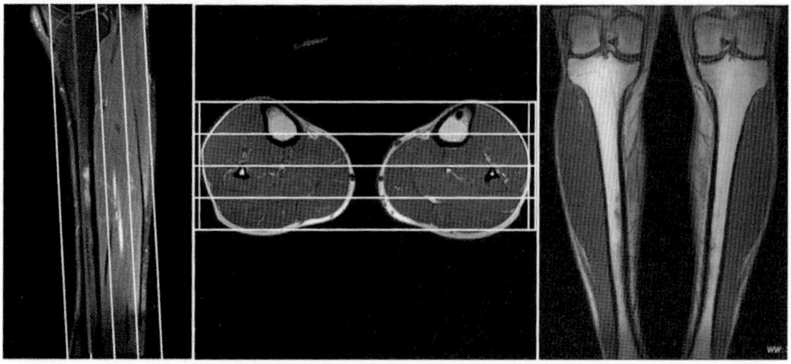

Figure 8.54 Coronal prescription from axial and sagittal images is shown.

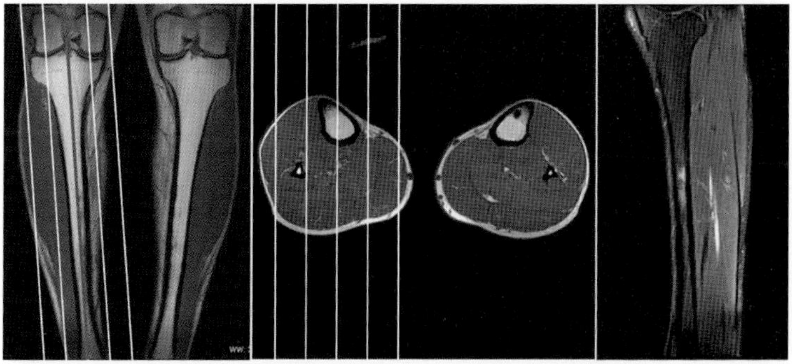

Figure 8.55 Sagittal prescription from axial and coronal images is shown.

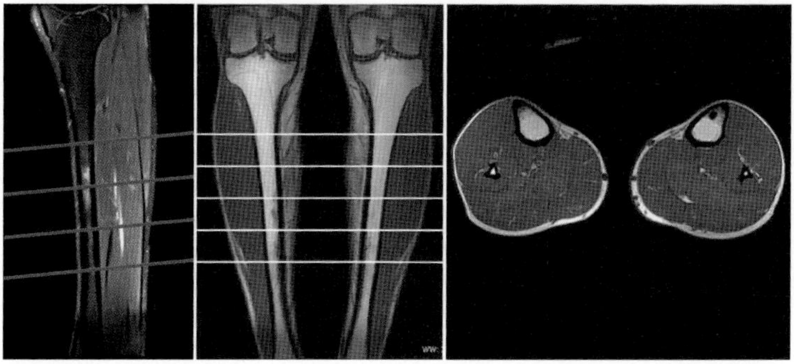

Figure 8.56 Axial planning from sagittal and coronal images is shown.

Chapter 9

Body Imaging: MRI Protocols, Imaging Parameters, and Graphical Prescriptions

Until recently, body imaging was the domain of multislice CT and ultrasound for most applications because of its very short acquisition time, higher resolution, and widespread availability. However, thanks to the recent sequence, coil and MR hardware advances, MR became a powerful imaging modality due to its inherent multiple tissue contrast, safer scanning ability, and its ability to visualize anatomy. The main disadvantage of MR imaging is longer scan time. However, with the multichannel coil structures and parallel imaging concept, both image quality and routine MR examination times improved significantly and will continue to improve.

In body imaging, the biggest challenge for MRI is the need to image moving organs. Gross organ motion creates significant artifacts in MRI and makes it difficult to get reliable diagnostic information. Therefore, the main strategy of body MR imaging is eliminating the gross cardiac and breathing-related motion artifacts by utilizing respiratory gating, cardiac gating, and/or breath holding. All the gating techniques as well as breath hold can make a great difference on the resulting image quality.

In this chapter, after introducing the key concepts of body imaging, we will describe the body imaging in pictures with sample protocols.

For the key concepts, we will start with parallel imaging and continue with gating techniques, which are frequently used for body imaging.

M. Elmaoğlu and A. Çelik, *MRI Handbook: MR Physics, Patient Positioning, and Protocols*, DOI 10.1007/978-1-4614-1096-6_9,

Parallel imaging: Parallel imaging is introduced to the MR community with sense in early 2000 and became an interesting option since then due to its ability to reduce the scan times significantly. Parallel imaging can be done with multichannel coils with multiple coil elements. In common parallel imaging techniques (SENSE, ASSET), before the actual scan, a calibration scan is needed to create a coil sensitivity map for each element in the coil. Then the MR images are acquired with an acceleration factor of 2–4 or more. The acceleration factor does give us the information on approximately how much faster we can go. For example, acceleration factor of 2 and 3 tells us that we will be almost 2 times faster or 3 times faster, respectively, than a nonparallel imaging acquisition with the same parameters. However, as you can expect, this acceleration does not come for free. With each acceleration factor, our SNR will be reduced in a rate directly proportional to the square root of acceleration factor. For example, 2 time acceleration will cost us 41% reduction in SNR. The parallel imaging option is going to acquire raw MR data in a way that it will collect less k-space data to reduce the total scan time. The missing k-space data will be recalculated by the machine by using the initial low resolution calibration image. Since we will collect less data in parallel imaging, we can go faster at the expense of SNR. The first-generation parallel imaging techniques such as SENSE, ASSET, and IPAT may require a separate calibration scan with breath hold for body applications. The newer parallel imaging techniques such as GRAPPA and ARC can create calibration images automatically from the actual image with parallel imaging and can make the job easier for all of us.

Parallel imaging can create its own specific MR artifacts and require a better attention to patient breath hold and FOV selection. For example, for parallel imaging with separate calibration, the patient breath hold of the actual scan should match to the calibration scan breath hold. In addition, FOV should be large enough to eliminate any potential folding artifacts since the aliased parts of the image can appear in the middle of the image rather than the edges.

Parallel imaging techniques are based on the similar principles for all vendors. However, the implementation can vary depending on your MR system. Therefore, we recommend you to follow the guidelines given by each respective company for the proper use of parallel imaging in the system. Parallel imaging is too important to ignore in MR imaging and you should be using it whenever possible.

ECG gating and electrode placement: The ECG electrodes can be placed in few different ways. Two alternative connection methods for standard cardiac gating are shown in Figs. 9.1a and 9.1b. If you have what is called vector gating,

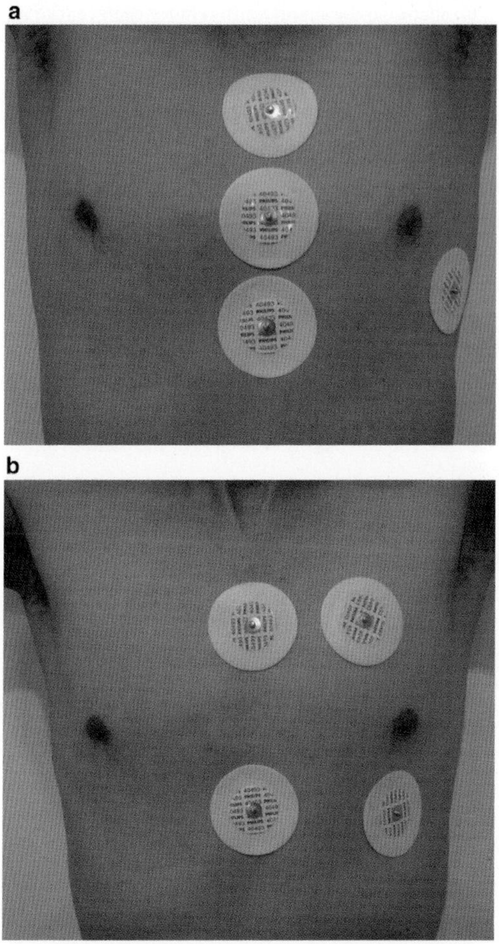

Figure 9.1 (a) Two samples of ECG electrode placement methods for thorax-related exams. The ECG placement can be different for different MR vendors. (b) Two samples of ECG electrode placement methods for thorax-related exams. The ECG placement can be different for different MR vendors.

then you can use vector gating by default since it provides a more reliable cardiac gating. As a golden rule, the electrodes should be placed on the chest to left side of sternum and on the tissue between the ribs. The skin should be cleaned well to remove the dead skin layer for better connectivity. The exact

ECG connection shape can be slightly different for each vendor and you should follow the proper connection guidelines given in your systems manual.

Peripheral cardiac gating and its placement: For body imaging in general, peripheral gating can be used as an alternative method to cardiac gating, because it is easier to connect and is a standard hardware tool on almost all MR scanners. Peripheral gating detects the cardiac way by means of an optical sensor placed at patient's finger. The detected cardiac wave from peripheral gating looks much broader than the ECG detected cardiac wave and occurs with a delay of approximately 200–300 ms. Therefore, peripheral gating should not be the first choice for cardiac MR examination even though it can be used successfully with body imaging applications. The optical sensor of peripheral gating tool is placed firmly on the patient's finger and locked in this position for the MR scan. We recommend thumb for PG placement as it has the widest surface in hand, but you can use other fingers of the hand as long as you receive the signal.

Respiratory gating and bellows placement: Respiratory bellows detects the motion of abdominal wall. Respiratory gating in MRI is one of the lifesaving options for patients unable to hold breath. However, they can also improve the image quality for T2 sequences due to longer TR and ability to do longer acquisition times. Respiratory waveform can be acquired with different methods such as air pressure sensitive (airsack) or stretch devices (bellows). The black bellows in Fig. 9.3 is respiratory gating device used to acquire the waveforms. Most of the T2 sequences can be used with respiratory gating option since the prolonged TR would not create any problems on the image. However, respiratory gating cannot be used with T1 weighted acquisitions. Because the significant increase in TR time with the respiratory gating can destroy the T1 contrast completely. Therefore, either respiratory compensation or prospective acquisition correction techniques (PACE) can be used for T1 weighted imaging.

Navigator gating: Navigator technique is based on detecting the abdominal wall motion using a 1D or 2D navigator slice. Therefore, it does not require any additional hardware for respirator monitoring. It has been used in cardiac imaging especially for coronary imaging but can also be used for abdominal imaging when respiratory triggering is needed. Navigator gating technique may provide superior image quality compared to respiratory gating devices but the scan time cannot be estimated.

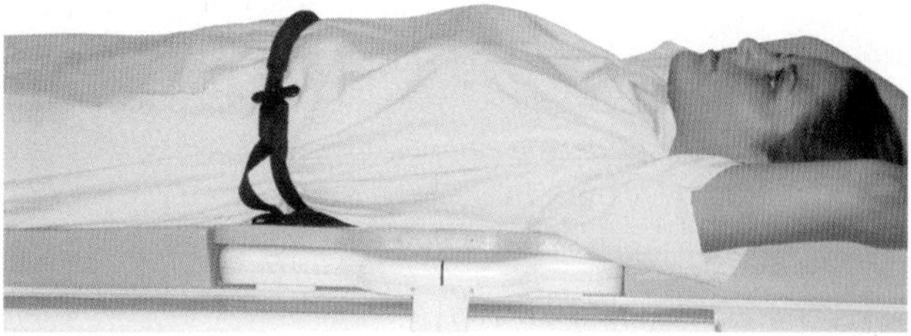

Figure 9.2 A sample feet first and supine patient thorax positioning in a multichannel phase array coil is shown.

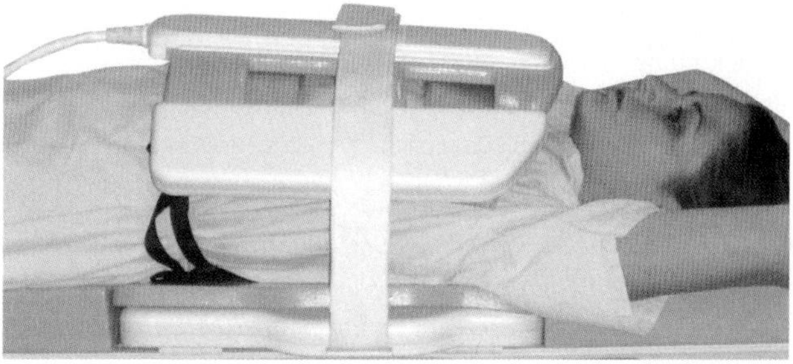

Figure 9.3 A sample feet first and supine patient thorax positioning in a multichannel phase array coil is shown.

Breath holding: Most of the T2 sequences can be used with respiratory gating option since the prolonged TR would not create any problems on the image. However, T1 weighted imaging requires short TR times and cannot be combined with respiratory triggering techniques easily. Breath-hold techniques can significantly reduce sequence times for T2 imaging and can be the only option for good-quality T1 weighted imaging. Breath holding can freeze the abdominal wall motion and enable us to image them almost motion free. Even though a routine breath-hold scan can be on the order of 20 s or so, the breath-hold times for elderly and sick patients would be considerably less. To maintain the quality of breath-hold scans, we strongly recommend practicing the breath holding on the MR table before the actual scan, so that the patient can understand what is required. Breath holding in inspiration or expiration seems to be a choice of each site depending on their experience. However, we recommend expiration breath hold for two reasons. Firstly, the patient would likely spend more energy to maintain and keep the breath in with inspiration breath holds and will cause a drift of abdominal wall. Secondly, inspiration breath holds will cause a significant chest wall difference between the calibration scans (inspiration) and respiratory triggered (expiration) scans when parallel imaging is used.

For longer breath holds, the patient can inhale oxygen if you have the setup in the room. The oxygen supplement can increase the breath holding ability of the patients.

Thorax Imaging

For an optimum thorax MR examination, cardiac gating options such as electrocardiography (ECG) and/or peripheral gating (PG) should be available and working on the MRI system. The cardiac gating option is required for what is called black blood and white blood imaging. Respiratory gating or navigator options are also critical for thorax and general body imaging.

Let us take a brief look at some of the key sequences and options critical to high-quality body imaging below:

Blood suppression (black blood) techniques: Blood suppression or black blood (BB) imaging techniques have been used for quite a long time. Currently used pulse sequence is fast spin echo based and can be used with cardiac gating to eliminate cardiac and flow artifacts by eliminating the signal from blood. This is done with two consecutive inversion pulses and is called double inversion. The first nonselective inversion pulse inverts all the spins in the broad range of anatomy and the second selective inversion pulse inverts nonmoving tissues back to initial state within the selected slice. This way, we will be able to recover the signal from the tissue, and blood signal will be void. Therefore, it is called black blood imaging or blood suppressed imaging. However, more classically gated SE pulse sequence has been used with additional two saturation pulses to suppress the fresh blood within the imaging slice. Due to longer scan time and inability of long breath holding, this technique has been abandoned.

With double inversion black blood imaging, the fat signal will be present. If we add a third inversion pulse very similar to STIR imaging pulse with the right TI inversion time, we will be able to get a triple inversion sequence suppressing the blood and fat signal. You can alternatively do a double inversion black blood imaging with a chemical fat saturation option if you prefer as well.

Bright blood techniques: General gradient echo–based sequences create bright blood images. Specifically, balanced imaging techniques such as Fiesta, True FISP, balanced FFE sequences provide a bright blood imaging and a good contrast between the blood and myocardium. These sequences are also known as ultrafast sequences and usually synchronized with a cardiac gating device. With the triggering signal, the sequence can either acquire multiple slices in the cardiac cycle or multiple cardiac phases of the same slice. The multiple cardiac cycles of the same slice can be displayed in CINE mode to see the tissue motion. The balanced sequences can be used for cardiac imaging with multiple breath holds. However, they are also used for body imaging, vascular visualization, and myelography due to their excellent anatomical information and speed.

Patient Preparation and Positioning

Patient preparation: The patient consent form should be given to the patient with a detailed explanation on the content. The form should be carefully read, all questions must be answered with clear answers such as “YES” or “NO” and additional clarifications should be written. It must be signed by the patient or legal guardians and confirmed by MR personnel. If there are any surgical implants, radiologist on duty has to make a decision based on implant type and MR compatibility. *If there is any suspicion or lack of information on the implant, do not take any risk with the patient safety and do not scan the patient.* If the form is complete with all the information, the patient should change to MR gown and remove any clothing with any metal. If you need to place the cardiac electrodes, the medical gown should have an opening on the chest to place electrodes and connect the cables. It is always a good practice to remove the jewellery as well. As the last line of patient safety, it is also a good practice to scan patient with a handheld metal detectors before taking the patient to MR room.

ECG or PG gating placement: Place the ECG electrodes or PG gating on outside of the MR room to save time or on the MR table as described earlier. ECG electrodes should be placed appropriately in patients who had been operated from chest or cardiac. The electrodes should be placed away from operation line in order to eliminate signal confusion from metallic clips or forceps.

Respiratory gating and bellows placement: Respiratory bellows or airsack should be placed at the level of diaphragm. Before you place the bellows, ask the patient to breathe normally and see the maximum abdominal wall motion region. Then place the bellow on the location where the maximum breathing motion occurs.

Breath hold: Instruct the patient how a proper breath holding should be done and do some practice before the exam. Recommend expiration breath holds for better results.

Patient positioning: Place the coil straight at the center of the MR table. Then you position the patient supine on the coil while the arms are raised above the head unless there is a physical restriction (pain, age, etc.). The ECG electrodes are placed on the chest and additional pads are placed between the coil and electrodes. The coil center should align with the center of breast mass for females and nipple for male patients. Place the respiratory bellows on the level of diaphragm.

Please make sure that you give the patient alarm bell and test it before sending in. After landmarking the center of coil using laser lights or touch sensors, you can send the patient in and start the exam. It is always recommended to let the patient know how long the scan is going to take and also keep communicating frequently to make them as comfortable as possible in the MR bore.

Sample Imaging Protocols

A sample imaging protocol for a patient referred to the MRI for thorax examination is given below (Tables 9.1 and 9.2).

Sample Imaging Parameters for 1.5T

Table 9.3.

Table 9.1 A sample thorax protocol for potential indications such as tumor, trauma, aneurysm, or bone lesion is given.

Sequences	Comments	Slice order
3 Plane localizer	Acquire five slices in each plane	
Coronal SSFSE	Prescribe straight coronal slices to cover the entire region of interest from axial and sagittal images (breath hold)	A–P
Axial T1–BB	The black blood sequence is breath hold and cardiac gated	S–I
Axial STIR BB	Same as above but used for fat suppression (triple IR)	S–I
Axial 3D LAVA–3D VIBE	Breath hold 3D T1spoiled gradient echo sequence with fat saturation (good breath holding is required)	S–I
Postcontrast	*If the contrast injection is required or decided*	
Axial 3D LAVA–3D VIBE	Prescribe with the same coverage as above with multiple phase (good breath holding is required)	S–I
Axial T1-BB-FS	Same as precontrast black blood imaging but with fat saturation	S–I

Table 9.2 A sample routine thorax protocol is given.

Sequences	Comments	Slice order
3 Plane localizer	Acquire five slices in each plane	
Coronal T2 RTR (SSFSE or FRFSE)	Prescribe straight respiratory triggered (RTR) coronal slices to cover the entire region of interest from axial and sagittal images	A–P
Axial T2 RTR (FRFSE/ RESTORE)	Prescribe straight respiratory triggered (RTR) axial slices to cover the entire region	S–I
Axial T1 dual echo (out-in phases)	Copy from previous axial. Breath holding is required	S–I
Axial 3D LAVA–3D VIBE	Breath hold 3D T1spoiled gradient echo sequence with fat saturation (good breath holding is required)	S–I
Postcontrast	*If the contrast injection is required or decided*	
Axial LAVA–VIBE	Prescribe with the same coverage as above with 3 phases	S–I

Table 9.3 A sample thorax imaging parameter is given for a multichannel coil at 1.5T.

	T2	T2	T1BB	STIR BB	Dual	LAVA	LAVA
Plane	Coronal	Axial	Axial	Axial	Axial	Axial	Coronal
Sequence type	SSFSE	FRFSE	FSE	FSE-IR	SPGR	SPGR	SPGR
TE	90	90	42	42	Dual	Min	Min
TR	Min	Auto	Auto	Auto	165	Auto	Auto
ETL		15	32	32			
BW	83.33	41.67	62.5	62.5	62.5	83.33	62.5
Slice thickness	8.0	8.0	8.0	8.0	8.0	8.0	6.0
Slice spacing	1.5	1.5	1.5	1.5	1.5	−4.0	−3.0
FOV	44	40	40	40	40	40	42
Matrix	384 × 224	320 × 256	352 × 256	288 × 256	320 × 192	320 × 224	320 × 160
NEX/NSA	1	4	1	1	1	1	1
Frequent direction	S–I	R–L	R–L	R–L	R–L	R–L	S–I
BB TI/TI			Auto	Auto/150			
Gating/FA	BH	RTR	BH	BH	BH/80	BH/10	BH
Parallel imaging	On	On	On	On	On	On	On

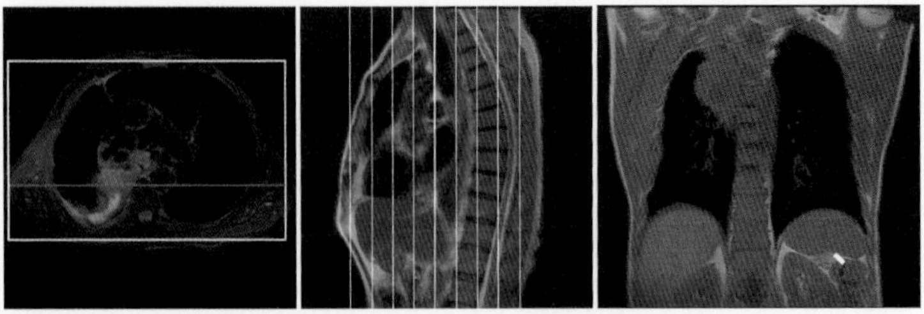

Figure 9.4 Coronal prescription from axial and sagittal images is shown.

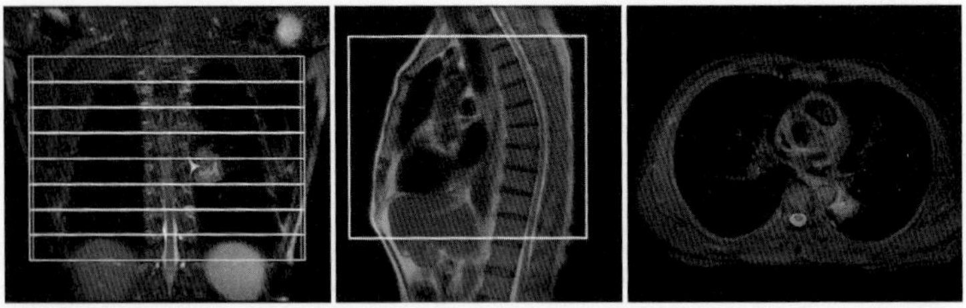

Figure 9.5 Axial planning from coronal and scout sagittal images is shown.

Graphical Prescription

Figures 9.4 and 9.5.

Routine and Dynamic Liver Imaging

For an optimum liver MR examination, respiratory triggering option should be used especially for the patient unable to hold breath. Multichannel coil elements can both improve the image quality and reduce the scan times by using parallel imaging efficiently.

Antispasmodic drugs may decrease the involuntary movement of small intestines, bowels, and stomach. However, these drugs cannot be used without radiologist decision.

Patient Preparation and Positioning

Patient preparation: The patient consent form should be given to the patient with a detailed explanation on the content. The form should be carefully read, all questions must be answered with clear answers such as "YES" or "NO," and additional clarifications should be written. It must be signed by the patient or legal guardians and confirmed by MR personnel. If there are any surgical implants, radiologist on duty has to make a decision based on implant type and MR compatibility. *If there is any suspicion or lack of information on the implant, do not take any risk with the patient safety and do not scan the patient.* If the form is complete with all the information, the patient should change to MR gown and remove any clothing with any metal. It is always a good practice to remove the jewellery as well. As the last line of patient safety, it is also a good practice to scan patient with a handheld metal detector before taking the patient to MR room.

Respiratory gating and bellows placement: Respiratory bellows or airsack should be placed at the level of diaphragm. Before you place the bellows, ask the patient to breathe normally and see the maximum abdominal wall motion region. Then place the bellow on the location where the maximum breathing motion occurs. If you are using respiratory bellows such as that shown in Fig. 9.6, you need to place pads just above and below the bellow. Otherwise, the coil may compress the respiratory bellow and disable its ability to accurately measure the respiratory waveforms.

Breath hold: Instruct the patient how a proper breath holding should be done and do some practices before the exam. Recommend expiration breath holds for better results.

Patient positioning: Place the coil straight at the center of the MR table. Then you position the patient supine on the coil while the arms are raised above the head unless there is a physical restriction (pain, age, etc.). The coil center should align with the lower tip of sternum (xiphoid process or xiphisternum). Place the respiratory bellows on the level of diaphragm.

Please make sure that you give the patient alarm bell and test it before sending in. After landmarking the center of coil using laser lights or touch sensors, you can send the patient in and start the exam. It is always recommended to let the patient know how long the scan is going to take and also keep communicating frequently to make them as comfortable as possible in the MR bore (Figs. 9.6 and 9.7).

Sample Imaging Protocols

A sample imaging protocol for a patient referred to the MRI for liver examination is given below (Table 9.4):

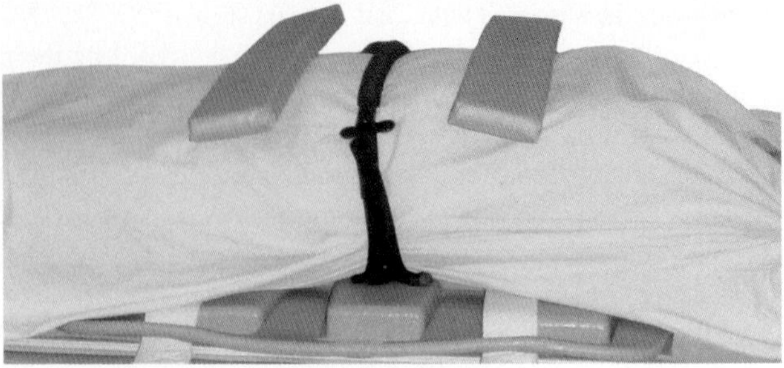

Figure 9.6 Respiratory bellow positioning is shown.

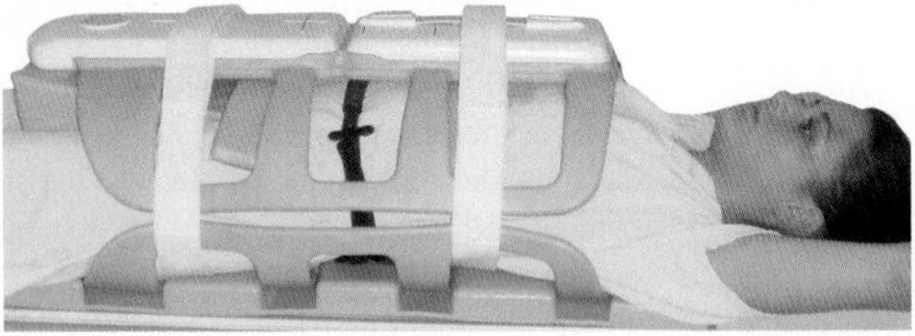

Figure 9.7 A sample feet first and supine patient liver positioning in a multichannel coil is shown.

Tips and Tricks

- Heavy T2 acquisition for liver imaging can help for differential diagnosis of the cysts and various pathologies such as hemangioma, liver adenoma, or metastases.
- Axial T2 sequences can be done either breath hold or respiratory triggered. However, triggered scans can provide higher resolution and better SNR.
- In-phase and out-of-phase images can help differentiating adrenal gland adenomas from tumors or metastases.
- The flow artifacts in 2D axial spoiled gradient echo–based T1 sequences can be reduced with application of superior and inferior saturation bands and/or flow compensation in slice direction.
- When the dual echo is acquired, there is no need to acquire SPGR T1, where the "in-phase" is already T1.

Table 9.4 A sample routine liver protocol.

Sequences	Comments	Slice order
3 Plane localizer	Acquire 5 slices in each plane with breath holding	
Coronal heavy T2	Prescribe straight breath hold coronal slices to cover the entire region of interest from sagittal and axial images. Heavy T2 will have longer TE times and use fast single shot sequence such as SSFSE, HASTE, or EXPRESS	A–P
Axial T2 BH	Prescribe straight axial breath hold slices only for the region of interest. Use SSFSE or FSE sequence	S–I
Axial T2 fat saturation RTR	Prescribe straight axial slices only for the region of interest. Use respiratory gated FRFSE or FSE sequence	S–I
Axial T1 BH	Prescribe same as above breath hold slices. Use an SPGR or FLASH sequence	S–I
Axial dual BH	Prescribe axial breath hold slices. The sequence is a dual echo (in-phase and out-of-phase)	S–I
Axial LAVA–VIBE	Prescribe axial thin slice, breath hold 3D T1 gradient echo sequence with fat saturation	S–I
Postcontrast	*If the contrast injection is desired by physician or radiologist*	
Axial LAVA–VIBE	Prescribe with the same coverage as above with 3–5 phases	S–I
Axial T1 FS BH	Same as precontrast axial T1 imaging but with fat saturation	S–I

- Out-of-phase TE time can be chosen as 2.3 ms or 6.9 ms for 1.5T and 1.15 ms or 3.45 ms for 3.0T.
- In-phase TE time can be chosen as 4.4 ms or 9.2 ms for 1.5T and 2.3 ms or 4.6 ms for 3.0T.
- 3D T1 sequences can provide better resolution and multiplanar reformatted images.

Sample Imaging Parameters for 1.5T

Table 9.5.

Table 9.5 A sample routine liver protocol parameter given for a multichannel parallel imaging compatible body coil.

	T2	T2	T2 fat saturation	T1	Dual echo	3D LAVA	T1 FS	3D LAVA
Plane	Coronal	Axial	Axial	Axial	Axial	Axial	Axial	Coronal
Sequence type	SSFSE	SSFSE	FRFSE	SPGR	FSPGR	FSPGR	FSPGR	FSPGR
TE	90	90	90	In phase	Dual	Min	In phase	Min
TR	Min	Min	Auto	200	165	Auto	275	Auto
ETL			14					
BW	83.33	83.33	50.00	41.67	41.67	62.50	31	62
Slice thickness	6–8	6–8	6–8	6–8	6–8	4–6	6–8	4.4
Slice spacing	1.5	1.5	1.5	1.5	1.5	−2.4	1.5	−2.2
FOV	42	40	40	40	40	40	40	42
Matrix	384 × 224	384 × 224	320 × 256	320 × 192	320 × 192	320 × 160	320 × 160	320 × 160
NEX/NSA	1	1	4	1	1	1	1	1
Frequent direction	S–I	R–L	R–L	R–L	R–L	R–L	R–L	S–I
SAT band				S–I	S–I			
Gating/FA	BH	BH	RTR	BH/80	BH/80	BH/12	BH/80	BH
Parallel imaging	On	On	On	On	On	On	On	On

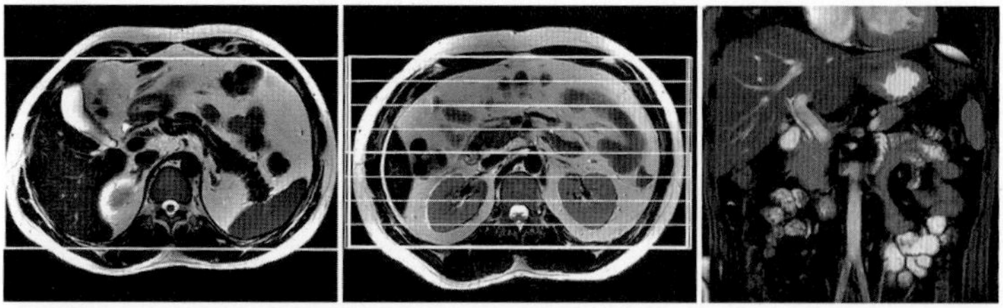

Figure 9.8 Coronal prescription from axial images is shown.

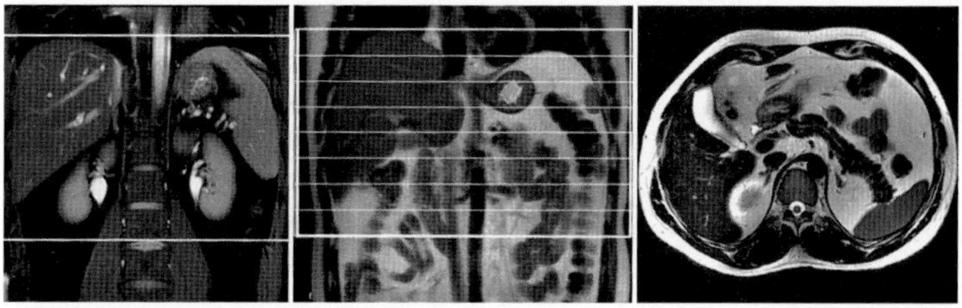

Figure 9.9 Axial planning from coronal images is shown.

Graphical Prescription

Figures 9.8 and 9.9.

Pancreas

Pancreas imaging can be done best with multichannel coils with smaller elements such as cardiac or abdomen coils. Pancreas imaging should be done with thin slices and high resolution T2 weighted sequences with respiratory triggering and breath hold T1 weighted sequences.

Patient Preparation and Positioning

Patient preparation: Patient preparation is same as liver imaging (previous section).

Respiratory gating and bellows placement: Respiratory bellows or airsack is placed exactly same as a routine liver imaging.

Breath hold: Instruct the patient how a proper breath holding should be done and do some practices before the exam. Recommend expiration breath holds for better results.

Patient positioning: The coil placement and patient positioning is identical to liver imaging.

Sample Imaging Protocols

A sample imaging protocol for a patient referred to the MRI for pancreas examination is given below (Table 9.6).

Tips and Tricks

- In-phase and out-of-phase (dual echo) images provide excellent delineation of pancreas anatomy and pathologies.
- Out-of-phase TE time can be chosen as 2.3 ms or 6.9 ms for 1.5T and 1.15 ms or 3.45 ms for 3.0T.
- In-phase TE time can be chosen as 4.4 ms or 9.2 ms for 1.5T and 2.3 ms or 4.6 ms for 3.0T.
- 3D dual echo (out-in phases) or 3D T1 fat saturation sequences (LAVA/VIBE) provide better spatial resolution and large coverage. Also they can be used to reconstruct images into other planes.

Table 9.6 A sample routine pancreas protocol.

Sequences	Comments	Slice order
3 Plane localizer	Acquire 5 breath hold slices in each plane	
Coronal T2	Prescribe straight breath hold coronal slices to cover the entire region of interest from axial images. Use 3–5 mm fast single shot sequences such as SSFSE, HASTE, or EXPRESS	A–P
Axial T2 RTR	Prescribe straight axial slices for pancreas region. Use FRFSE or TSE sequence with respiratory gating	S–I
Axial T1 BH	Prescribe same as above breath hold slices. Use an FSPGR or Turbo FLASH sequence	S–I
Axial dual BH	Prescribe axial breath hold slices. The sequence is a dual echo (in-phase and out-of-phase)	S–I
Axial LAVA–VIBE	Prescribe axial thin slices, breath hold 3D T1 gradient echo sequence with fat saturation (LAVA/VIBE)	S–I
Postcontrast	*Usually contrast injection is needed (confirmation of radiologist is essential)*	
Axial LAVA–VIBE	Prescribe with the same coverage as above with 3 phases	S–I
Axial T1 FS BH	Same as precontrast axial T1 imaging but with fat saturation	S–I

- Axial T2 BH sequences provide low SNR and poor spatial resolution and therefore should be avoided in pancreas imaging. The flow artifacts in 2D axial spoiled gradient echo–based T1 sequences can be reduced with application of superior and inferior saturation bands and/or flow compensation in slice direction.
- Diffusion can be applied as an additional sequence with multiple *b* values.

Sample Imaging Parameters for 1.5T

Table 9.7.

Graphical Prescription

Figures 9.10 and 9.11.

Table 9.7 A sample routine pancreas protocol parameter given for a multichannel parallel imaging compatible body coil.

	T2/T1	T2	T1	Dual	LAVA	T1 FS	Diffusion
Plane	Coronal	Axial	Axial	Axial	Axial	Axial	Axial
Sequence type	Fiesta	FRFSE	SPGR	SPGR	FSPGR	SPGR	EPI
TE	MinFull	90	In phase	Dual	Min	In phase	Min
TR	Auto	Min	200	170	Auto	275	4000
ETL		14					
BW	83.33	50.00	41.67	41.67	41.67	31.25	Auto
Slice thickness	4.0	4.0	4.0	4.0	4.0	4.0	4.0
Slice spacing	0.4	0.4	0.4	0.4	−2.0	0.4	0.4
FOV	40	40	40	40	40	40	40
Matrix	256 × 320	320 × 224	320 × 192	320 × 224	320 × 160	256 × 160	160 × 160
NEX/NSA	1	4	1	1	1	1	8
Frequent direction	S–I	R–L	R–L	R–L	R–L	R–L	R–L
SAT band		S–I	S–I	S–I			
Gating/FA	BH/75	RTR	BH/80	BH/80	BH/12	BH/80	
Parallel imaging	On	On	On	On	On	On	On

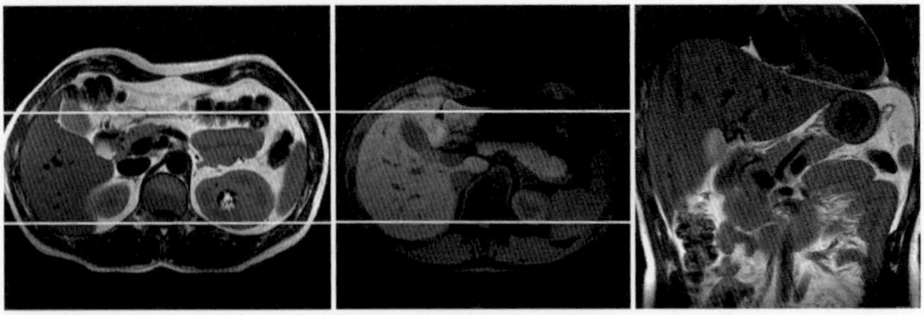

Figure 9.10 Coronal prescription from axial images is shown.

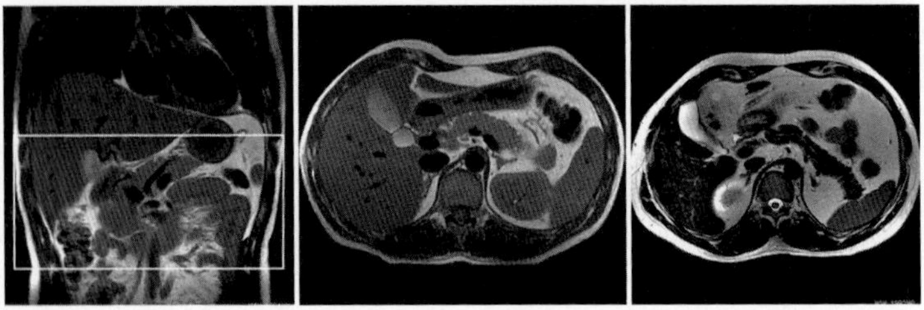

Figure 9.11 Axial planning from coronal images is shown.

Magnetic Resonance Colangio Pancreatography

Magnetic resonance colangio pancreatograpgy (MRCP) is a technique that can be used as a noninvasive alternative to endoscopic retrograde cholangiopancreatography (ERCP). MRCP scans can be done with breath hold or respiratory triggered. Antispasm medicines can be used to reduce the intestinal motion artifacts under the control of radiologist.

Patient Preparation and Positioning

Patient preparation: Usually, 4–6 h fasting is required prior to MRCP exams. Additionally, a glass of pineapple juice may be used to decrease the T2 time of the fluid within the stomach and duodenum. The patient consent form should be given to the patient with a detailed explanation on the content. The form should be carefully read, all questions must be answered with clear answers such as "Yes" or "No," and additional clarifications should be written. It must be signed by the patient or legal guardians and confirmed by MR personnel.

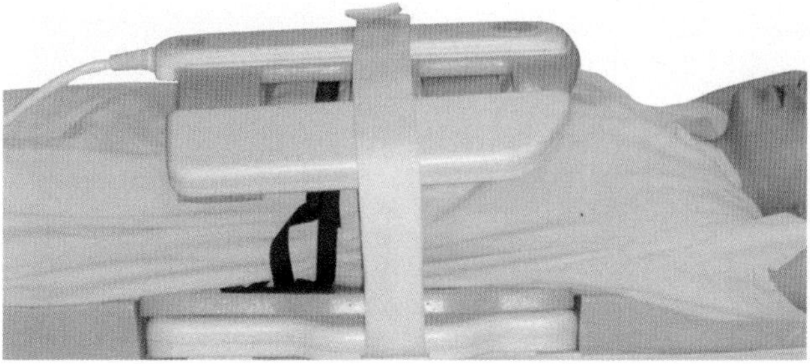

Figure 9.12 A sample MRCP patient positioning for a multichannel coil is shown.

If there are any surgical implants, radiologist on duty has to make a decision based on implant type and MR compatibility. *If there is any suspicion or lack of information on the implant, do not take any risk with the patient safety and do not scan the patient.* If the form is complete with all the information, the patient should change to MR gown and remove any clothing with any metal. It is always a good practice to remove the jewellery as well. As the last line of patient safety, it is also a good practice to scan patient with a handheld metal detector before taking the patient to MR room.

Respiratory gating and bellows placement: Respiratory bellows or airsack is placed exactly same as a routine liver imaging.

Patient positioning: The coil placement and patient positioning is identical to liver imaging. An additional patient positioning with cardiac coil is shown below (Fig. 9.12).

Sample Imaging Protocols

A sample imaging protocol for a patient referred to the MRI for MRCP examination is given below (Table 9.8).

Tips and Tricks

- Long TE scans producing heavy T2 weighting or balanced sequences (Fiesta, TrueFISP, bFFE) can be very useful to delineate cystic lesions, gallbladder, and biliary canal stones.
- 3D T2 sequence with FRFSE or RESTORE type sequences can be very useful for high-resolution MRCP imaging. Respiratory triggering and parallel imaging should be preferred for better image quality.

Table 9.8 A sample routine MRCP protocol with contrast injection.

Sequences	Comments	Slice order
3 Plane localizer	Acquire 5 breath hold slices in each plane	
Coronal T2	Prescribe straight breath hold coronal slices to cover the entire anatomy from sagittal and axial images. Use 4–5 mm slice thickness (SSFSE, HASTE, or EXPRESS)	S–I
Axial heavy T2	Prescribe straight axial with long TE (150–190 ms) for heavy T2 contrast with breath hold. You can use one of the single shot techniques	S–I
Axial dual echo	Prescribe axial breath hold slices with 4–5 mm thickness. The sequence is a dual echo (in-phase and out-of-phase)	S–I
Radial heavy T2 thick slice	Prescribe radial slices to start from pancreatic canal up to gallbladder. Place the radial slices from the axial image above with a slice thickness of 50–70 mm with a breath hold for each scan. Wait minimum 10 s before the next slice	Clockwise
Coronal 3D T2 RTR or BH	Prescribe straight coronal slices to cover pancreas and gallbladder with 1–2 mm slice thickness. Acquire either breath hold or respiratory triggered images	A–P
Axial LAVA/VIBE	Prescribe axial 3–4 mm slices, breath hold 3D T1 SPGR sequence with fat saturation	S–I
Postcontrast	If the contrast injection is required and decided by radiologist	
Axial LAVA/VIBE	Prescribe with the same coverage as above with 3 phases	S–I
Coronal LAVA/VIBE	Prescribe coronal slices with 2–3 mm slice thickness with 3 phases	A–P

- In-phase and out-of-phase images can help differentiating fatty infiltration of the liver infections, cystic and metastatic lesions, surrenal adenomas, and tumors.
- 3D T1 sequences can provide better spatial resolution and can be used to reconstruct images into other planes.

Sample Imaging Parameters for 1.5T

Table 9.9.

Graphical Prescription

Figures 9.13–9.15.

Table 9.9 A sample routine MRCP protocol for a multichannel abdomen coil is given.

	T2	Heavy T2	Dual echo	Thick slab	3D T2	3D T1 fat saturation
Plane	Coronal	Axial	Axial	Radial	Coronal	Axial
Sequence Type	SSFSE	SSFSE	SPGR	SSFSE	FRFSE	LAVA/VIBE
TE	85	200–↑	Dual	Auto (800–↑)	Auto	Min
TR	Min	Min	175	Auto	Auto	Min
ETL		Auto		Auto	Auto	
BW	83.33	83.33	62.50	31.2	31.2	62.50
Slice Thickness	5.0	5.0	5.0	40.0	1.6	4.0
Slice Spacing	1.0	1.0	1.0	–	−0.8	−2.0
FOV	35	35	35	32	32	35
Matrix	384 × 256	384 × 224	320 × 160	416 × 256	320 × 320	320 × 224
NEX/NSA	1	1	1	1	1	1
Frequent Direction	S–I	R–L	R–L	S–I	S–I	R–L
SAT Band			S–I			
Gating/FA	BH	BH	BH	BH	RTR	BH/12
Parallel imaging	On	On	On	On	On	On

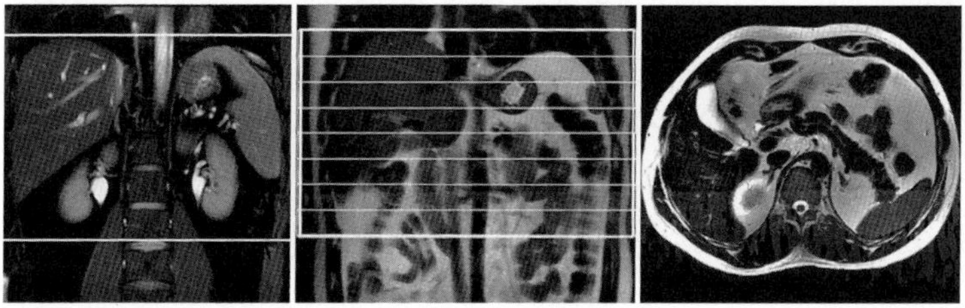

Figure 9.13 Axial planning from coronal images is shown.

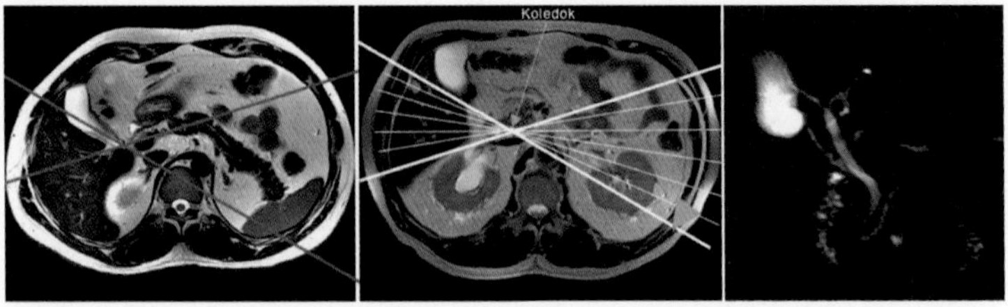

Figure 9.14 Radial planning from axial images is shown.

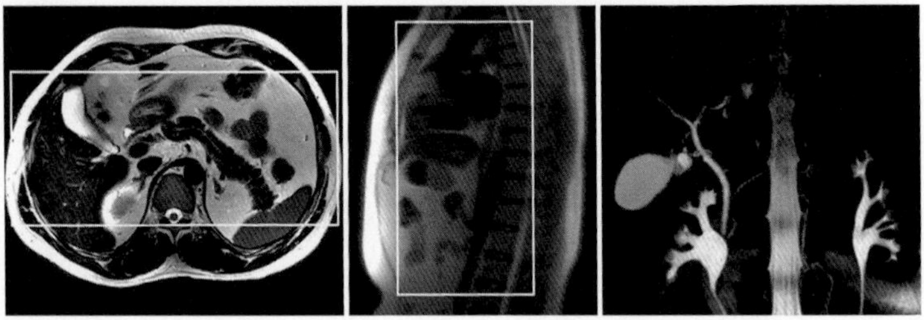

Figure 9.15 Coronal 3D T2 prescription from axial and sagittal images is shown.

Magnetic Resonance Urography

Magnetic resonance urography (MRU) can be described as MR imaging of urinary tracts. MR urography is somewhat an uncommon MR request due to longer acquisition times, need for more high-end MR systems, and technical challenges of getting consistent image quality. However, with the right MR options and better education, the success rate of MR urography can be improved significantly. MR urography sequences are pretty similar to MRCP sequences and may require respiratory triggering with 2D- and 3D-based sequences.

Sample protocols and optimized imaging practices for MRU will be given in this section. It is recommended for the patient to use antigas medicines 1–2 days before the exam. In addition, antispasm drugs can be given to the patient on the MR table just before the exam intravenously of 15 min before the exam intramuscularly. Diuretic drugs are also used for increasing the urine secretion when the ureteries are not visualized in MRI (application of these additional medicines require radiologist permission or legal confirmation).

Patient Preparation and Positioning

Patient preparation: It is identical to patient preparation for MRCP. Additionally, patient should go to the restroom before the exam in order to start the exam with empty bladder. This is quite important for MRU, because diuretic drugs will significantly increase the urine secretion.

Respiratory gating and bellows placement: Respiratory bellows or airsack is placed exactly same as a routine liver imaging.

Breath holding: Instruct the patient how a proper breath holding should be done and practice before the exam. Recommend expiration breath holds for better results.

Patient positioning: Place the coil straight at the center of the MR table. Then you position the patient supine on the coil while the arms are raised above the head unless there is a physical restriction (pain, age, etc.). The coil center should align with the belly button. Place the respiratory bellows on the level of diaphragm.

Please make sure that you give the patient alarm/buzzer to patient's hand and test it. After landmarking the center of coil using laser lights or touch sensors, you can send the patient in and start the exam. It is always recommended to let the patient know how long the scan is going to take and also keep communicating frequently to make them as comfortable as possible in the MR bore.

Sample Imaging Protocols

A sample imaging protocol for a patient referred to the MRI for MRU examination is given below (Table 9.10).

Tips and Tricks

- Long TE scans producing heavy T2 weighting can be very useful to delineate urinary tract stones and/or tumors in the region. Especially, 3D T2 imaging with thin slices can be used for better resolution and quality.
- Parallel imaging is used for MRU as well to accelerate the acquisition and reduce the blurring with single shot–based techniques.
- Respiratory triggering always provides better image quality than breath-hold techniques.
- 3D T1 postcontrast sequences provide better spatial resolution and allow multiplanar reformat and MIP images.
- Subtracted images of functional studies provide better visualization of ureters.

Table 9.10 A sample routine MRU protocol including functional study is given.

Sequences	Comments	Slice Order
3 Plane localizer	Acquire 5 breath hold slices in each plane	
Axial heavy T2	Prescribe straight breath hold axial slices. Use 4–5 mm slice thickness with SSFSE, HASTE, or EXPRESS sequences	S–I
Sagittal heavyT2 thick slice	Prescribe 50 mm sagittal slices separately for each ureter	R–L
Coronal 3D T2 RTR	Prescribe oblique coronal slices to cover urinary tracts with 1 or 2 mm slice thickness. Acquire either breath hold or respiratory triggered images	A–P
Coronal heavy T2 thick slice	Prescribe breath hold 40–50 mm coronal slices separately for urinary tracts	S–I
Coronal heavy T2 thin slice	Prescribe breath hold 4–5 mm coronal slices separately for urinary tracts	S–I
Postcontrast	If needed due to infection or tumor or functional study	
Coronal 3D T1 FSPGR (functional study)	Prescribe a multiphase coronal 3D T1 FSPGR for MRU and acquire precontrast phase to check the image quality. Then repeat in every 1 minute until you see both the ureters in postcontrast acquisitions	A–P
Axial LAVA/VIBE	Prescribe axial LAVA with 3–4 mm slice thickness for anatomical delineation	S–I

Sample Imaging Parameters for 1.5T

Table 9.11.

Graphical Prescription

Figures 9.16–9.18.

Table 9.11 A sample routine MRU protocol for a multichannel parallel imaging compatible abdomen coil is given.

	Thin slice T2	Thick slice T2	3D T2 RTR	Thick slice T2	Thin slice T2	3D CE	3DT1 FS
Plane	Axial	Sagittal	Coronal	Coronal	Coronal	Coronal	Axial
Sequence type	SSFSE	SSFSE	FRFSE	SSFSE	SSFSE	SPGR	LAVA
TE	85	1000	Auto	1000	550	Min	Min
TR	Min	Auto	Auto	3000	6000	Auto	Auto
ETL			Auto				
BW	83.33	31.25	31.25	31.25	83.33	62.50	62.50
Slice thickness	8.0	50	1.6	40	4.0	2.8	5.0
Slice spacing	1.0	–	−0.8	−30	1.0	−1.4	−2.5
FOV	40	40	40	40	40	40	40
Matrix	384 × 224	416 × 256	320 × 320	416 × 256	384 × 224	352 × 192	320 × 160
NEX/NSA	1	1	1	1	1	0.75	1
Frequent direction	R–L	S–I	S–I	S–I	S–I	S–I	R–L
Gating/FA	BH	BH	RTR	BH	RTR	BH	BH
ASSET/SENSE/IPAT	On	On	On	On	On	On	On

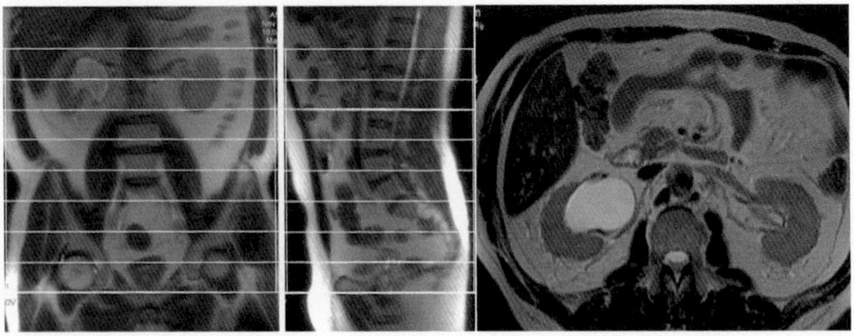

Figure 9.16 Axial planning from scout coronal and sagittal images is shown.

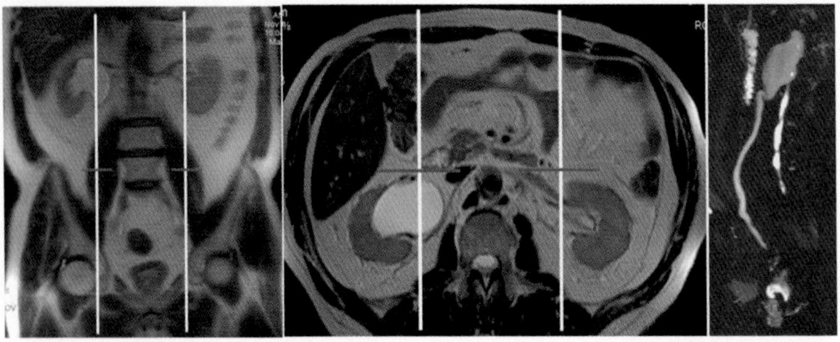

Figure 9.17 Sagittal thick slice MRU prescription from coronal and axial images is shown.

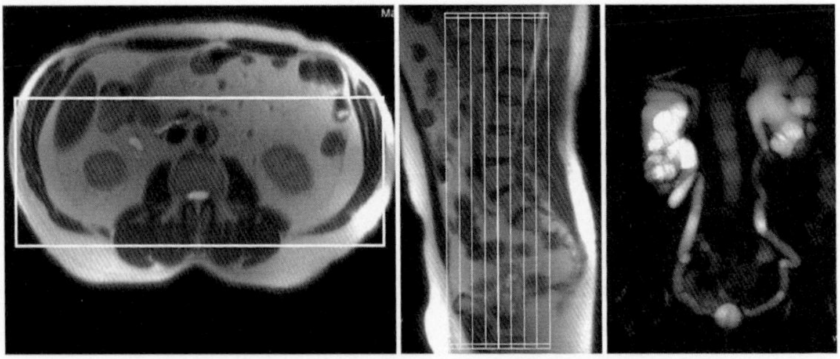

Figure 9.18 Coronal prescription from axial and sagittal images is shown.

Pelvis

Pelvis MR imaging should be done in high spatial resolution (smaller FOV, higher matrixes, and thinner slices). Parallel imaging is also recommended for pelvis imaging. However, you may need to increase your FOV with certain parallel imaging applications (SENSE or ASSET) to prevent artifacts specific to parallel imaging technique you are using. Multichannel coils with smaller coil elements such as cardiac coil can provide better image quality for pelvis imaging. Antispasm drugs can be given to reduce the involuntary gross organ motion-related artifacts.

Patient Preparation and Positioning

Patient preparation: We don't recommend starting the pelvis exam with totally full or empty bladder. Patient should be in a condition that he/she can easily tolerate a 20-min exam. The patient consent form should be given to the patient with a detailed explanation on the content. The form should be carefully read, all questions must be answered with clear answers such as "Yes" or "No," and additional clarifications should be written. It must be signed by the patient or legal guardians and confirmed by MR personnel. If there are any surgical implants, radiologist on duty has to make a decision based on implant type and MR compatibility. *If there is any suspicion or lack of information on the implant, do not take any risk with the patient safety and do not scan the patient.* If the form is complete with all the information, the patient should change to MR gown and remove any clothing with any metal. It is always a good practice to remove the jewellery as well. As the last line of patient safety, it is also a good practice to scan patient with a handheld metal detector before taking the patient to MRI room.

Patient positioning: Place the coil straight at the center of the MR table. Then you position the patient supine on the coil and arms can be placed at sideways above the coil level. The coil center should be around 10 cm below the iliac crest. If you have a body coil with long coverage, we recommend the top of the coil at the level of iliac crest. By this way, you can eliminate or decrease breathing-related artifacts significantly.

Please make sure that you give the patient alarm bell and test it before sending in. After landmarking the center of coil using laser lights or touch sensors, you can send the patient in and start the exam. It is always recommended to let the patient know how long the scan is going to take and also keep communicating frequently to make them as comfortable as possible in the MR bore (Figs. 9.19 and 9.20).

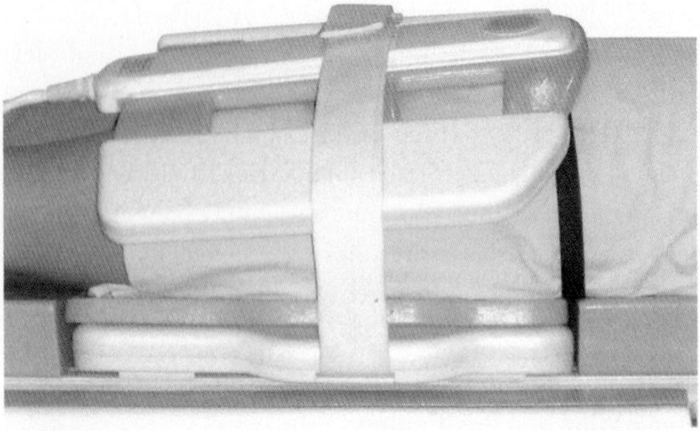

Figure 9.19 A sample patient positioning for pelvic MRI in a multichannel coil is shown.

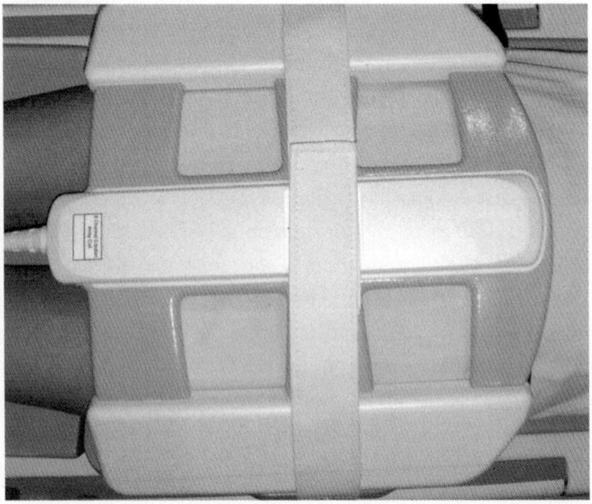

Figure 9.20 A sample patient positioning for pelvic MRI in a multichannel coil is shown.

Sample Imaging Protocols

A sample imaging protocol for a patient referred to the MRI for MRU examination is given below (Table 9.12).

Sample Imaging Parameters for 1.5T

Table 9.13.

Table 9.12 A sample routine pelvis protocol.

Sequences	Comments	Slice order
3 Plane localizer	Acquire 5 slices in each plane	
Sagittal T2	Prescribe straight 3–5 mm sagittal slices to cover both ovarium or the region between the femoral heads	R–L
Axial T2	Prescribe straight 3–5 mm axial slices to cover from iliac crest to pubic bone (pubic symphisis)	S–I
Axial T1	Same as axial T2 above	S–I
Axial dual BH	Same as axial above	S–I
Coronal T2 FS	Prescribe straight coronal for males or oblique coronal for females parallel to uterus angle	A–P
Axial LAVA–VIBE	Prescribe 3–4 mm 3D T1 gradient echo sequence with fat saturation	S–I
Postcontrast	*If the contrast injection is desired by radiologist*	
Axial LAVA–VIBE	Prescribe with the same coverage as above with minimum 3 phases	S–I
Sagittal T1 fat saturation	Same prescription as precontrast T2	R–L

Table 9.13 A sample routine pelvis protocol for a multichannel cardiac coil is given.

	T2	T2	T1	T2 FS	LAVA	T1 FS	T1 FS
Plane	Sagittal	Axial	Axial	Coronal	Axial	Sagittal	Axial
Sequence type	FRFSE	FRFSE	FSE	FRFSE	SPGR	SPGR	FSE
TE	100	100	MinFull	68	In phase	In phase	MinFull
TR	5340	5340	640	5140	Auto	200	675
ETL	21	21	3	19			2
BW	31.25	31.25	41.67	31.25	62.50	62.50	31.25
Slice thickness	5.0	5.0	5.0	5.0	5.0	5.0	5.0
Slice spacing	1.0	1.0	1.0	1.0	−2.5	1.0	1.0
FOV	24	32	32	32	35	32	32
Matrix	320 × 256	320 × 288	384 × 288	320 × 256	288 × 192	320 × 224	352 × 224
NEX/NSA	4	2	2	3	1	2	2
Frequent direction	A–P	R–L	R–L	S–I	R–L	S–I	R–L
Flip angle					12	80	
Parallel imaging	Off	Off	Off	Off	On	Off	Off

Graphical Prescription

Figures 9.21–9.23.

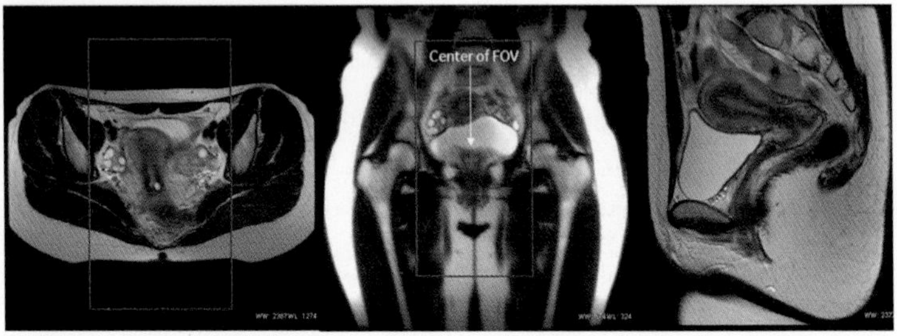

Figure 9.21 Sagittal prescription from axial and coronal images is shown.

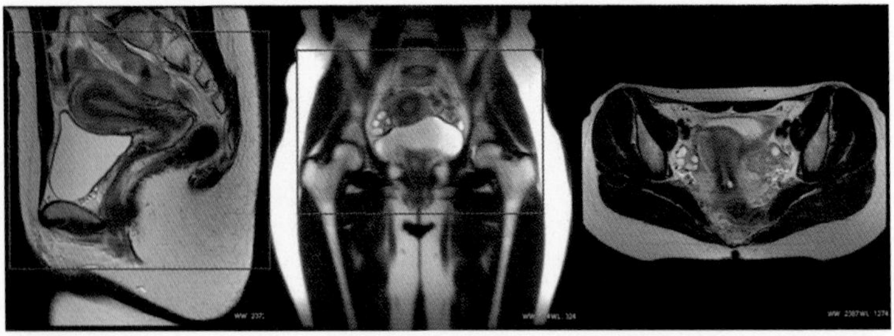

Figure 9.22 Axial planning from sagittal and coronal images is shown.

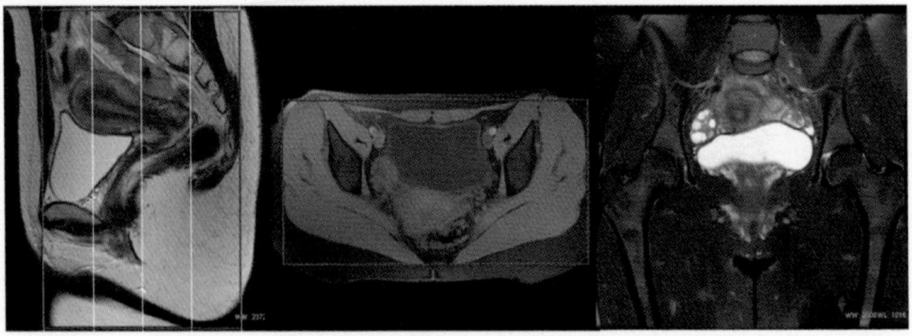

Figure 9.23 Coronal prescription from sagittal and axial images is shown.

Chapter 10

Cardiovascular Imaging: MRI Protocols, Imaging Parameters, and Graphical Prescriptions

Cardiac and vascular imaging applications are usually combined under the more general title of cardiovascular imaging applications. Vascular MR application is done with a variety of pulse sequences to create MR angiography (MRA). Most of the MRA applications provide the best quality image with contrast injection due to T1 shortening of contrast agents. However, due to nephrogenic systemic fibrosis (NSF) case reported within the last few years, there is a renewed interest in noncontrast enhanced MRA applications and all vendors made significant progress creating excellent MRA images without contrast agent. At the same time, new techniques made it possible to produce high-quality MRA images with even lesser contrast injection. Even though multislice CT has an advantage over MRI with its higher resolution and shorter scan times, it requires a higher dose of contrast injection. The hardware and software advances in MRI make vascular MR imaging a very interesting application.

Cardiac MR imaging is still a relatively small portion of routine clinical MR imaging. However, recent hardware and software developments bring more exposure to cardiac imaging in both radiology and cardiology departments. Tissue viability and perfusion imaging the main strengths of cardiac MRI and MR ejection fraction measurement are considered to be the gold standard as of today. Coronary MR imaging also made significant progress and produces very impressive images. We believe that cardiac MR imaging application will be more common in near future with more interdepartmental collaboration.

M. Elmaoğlu and A. Çelik, *MRI Handbook: MR Physics, Patient Positioning, and Protocols*, DOI 10.1007/978-1-4614-1096-6_10,

In this chapter, cardiac and vascular application will be covered with the same structure given in earlier chapters for easier organization and follow-up. For each section, we will discuss patient preparation, patient positioning, imaging protocols, graphical prescriptions, and sample imaging parameters.

Cardiac MR Imaging

Cardiac MR imaging can be performed in part using sequences available at most of the new scanners. However, full cardiac imaging requires special sequences purchased for cardiac examinations. ECG gating and PG gating options should be available as well. The main difficulty of cardiac MR examinations is the need for repeated breath holds due to the obvious need of eliminating the respiratory artifacts. Parallel imaging, similar to abdominal imaging, is also used often for cardiac imaging to reduce the breath holding time and relatively total scan time. Cardiac imaging is a relatively long MRI exam. You may expect a full cardiac exam anywhere from 30 min to 1 h depending on the suspected pathology.

Before we start the cardiac exam preparation and planning, we would like to review the key cardiac concepts and sequences below:

- *Cardiac slice prescription*: Cardiac imaging requires multiple breath holds to obtain good image quality. Due to the shape of the heart, cardiac planes are separated into long axis and short axis acquisitions. Long axis scans are generally either 2 chamber view (2CV) showing one ventricle and one atrium or 4 chamber view (4CV) showing all four chambers (left ventricle, left atrium, right ventricle, and right atrium) of the heart. However, multiple orientations to look at valves, outflow tracts, and coronary imaging planes can be required for a detailed cardiac exam depending on the suspected pathology.
- *Real-time imaging*: Cardiac imaging requires an accurate localization of long axis and short axis planes. This can be achieved with non-breath holds balanced sequence (Fiesta, TrueFISP, and b-FFE) examinations in axial view, 2CV, 4CV, and short axis views. However, gradient echo or balanced gradient echo based real-time imaging can significantly shorten the cardiac plane localization with free breathing.
- *Function or morphology*: Fast imaging techniques, especially, balanced gradient sequences such as Fiesta, can provide excellent image quality for cardiac imaging. These sequences are called as bright blood sequences since the blood has hyper signal. They provide excellent contrast between blood

pool and myocardial tissue. Therefore, they are used very frequently for morphological imaging to visualize the cardiac anatomy. They are also used in CINE mode to rapidly acquire multiple cardiac phases of the same slice location. With more than ten images per second per frame visual assessment of functional myocardial defects (myocardial wall motion abnormalities) can be done with this sequence. Ejection fraction measurement in MRI can be done in CINE mode with fiesta-like sequences. For ejection fraction, the short axis slices to cover the entire left ventricle from base to apex has to be covered. Depending on the patient condition, parallel method, and protocol, entire heart can be covered within a single breat hold or multiple breath holds.

- *Perfusion*: MR imaging of the heart can be done dynamically (multiple times) during the passage of contrast agent. This technique is called time course imaging or perfusion imaging. The dynamic perfusion images are used to visualize the myocardiac perfusion defects. Specifically, healthy myocardiac tissue signal will be hyperintense due to contrast presence while the infarcted tissue signal will be hypointense due to lack of contrast presence. Contrary to T2 weighted in brain dynamic time course imaging with EPI sequences, cardiac perfusion imaging is a T1 weighted technique and can be done with fast gradient echo techniques employing a single echo (FGRE) or multiple echoes (FGRE-ET). Cardiac perfusion imaging is done usually with 30–40 repetitions (around 60 s total time) with a 2 s temporal resolution. A single dose of contrast injection is performed 6–8 s after the starting time of the sequence to acquire some precontrast images. For the perfusion exam, shallow breathing or breath holds are recommended. Shallow breathing is preferred if the patient is unable to hold breath at all and requires shallow breathing for the duration of perfusion exam. For the breath hold perfusion exams, the patient holds the breath as long as he/she can and then breathes shallowly until to the end. The contrast injection for myocardial perfusion should be done fast (4–5 mL/s).
- *Myocardial delayed enhancement (MDE) or viability imaging*: Myocardial delayed enhancement sequences are designed to show the myocardial infarct enhancement postcontrast. Fast gradient echo sequences with an additional inversion pulse are used for viability or MDE imaging. The inversion pulses in MDE sequences are used to suppress healthy myocardial tissue using a user selected inversion time (TI) as shown in Fig. 10.1. The injected contrast agent will wash in and wash out the infarcted tissue much later than the healthy myocardial tissue. Therefore, 5–10 min after the

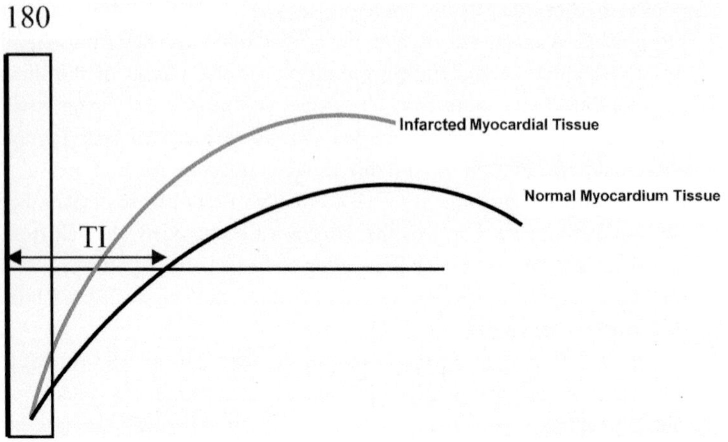

Figure 10.1 Signal enhancement of normal and infracted myocardial tissue after an inversion recovery pulse for viability imaging.

contrast injection, the normal myocardium can be suppressed and only the myocardiac infract, having higher contrast concentration, can be visualized effectively with the MDE sequences. MDE sequences require an optimum selection of TI time to fully suppress the health myocardium. Otherwise, visualization of the infarct would be more difficult. As a general guideline, the TI time can be around 220 ms 10 min postcontrast for a double dose injection. Optimum TI time can be selected using one of the TI sweeping sequences acquiring multiple TI times in a single breath hold. However, if your scanner does not have this type of sequence, you may have to scan a single slice with different TI times to find out the optimum value. MDE sequences can be either 2D or 3D, you can use either sequence for MDE imaging. MDE imaging can be done both in short and long axis for a better localization of the infarct and its extension.

In Fig. 10.2, MDE sequence acquired with different TI times are shown. The images on the top row show an optimum TI time of 200 ms to suppress the healthy myocardium and perfectly delineate the infarct area shown (pointed with the arrow). Some hospitals also use what is called a short TI time to invert the contrast of infarcted tissue to eliminate potential artifacts. For example, if you use a TI time of 100 ms as shown on bottom row of Fig. 10.2, you can

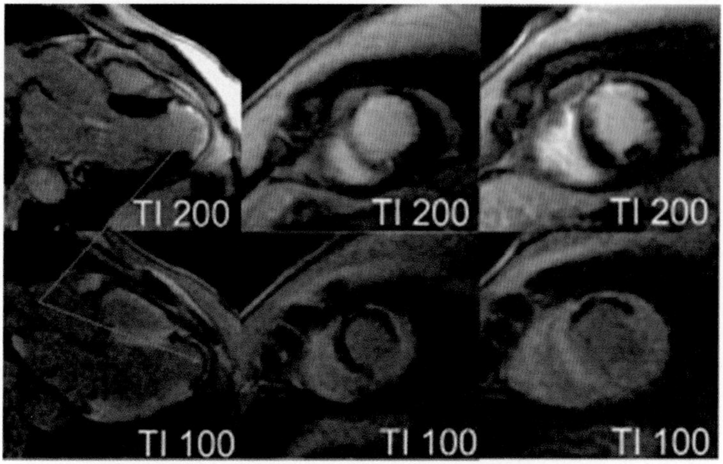

Figure 10.2 Optimal TI time and short TI acquisition images are shown.

end up with hypointensity infarcted signal. This method is helpful to correlate the infarcted myocardial tissue and papillary muscles where the contrast agent itself may mimic the pathology particularly for endocardium.

Patient Preparation and Positioning

Patient preparation: The patient consent form should be given to the patient with a detailed explanation on the content. The form should be carefully read, all questions must be answered with clear answers such as "YES" or "NO," and additional clarifications should be written. It must be signed by the patient or legal guardians and confirmed by MR personnel. If there are any surgical implants, radiologist on duty has to make a decision based on implant type and MR compatibility. *If there is any suspicion or lack of information on the implant, do not take any risk with the patient safety and do not scan the patient.* If the form is complete with all the information, the patient should change to MR gown and remove any clothing with any metal. If you need to place the cardiac electrodes, the medical gown should have an opening on the chest to place electrodes and connect the cables. It is always a good practice to remove the jewelry as well. As the last line of patient safety, it is also a good practice to scan patient with a handheld metal detector before taking the patient to MR room.

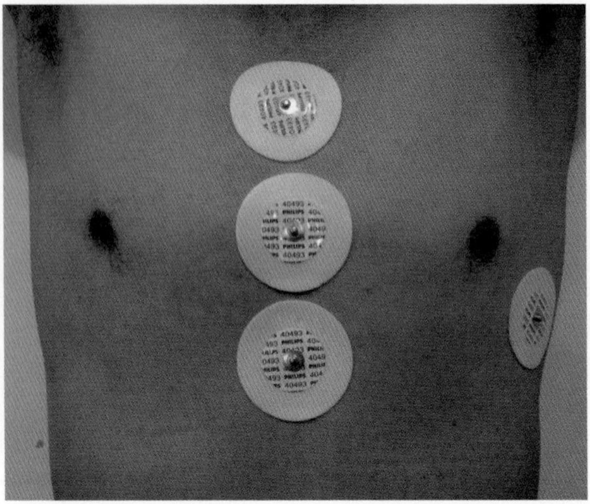

Figure 10.3 Sample ECG connection methods for cardiac gated exams. The ECG placement can be different for different MR vendors.

ECG gating and electrode placement: The ECG electrodes can be placed in a few different ways. Two alternative connection methods for standard cardiac gating are shown in Figs. 10.2 and 10.3. If you have what is called vector gating, then you can use vector gating by default since it provides a more reliable cardiac gating. As a golden rule, the electrodes should be placed on the chest to left side of sternum and on the tissue between ribs. The skin should be cleaned well to remove the dead skin layer for better connectivity. The exact ECG connection shape can be slightly different for each vendor and you should follow the proper connection guidelines given in your systems manual (Fig. 10.4).

Navigator gating: Navigator technique is based on detecting the abdominal wall motion using a 1D or 2D navigator slice. Therefore, it does not require any additional hardware for respirator monitoring. It has been used in cardiac imaging especially for coronary imaging.

Breath hold: Instruct the patient how a proper breath holding should be done and do some practices before the exam. Recommend expiration breath holds for better results.

Patient positioning: Place the coil straight at the center of the MR table. Then you position the patient supine on the coil while the arms are raised above the head unless there is a physical restriction (pain, age, etc.). The coil center should align with the center of breast mass for females and nipple for male patients.

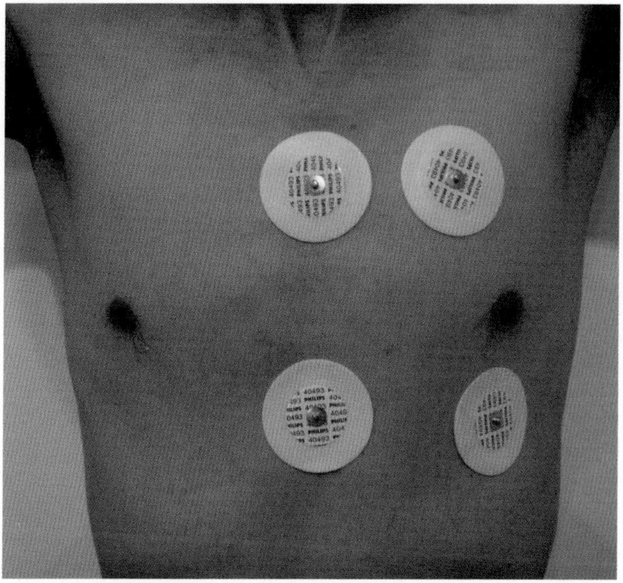

Figure 10.4 Sample ECG connection methods for cardiac gated exams. The ECG placement can be different for different MR vendors.

Please make sure that you give the patient alarm/buzzer to patient's hand and test it before sending in. After landmarking the center of coil using laser lights or touch sensors, you can send the patient in and start the exam. It is always recommended to let the patient know how long the scan is going to take and also keep communicating frequently to make them as comfortable as possible in the MR bore.

Sample Imaging Protocols

A sample imaging protocol for a patient referred to the MRI for cardiac examination is given below (Table 10.1 and Fig. 10.5).

Sample Imaging Parameters for 1.5T

Table 10.2.

Table 10.1 A sample routine cardiac protocol.

Sequences	Comments	Slice order
3 Plane localizer	Acquire 5 breath hold slices in each plane	
Real Time	Free breathing real time sequence is used to acquire multiple plane's cardiac scout images	
Axial T1-BB	Prescribe straight axial slices only for the region of interest. The black blood sequence is breath hold and cardiac gated	S–I
Axial STIR BB	Same as above	S–I
2D Fiesta long axis	Prescribe 2D Fiesta sequence for long axis morphological imaging such as 2, 3, or 4 chamber views	–
2D Fiesta short axis	Prescribe 2D Fiesta sequence for short axis morphological (functional) imaging for ejection fraction calculation	–
FGRE-ET time course	Multiphase time course imaging is used for cardiac perfusion	–
2D MDE	Prescribe short axis or long axis viability sequence	–

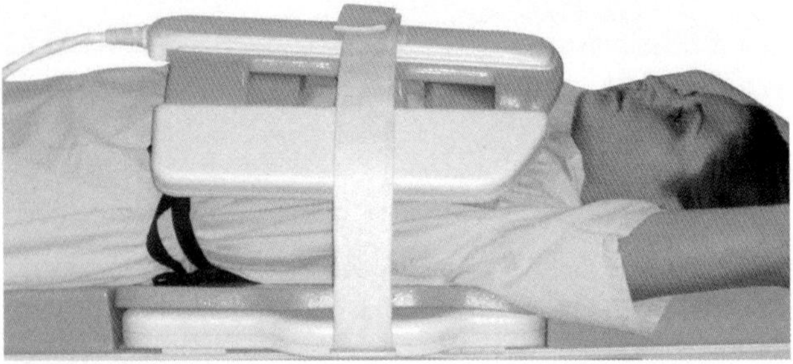

Figure 10.5 A sample feet-first and supine patient cardiac exam positioning in a multichannel coil is shown.

Table 10.2 Sample cardiac imaging parameters are given for a multichannel cardiac coil.

	T1 BB	STIR BB	Cine	Perfusion	2D MDE	T1BB FS	Flow
Plane	Oblique	Oblique	SA	SA	SA	Oblique	Oblique
Sequence	FSE	FSE	Fiesta	FGRE	FGRE-IR	FSE	2D PC
TE	42	42	MinFull	Min	Min	MinFull	MinFull
TR	Auto	Auto	Auto	Auto	Auto	Auto	Auto

(continued)

Table 10.2 (continued)

	T1 BB	STIR BB	Cine	Perfusion	2D MDE	T1BB FS	Flow
ETL	32	32		4		4	
BW	62.5	62.5	125	125	31.25	62.5	15.63
Slice thickness	8.0	8.0	8.0	8.0	8.0	8.0	10.0
Slice spacing	1.0	1.0	0.0	1.0	1.0	1.0	0.0
FOV	40	40	35	35	35	35	40
Matrix	352 × 256	288 × 256	256 × 256	128 × 128	224 × 160	288 × 224	256 × 128
NEX/NSA	1	1	1	1	2	1	1
Frequent direction	R–L	R–L	R–L	S–I	S–I	R–L	R–L
TI/TI	Auto	Auto/150					
Gating/FA	Acık/BH	Acık/BH	BH/45	BH/25	BH/20	BH	BH
Parallel imaging	On	Off	On	Off	Off	On	Off

Graphical Prescription

See Fig. 10.6.

Brain MR Angiography

Brain MRA can be done with either noncontrast enhanced or contrast enhanced imaging techniques. Noncontrast enhanced MRA techniques can be based on either time-of-flight (TOF) effect or phase contrast (PC). Noncontrast MRA techniques can be either 2D or 3D acquisition modes. Contrast enhanced MR angiography (CE-MRA) techniques can be either modified 3D fast gradient echo based (FSPGR, TURBO FLASH, or fast field echo) or so-called 4D imaging sequences such as TRICKS, TWIST, or CENTRA. Before we start patient positioning, let us review the main MRA sequences and how they do work.

Time-of-Flight MR Angiography

TOF sequences are one of the most commonly used sequences for noncontrast MRA. 2D and 3D TOF technique is used to differentiate the stationary tissue and moving protons inside the blood vessels. This can be accomplished saturating the background signal in the slice that is to be imaged with rapid RF pulses. Since the fresh incoming blood supplies a significant amount of spins which has not *seen* the rapid RF pulses, the blood vessels would have a quite bright signal while the stationary tissue signal is almost completely eliminated.

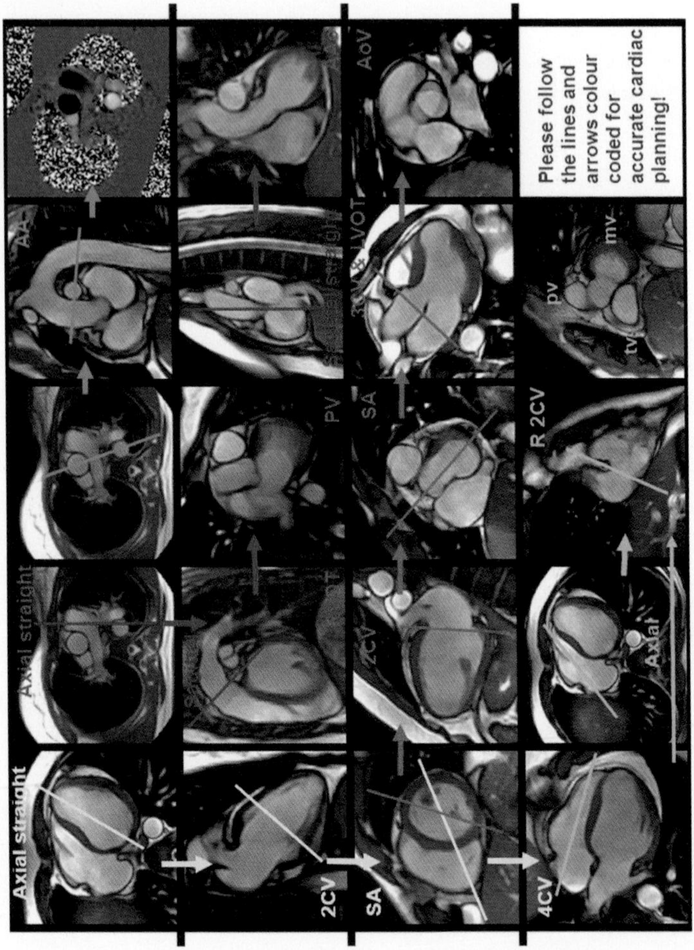

Figure 10.6 Various imaging planes for cardiovascular MR Exams are shown.

TOF sequences almost always use gradient echo pulse sequence family with relatively small flip angle to be able to create a series of *rapid RF pulses.* As it can be obvious to some of the readers, we can maximize the signal from blood if we choose the slice orientation perpendicular to the blood vessels. In this case, the time of travel (or TOF) of blood vessels will be the shortest and they will see only very few RF pulses during their travel within the slice. If we choose a slice orientation parallel to the blood vessel, the TOF of blood spins will be the longest and they too will be saturated by the rapid RF pulses.

One of the biggest advantages of TOF technique is that it can be used to visualize veins, arteries, or both. To selectively visualize arteries or veins, the user is requested to place a saturation band. For example, if you want to visualize Circle of Willis (COW) polygon, you need to put a saturation band superior to the 3D slab of interest. However, due to considerably slower blood in veins, TOF techniques do not produce very good image quality. Even though 2D TOF techniques are used for sagittal and transverse sinus imaging, other techniques including phase contrast and contrast enhanced 3D techniques provide superior image quality.

3D TOF techniques in the brain can be used with fat sat and magnetization transfer options. Fat sat improves the vascular visualization in orbital regions. MT pulse can be used to further suppress the stationary brain tissue and provide better contrast between blood and stationary tissue. However, both these options increase the scan time. Flow compensation option and spatial resolution interpolations such as ZIP2, ZIP4, ZIP 512, or ZIP 1024 or REM (resolution extended matrix) can provide a better image quality at no time penalty. Parallel imaging techniques can be used to further reduce the scan time as well.

Phase Contrast MR Angiography

Phase contrast MR angiography (PC MRA) has been known and used since the early days of MRI. Phase contrast technique is based on the principle that *flowing blood in the body produces a different phase than stationary tissue and this phase is proportional to the direction and velocity of the flow.* Therefore, phase contrast angiography can be used to visualize arteries and veins of the brain by eliminating signal from stationary tissues in the background using the phase information. However, in phase contrast techniques, the user should have an estimate of velocity of the vessels of interest for best image quality. This value as called velocity encoding (VENC) is required to optimize the dynamic range of phase information we will get with phase contrast techniques. Due to renewed interest in noncontrast MRA applications, phase contrast technique has been used more commonly in clinical practice now.

Contrast Enhanced MR Angiography

Let us remind you again that CE-MRA imaging requires the off-label use of contrast agents. Contrast enhanced MR angiography (CE-MRA) techniques for brain vasculature can be either 3D or 4D. 3D CE-MRA is not used often for brain MRA. However, 4D techniques can be used for especially brain arterio-venous malformations (AVM) due to their superior temporal resolution, which can be around a fraction of a second.

Patient Preparation and Positioning

Patient preparation: The patient consent form should be given to the patient with a detailed explanation on the content. The form should be carefully read, all questions must be answered with clear answers such as "YES" or "NO," and additional clarifications should be written. It must be signed by the patient or legal guardians and confirmed by MR personnel. If there are any surgical implants, radiologist on duty has to make a decision based on implant type and MR compatibility. *If there is any suspicion or lack of information on the implant, do not take any risk with the patient safety and do not scan the patient.* If the form is complete with all the information, the patient should change to MR gown and remove any clothing with any metal. It is always a good practice to remove the jewelry as well. As the last line of patient safety, it is also a good practice to scan patient with a handheld metal detector before taking the patient to MR room.

Patient positioning: Place the coil on the table and position the patient like a routine brain imaging.

Please make sure that you give the alarm/buzzer to patient's hand and test it before sending in. After landmarking the center of coil using laser lights or touch sensors, you can send the patient in and start the exam. It is always recommended to let the patient know how long the scan is going to take and also keep communicating frequently to make them as comfortable as possible in the MR bore (Fig. 10.7).

Sample Imaging Protocols

A sample imaging protocol for a patient referred to the MRI for brain MRA examination is given below (Table 10.3).

Sample Imaging Parameters for 1.5T

Table 10.4.

Graphical Prescription

See Figs. 10.8–10.11.

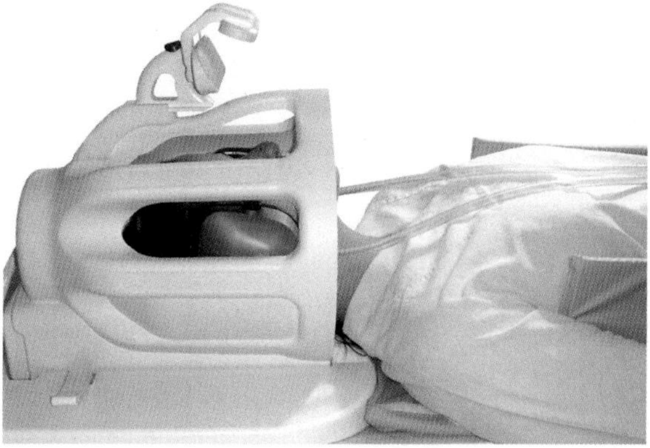

Figure 10.7 A sample patient positioning in a multichannel brain coil.

Table 10.3 Routine brain MRA protocols and prescription planes for multiple MRA techniques. Depending on the MRA request, these MRA sequences can be applied separately or in combination.

Sequences	Comments	Slice order
3 Plane localizer	Acquire 5 slices in each plane	
Axial 3D TOF	Prescribe straight axial slices. Place saturation band superiorly outside the slab for arterial imaging	S–I
Coronal 2DTOF	Prescribe coronal thin slices especially for sagittal sinus venography. Place inferior SAT band	P–A
Sagittal 2D PC MRA	Prescribe a single thick slice parallel to midbrain line. Choose a venc of 15–25 cm/s	
Axial 3D PC MRA	Prescribe an axial 3D slab to cover the transverse sinuses. Choose a venc of 15–25 cm/s	S–I
Axial TRICKS	Prescribe axial slices for the region of interest. Smaller coverage provides better temporal resolution. Choose 15–20 phases minimum	S–I
Coronal TRICKS	Prescribe coronal slices to cover carotids for 9–15 phases	A–P
Sagittal 3D CE-MRV	Prescribe sagittal slices to cover the whole brain	R–L

Table 10.4 Sample of brain MRA parameters in a multichannel brain coil is given.

	3D TOF arterial	2D TOF venous	3D PC arteries/ venous	2D PC venous	TRICKS/ CENTRA	3D CE MRA	3D CE MRV
Plane	Axial	Coronal	Axial	Sagittal	Axial	Coronal	Sagittal
Sequence	TOF	TOF	PC	PC	TRICKS	FSPGR	FSPGR
TE	Min	Min	Min	Min	Min	Min	MinFull
TR	Min	Min	20	50	Auto	Auto	Auto
BW	31.25	31.25	15.63	15.63	83.33	62.50	31.25
Slice thickness	1.2	1.5	3	60	2.2	1.8	1.4
Slice spacing	−0.6	0	0	0	−1.1	−0.9	−0.7
FOV/phase FOV	20	22	22	22	25	26/0.75	24.0
Matrix	544 × 352	320 × 160	256 × 192	256 × 192	256 × 160	352 × 256	320 × 320
NEX/NSA	1	1	1	4	0.75	1	1
Frequent direction	A–P	S–I	A–P	S–I	A–P	S–I	S–I
VENC/number of temporal phase			80–20	Venc:20	9 Phases	2 Phases	
Gating/FA	25	45	PG/20	PG/20	30	30	30
k-space order						Elliptical centric	Elliptical centric

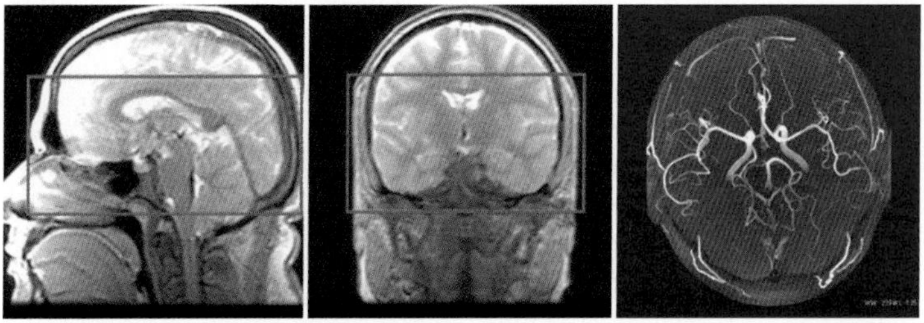

Figure 10.8 Axial 3D TOF brain MRA planning from sagittal and coronal images is shown.

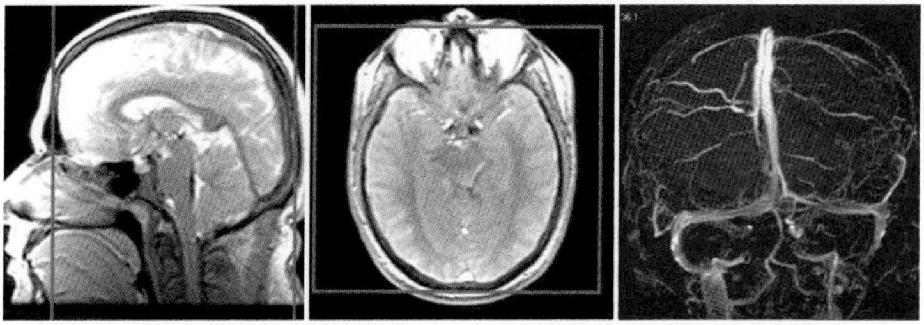

Figure 10.9 Coronal 2D TOF venous MRA planning from sagittal and axial images is shown.

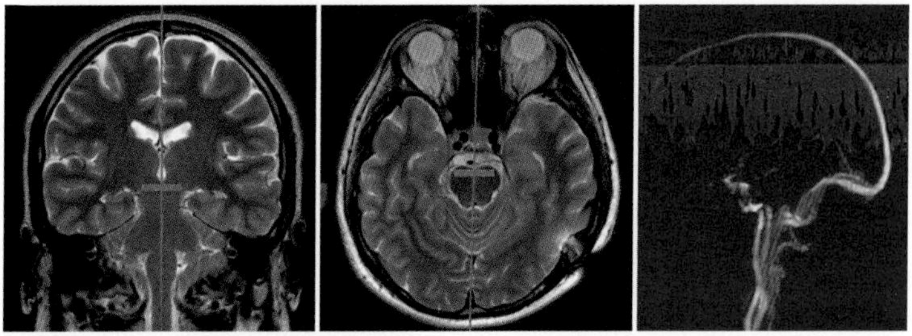

Figure 10.10 Sagittal PC MRA planning from coronal and axial images is shown.

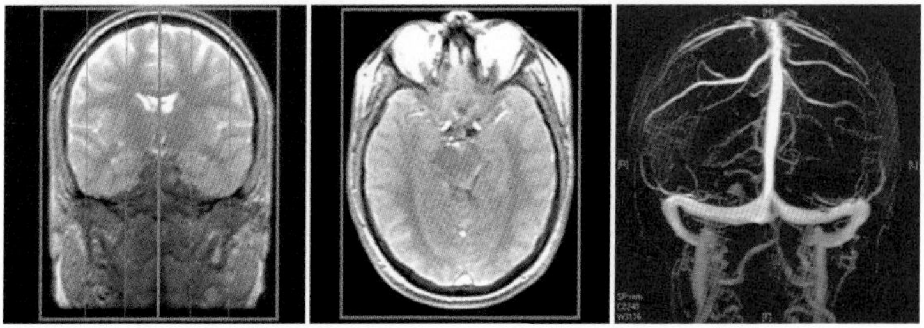

Figure 10.11 Sagittal 3D CE-MRV planning from coronal and axial images is shown.

Carotid MR Angiography

Carotid MRA can be done using the same sequences used for brain MRA. 3D time-of-flight MR angiography (TOF MRA) should be prescribed with multiple overlapping of thin slab acquisitions (MOTSA) to get better image quality. Due to faster blood flow in the carotids and turbulent flow pattern at bifurcation, TOF sequences are more prone to TOF artifacts in carotid MRA. Therefore, 3D CE-MRA and/or TRICKS like sequences are used more commonly for carotid imaging. The recently developed Non Contrast Enhanced (NCE) MRA techniques can also provide impressive results for carotid MRA imaging. If your machine has those new sequences, you can also use the vendor recommended protocols.

Patient Preparation and Positioning

Patient preparation: The patient consent form should be given to the patient with a detailed explanation on the content. The form should be carefully read, all questions must be answered with clear answers such as "YES" or "NO," and additional clarifications should be written. It must be signed by the patient or legal guardians and confirmed by MR personnel. If there are any surgical implants, radiologist on duty has to make a decision based on implant type and MR compatibility. *If there is any suspicion or lack of information on the implant, do not take any risk with the patient safety and do not scan the patient.* If the form is complete with all the information, the patient should change to MR gown and remove any clothing with any metal. It is always a good practice to remove the jewelry as well. As the last line of patient safety, it is also a good practice to scan patient with a handheld metal detector before taking the patient to MR room.

Patient positioning: For carotid MRA imaging, neurovascular coils covering the anterior and posterior portions of the neck or volume neck coils should be used. If your site does not have a specific coil for this purpose, cervical spine coil can be used with some anterior signal loss penalty. Proper patient positioning for the neurovascular coil is shown below.

Please make sure that you give the alarm/buzzer to patient's hand and test it before sending in. After landmarking the center of coil using laser lights or touch sensors, you can send the patient in and start the exam. It is always recommended to let the patient know how long the scan is going to take and also keep communicating frequently to make them as comfortable as possible in the MR bore (Fig. 10.12).

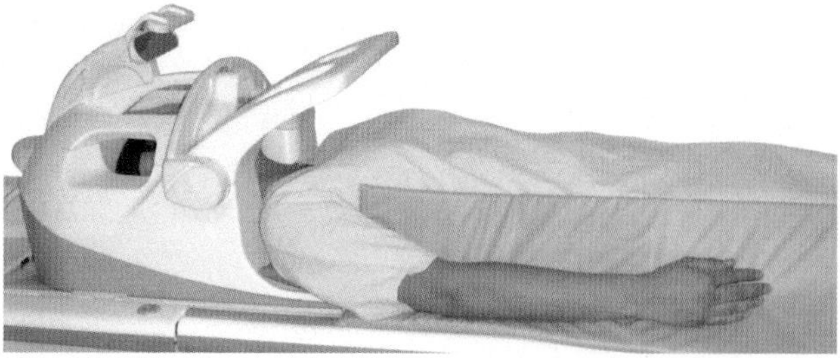

Figure 10.12 **A sample carotid MRA patient positioning in a multichannel neurovascular coil is shown.**

Table 10.5 Routine carotid MRA protocols and prescription planes for multiple MRA techniques are shown.

Sequences	Comments	Slice order
3 Plane localizer	Acquire 9–11 slices in each plane	
Axial 3D TOF	Prescribe multislab axial slices. Place saturation band superiorly outside the slab for arterial imaging	S–I
Axial 2D TOF	Prescribe axial slices without gating for carotid MRA. Use concatenated saturation pulse superiorly if available	S–I
Axial 2D TOF venous	Prescribe axial slices for venous imaging. Place the saturation band inferiorly	I–S
Coronal 3D PC MRA	Prescribe coronal slices to cover the carotids. Choose a venc of 60–80 cm/s for arteries and 15–25 for venous	A–P
Coronal TRICKS	Prescribe coronal slices to cover carotids for 10–15 phases	A–P
Coronal 3D CE	Prescribe coronal slices to cover carotids with 1.0–2.0 mm slice thickness	A–P

Sample Imaging Protocols

A sample imaging protocol for a patient referred to the MRI for carotid MRA examination is given below (Table 10.5).

Sample Imaging Parameters for 1.5T

Table 10.6.

Graphical Prescription

See Figs. 10.13 and 10.14.

Table 10.6 Routine carotid MRA imaging parameters for a multichannel neurovascular coil is given.

	3D TOF arterial	2D TOF arterial	3D PC arteries/ venous	2D PC arterial	TRICKS (CE)	3D CE MRA
Plane	Axial	Axial	Coronal	Coronal	Coronal	Coronal
Sequence	TOF	TOF	PC	PC	TRICKS	FSPGR
TE	6.9	Min	Min	Min	Min	Min
TR	Min	Min	20	33	Auto	Auto
BW	15.63	31.25	15.63	15.63	83.33	62.5
Slice thickness	2.4	2.0	3.0	20	2.8	1.8
Slice s pacing	−1.2	0.0	0.0	0	−1.4	−0.9
FOV	20	20	27	28	27	32
Matrix	256 × 160	256 × 160	256 × 192	256 × 160	288 × 160	352 × 320
NEX/NSA	1	1	1	4	0.75	1
Frequent direction	R–L	R–L	S–I	S–I	S–I	S–I
Venc/number of phases			Arteries: 70–80; Venous: 15–25	60/	/13	/2
Gating/FA	FA:20	45	PG/20	PG/20	30	30
k-space					4D	Elliptical centric

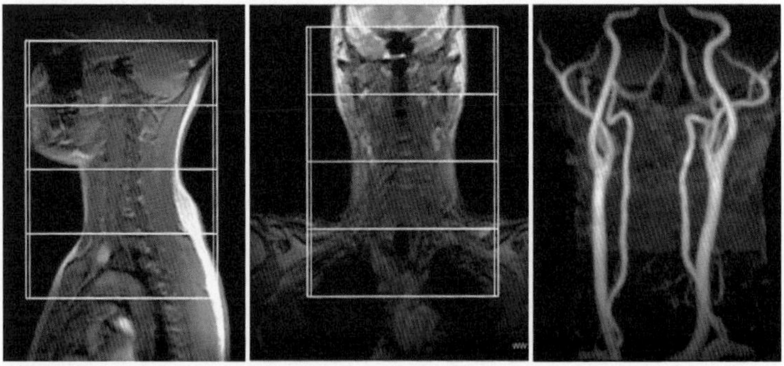

Figure 10.13 Axial multislab 3D TOF carotid MRA planning from sagittal and coronal images is shown.

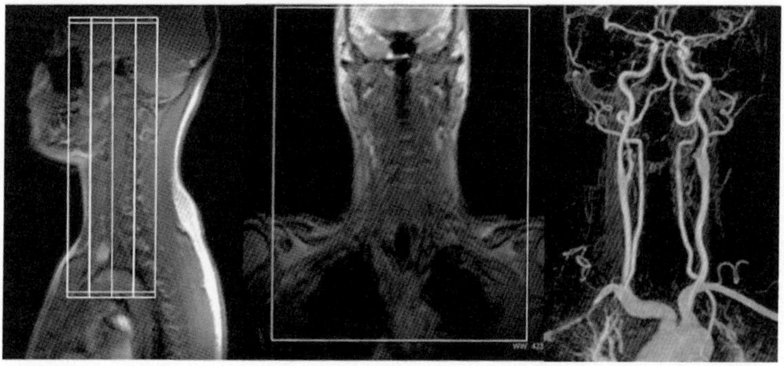

Figure 10.14 Coronal 3D CE carotid MRA planning from sagittal and coronal scout images is shown.

Pulmonary Angiography

Pulmonary MRA can be done either with 3D CE-FSPGR techniques or with 4D techniques such as TRICKS/TWIST/CENTRA. Both techniques can provide very nice image quality. However, 4D CE-MRA techniques are more powerful due to additional dynamic information they provide.

Let's take a quick look at these two techniques and how they are applied: *TRICKS/TWIST/CENTRA*: Pulmonary MRA is commonly prescribed in coronal plane to cover pulmonary vessels of the chest. These techniques are so called view sharing techniques manipulating k-space data ordering and sharing the k-space between different acquisitions. They acquire a noncontrast mask image to acquire the full data and k-space and the system pauses for contrast injection. Then the contrast injection starts and within the few seconds of breath hold, multiphase 4D MRA acquisition starts. In this operation, MR operator has to be careful with the timings of breath hold and contrast injection. 4D-based techniques can provide automatic MIP images of every single postcontrast phase with either background subtraction or no subtraction.

3D FSPGR CE: If you are using one of the contrast detection approaches such as smart prep, the tracker should be placed at pulmonary aorta. Due to the fast blood flow in pulmonary vessels, the breath hold instructions are given right after the injection, so that the system starts acquiring data right after the contrast detection. Real-time contrast triggering techniques such as fluoro triggering may require more experience. Some users may use a fixed delay time for postinjection such as 8–9 s and start the breath hold acquisition in the fixed time frame. However, fixed time delays are problematic with different pathologies. The acquisition time for 3D CE-MRA sequences should be less than 18 s or less for optimal quality.

The contrast injection amount and rate is also important for CE-MRA and will be discussing the contrast injection dynamics later in the chapter.

Patient Preparation and Positioning

Patient preparation: The patient consent form should be given to the patient with a detailed explanation on the content. The form should be carefully read, all questions must be answered with clear answers such as "YES" or "NO," and additional clarifications should be written. It must be signed by the patient or legal guardians and confirmed by MR personnel. If there are any surgical implants, radiologist on duty has to make a decision based on implant type and MR compatibility. *If there is any suspicion or lack of information on the implant, do not take any risk with the patient safety and do not scan the patient.* If the form is complete with all the information, the patient should change to MR gown and remove any clothing with any metal. It is always a good practice to remove the jewelry as well. As the last line of patient safety, it is also a good practice to scan patient with a handheld metal detector before taking the patient to MR room.

Patient positioning: For pulmonary MRA imaging, place the body or cardiac coil straight at the center of the MR table. Then you position the patient supine on the coil while the arms are raised above the head unless there is a physical restriction (pain, age, etc.). The coil center should align with the center of sternum.

Please make sure that you give the alarm/buzzer to patient's hand and test it before sending in. After landmarking the center of coil using laser lights or touch sensors, you can send the patient in and start the exam. It is always recommended to let the patient know how long the scan is going to take and also keep communicating frequently to make them as comfortable as possible in the MR bore (Fig. 10.15).

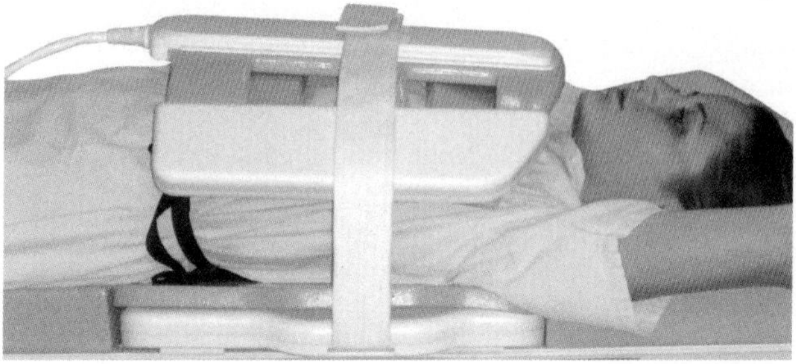

Figure 10.15 **Patient positioning for pulmonary MRA in a multichannel coil is shown.**

Table 10.7 Routine pulmonary MRA protocols and prescription planes for multiple MRA techniques are shown.

Sequences	Comments	Slice order
3 Plane localizer	Acquire 5–7 slices in each plane	
Axial 2D TOF Scout	Prescribe axial slices without gating for localizer pulmonary MRA. Use MIPs for coronal planning	S–I
Coronal TRICKS/TWIST/CENTRA	Prescribe coronal slices to cover pulmonary vessels for 9–15 phases depending on patient's breath hold ability. Use 2D TOF MIP as well as scout	A–P
3D FSPGR CE-MRA	Prescribe coronal slices to cover pulmonary vessels	A–P

Sample Imaging Protocols

A sample imaging protocol for a patient referred to the MRI for pulmonary MRA examination is given below (Table 10.7).

Sample Imaging Parameters for 1.5T and 3.0T

Table 10.8.

Graphical Prescription

See Fig. 10.16.

Table 10.8 Routine pulmonary MRA parameters for different sequences in a multichannel coil for 1.5 and 3.0T are given.

	1.5T	1.5T	3.0T	3.0T
	TRICKS/TWIST/ CENTRA	3D FSPGR CE	TRICKS/TWIST/ CENTRA	3D FSPGR CE
Plane	Coronal	Coronal	Coronal	Coronal
Sequence	TRICKS	FSPGR	TRICKS	FSPGR
TE	Min	Min	Min	Min
TR	Auto	Auto	Auto	Auto
BW	125.00	62.5	83.33	83.33
Slice thickness	4	3.0	3.0	3.2
Slice spacing	−2	−1.5	−1.5	−1.6
FOV	40	40	35	35
Matrix	288×160	320×160	320×160	384×224
NEX/NSA	0.75	1	0.75	1
Frequent direction	S–I	S–I	S–I	S–I
Number of phases	9	2	13	2
FA	10	35	30	25
k-space	4D	Elliptical centric	4D	Elliptical centric
Parallel imaging	OFF	ON	ON	ON

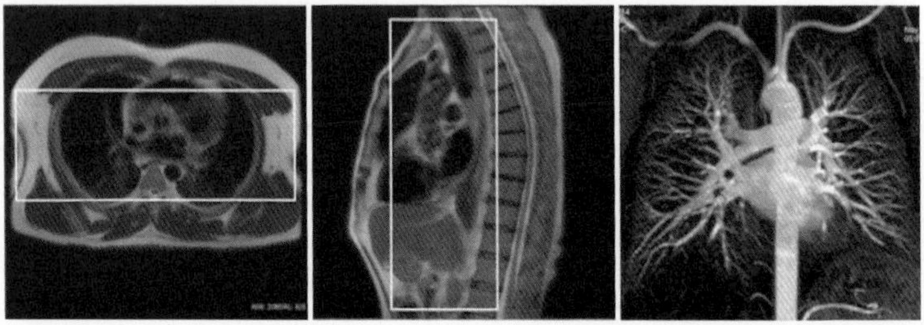

Figure 10.16 Coronal 3D CE pulmonary MRA planning from axial and sagittal images is shown.

Aorta Angiography

Aorta MRA is quite similar for thoracic aorta and abdominal aorta except the contrast timing differences. A majority of aortic MRA techniques use contrast injection even though phase contrast MRA and/or balanced SSFP sequence images can also be used. 2D SSFP techniques such as Fiesta are quite successful for visualizing aortic dissection and/or aneurysm. Non Contrast Enhanced MRA techniques should be used whenever there is a contraindication for contrast injection.

Patient preparation: The patient consent form should be given to the patient with a detailed explanation on the content. The form should be carefully read, all questions must be answered with clear answers such as "YES" or "NO," and additional clarifications should be written. It must be signed by the patient or legal guardians and confirmed by MR personnel. If there are any surgical implants, radiologist on duty has to make a decision based on implant type and MR compatibility. *If there is any suspicion or lack of information on the implant, do not take any risk with the patient safety and do not scan the patient.* If the form is complete with all the information, the patient should change to MR gown and remove any clothing with any metal. It is always a good practice to remove the jewelry as well. As the last line of patient safety, it is also a good practice to scan patient with a handheld metal detector before taking the patient to MR room.

Patient positioning: For pulmonary MRA imaging, place the body or cardiac coil straight at the center of the MR table. Then you position the patient supine on the coil while the arms are raised above the head unless there is a physical restriction (pain, age, etc.). The coil center should align with the center of sternum or to the section of aorta to be imaged.

Please make sure that you give the alarm/buzzer to patient's hand and test it. After landmarking the center of coil using laser lights or touch sensors, you can send the patient in and start the exam. It is always recommended to let the patient know how long the scan is going to take and also keep communicating frequently to make them as comfortable as possible in the MR bore (Fig. 10.17).

Sample Imaging Protocols

Sample imaging protocols for aorta MRA examinations are given below (Table 10.9).

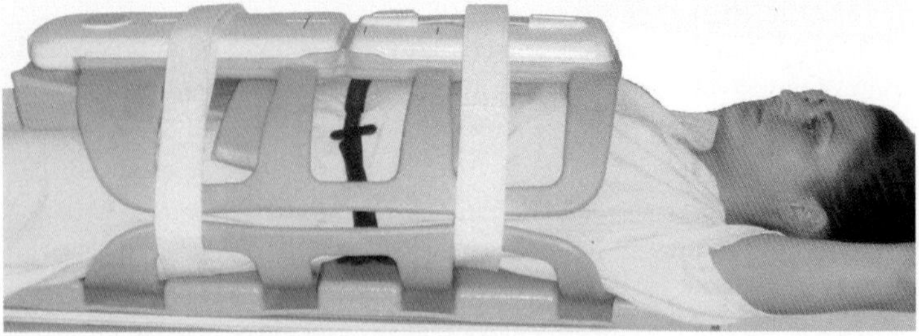

Figure 10.17 A sample aortic MRA patient positioning in a multichannel coil is shown.

Table 10.9 Noncontrast enhanced aorta MRA protocol and prescription planes for aortic dissection and/or aneurysm are shown.

Sequences	Comments	Slice order
3 Plane localizer	Acquire 5–10 slices in each plane	
Axial 2D fiesta	Prescribe axial slices for bright blood imaging	S–I
Sagittal 2D fiesta	Prescribe oblique sagittal slices for thoracic aorta and straight sagittal slices for abdominal aorta	R–L
Coronal 2D fiesta	Prescribe oblique coronal slices parallel to aorta	A–P

Table 10.10 Contrast enhanced aorta MRA protocols and prescription planes for aortic dissection and/or aneurysm are shown.

Sequences	Comments	Slice order
3 Plane localizer	Acquire 5–10 slices in each plane	
Axial 2D TOF scout	Prescribe axial slices without gating as a localizer for aorta MRA. Use MIPs for coronal planning	S–I
3D FSPGR CE	Prescribe coronal slices to cover aorta	A–P

Sample Imaging Parameters for 1.5T

Tables 10.10 and 10.11.

Graphical Prescription

See Table 10.12 and Figs. 10.18 and 10.19.

Table 10.11 Alternative phase contrast–based noncontrast enhanced aorta MRA protocol is shown.

Sequences	Comments	Slice order
3 Plane localizer	Acquire 5–10 slices in each plane	
Axial 2D fiesta	Prescribe axial slices for bright blood imaging	S–I
Sagittal 2D PC	Prescribe sagittal slices for the region of interest and enter a venc value	S–I
Coronal 2D PC	Prescribe coronal slices for the region of interest and enter a venc value	A–P

Table 10.12 Aortic MRA parameters for a multichannel body coil are given.

	Fast TOF	3D CE MRA	2D TOF artery	3D PC arteries/ venous	2D PC Arteries	TRICKS/ TWIST/ CENTRA	2D Fiesta AXIAL, SAGITTAL, Coronal
Plane	Axial	Coronal	Axial	Axial/ coronal	Axial/ coronal	Coronal	Axial
Sequence	TOF	FSPGR	TOF	PC	PC	TRICKS	Fiesta
TE	Min	Min	Min	Min	Min	Min	MinFull
TR	Min	Auto	Min	20	33	Auto	Auto
BW	15.63	41.67	31.25	15.63	15.63	83.33	125.00
Slice thickness	5	3.2	3.0	3.0	20–30	2.8	5.0
Slice spacing	0	−1.6	−1.0	0.0	0.0	−1.4	0.0
FOV	40	40	35	35	35	35	35
Matrix	256×128	352×192	256×160	256×192	256×160	288×160	256×256
NEX/NSA	0.75	0.75	1	1	4	0.75	0.75
Frequent direction	R–L	S–I	A–P	R–L/S–I	R–L/S–I	S–I	R–L
Venc/num ber of phases		/2		70/15	60/	/13	PG/ECG
Gating/FA	45	BH/30	45	PG/20	PG/20	30	45
k-space order		Centric				4D	

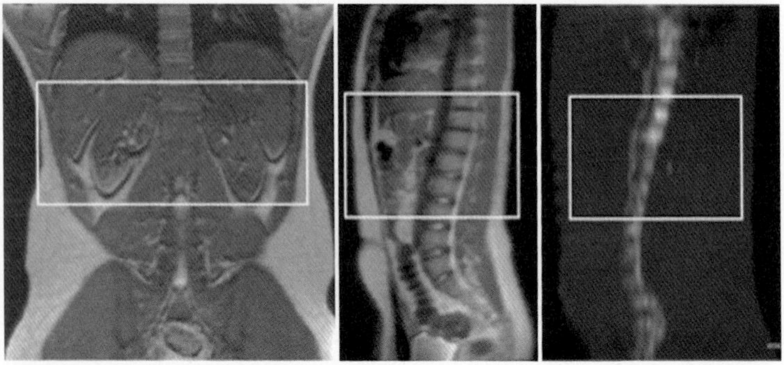

Figure 10.18 Axial 2D PC or 3D PC MRA planning from coronal and sagittal images is shown.

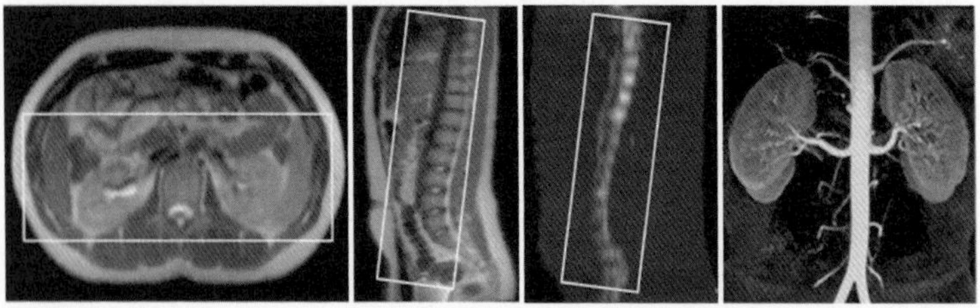

Figure 10.19 3D coronal CE-MRA planning from axial, sagittal, and scout 2D TOF MIP images for abdominal aorta is shown.

Renal MR Angiography

Renal MR angiography procedure is pretty similar to abdominal aorta MRA. A majority of renal MRA techniques uses contrast injection techniques and/or older phase contrast MRA techniques. However, due to higher NSF risk for the patients with renal insufficiency, the recently developed noncontrast MRA techniques using balanced 3D sequences can provide very impressive image quality. Therefore, they open new opportunities for renal MRA and may be applied with respiratory triggering for better patient comfort. We strongly recommend noncontrast-based renal MRA techniques for clinical use. For contrast enhanced renal MRA, 3D fast SPGR techniques are used during the breath hold and provides very good image quality if the patient can hold the breath. 4D dynamic contrast enhanced techniques can also be used for limited applications limited by the patient's ability to hold the breath as well.

Patient preparation: The patient consent form should be given to the patient with a detailed explanation on the content. The form should be carefully read, all questions must be answered with clear answers such as "YES" or "NO," and additional clarifications should be written. It must be signed by the patient or legal guardians and confirmed by MR personnel. If there are any surgical implants, radiologist on duty has to make a decision based on implant type and MR compatibility. *If there is any suspicion or lack of information on the implant, do not take any risk with the patient safety and do not scan the patient.* If the form is complete with all the information, the patient should change to MR gown and remove any clothing with any metal. It is always a good practice to remove the jewelry as well. As the last line of patient safety, it is also a good practice to scan patient with a handheld metal detector before taking the patient to MR room.

Patient positioning: For renal MRA imaging, place the body straight at the center of the MR table. Then you position the patient supine on the coil while the arms are raised above the head unless there is a physical restriction (pain, age, etc.). The coil center should align between the lower end of sternum and belly button. Please make sure that you give the alarm/buzzer to patient's hand and test it. After landmarking the center of coil using laser lights or touch sensors, you can send the patient in and start the exam. It is always recommended to let the patient know how long the scan is going to take and also keep communicating frequently to make them as comfortable as possible in the MR bore (Fig. 10.20).

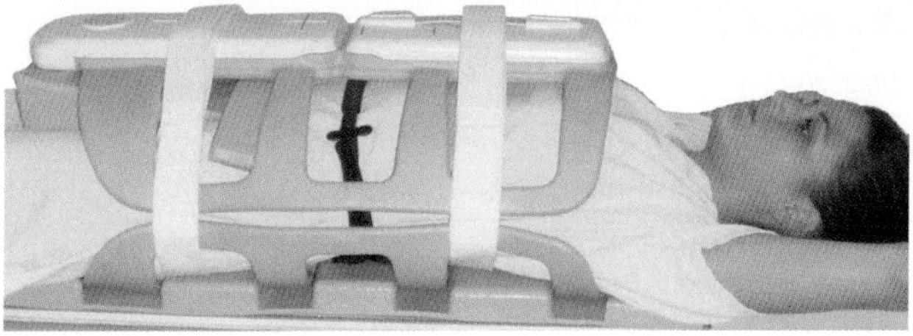

Figure 10.20 A sample renal MRA patient positioning in a multichannel coil is shown.

Sample Imaging Protocols

Sample imaging protocols for renal MRA examination are given below (Tables 10.13–10.15).

Sample Imaging Parameters for 1.5T

Table 10.16.

Table 10.13 A sample of Non Contrast Enhanced (NCE) MRA Protocol and prescription planes for aortic dissection and/or aneurysm are shown.

Sequences	Comments	Slice order
3 Plane localizer	Acquire 5–10 slices in each plane	
Axial 2D TOF scout	Prescribe axial slices without gating as a localizer renal MRA. Use MIPs for coronal planning	S–I
Axial 2D fiesta	Prescribe axial slices for bright blood imaging	S–I
Sagittal 2D fiesta	Prescribe oblique sagittal slices for thoracic aorta and straight sagittal slices for abdominal aorta	R–L
Coronal 2D fiesta	Prescribe oblique coronal slices parallel to aorta	A–P

Table 10.14 A sample of contrast enhanced renal MRA is shown.

Sequences	Comments	Slice order
3 Plane localizer	Acquire 5–10 slices in each plane	
Axial 2D TOF scout	Prescribe axial slices without gating as a localizer aorta MRA. Use MIPs for coronal planning	S–I
3D FSPGR CE	Prescribe coronal slices to cover aorta	A–P
TRICKS/CENTRA	Prescribe coronal slices to cover aorta	A–P

Table 10.15 Alternative phase contrast–based NCE aorta MRA protocols are shown.

Sequences	Comments	Slice order
3 Plane localizer	Acquire 5–10 slices in each plane	
Axial 2D fiesta	Prescribe axial slices for bright blood imaging	S–I
Coronal 2D fiesta	Prescribe coronal slices for bright blood imaging	
Axial 2D TOF	Prescribe axial slices for the region of interest	S–I
Coronal 2D/3D PC	Prescribe coronal slices for the region of interest and enter a venc value	A–P
Axial Inhance/Native	Prescribe axial slices using the new NCE-MRA techniques if available on your system	A–P

Table 10.16 Renal MRA imaging parameters for a multichannel body coil are given.

	2D Fiesta	Fast 2D TOF localizer	3D FSPGR CE	2D TOF Artery	3D PC arteries/venous	2D PC arteries	TRICKS/TWIST/CENTRA
Plane	Ax, Cor, Sag	Axial	Coronal	Axial	Axial/coronal	Coronal	Coronal
Sequence	Fiesta	TOF	FSPGR	TOF	PC	PC	TRICKS
TE	MinFull	Min	Min	Min	Min	Min	Min
TR	Auto	Min	Auto	Min	20	33	Auto
BW	125.00	15.63	41.67	31.25	15.63	15.63	83.33
Slice thickness	4.0	5.0	3.2	2.0	3.0	20	2.8
Slice spacing	0.0	0.0	−1.6	0.0	0.0	0.0	−1.4
FOV	35	40	40	35	35	35	35
Matrix	256 × 256	256 × 128	352 × 192	256 × 160	256 × 192	256 × 160	288 × 160
NEX/NSA	0.75	0.75	0.75	1	1	4	0.75
Frequent direction	R–L	R–L	S–I	R–L	R–L/S–I	S–I	S–I
Venc	PG				70	60	
Number of phases	ECG		2		15		13
Gating/FA	45	45	BH/30	45	PG/20	PG/20	30
k-space order			Centric				4D

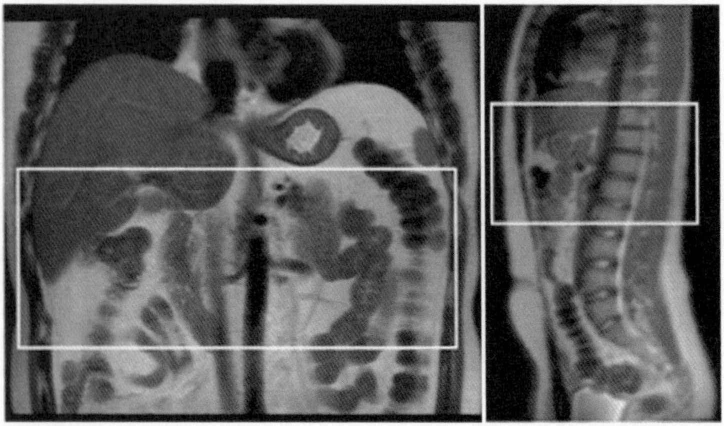

Figure 10.21 Axial 2DTOF, 3D PC or 3D NCE Renal MRA planning from coronal and sagittal images is shown.

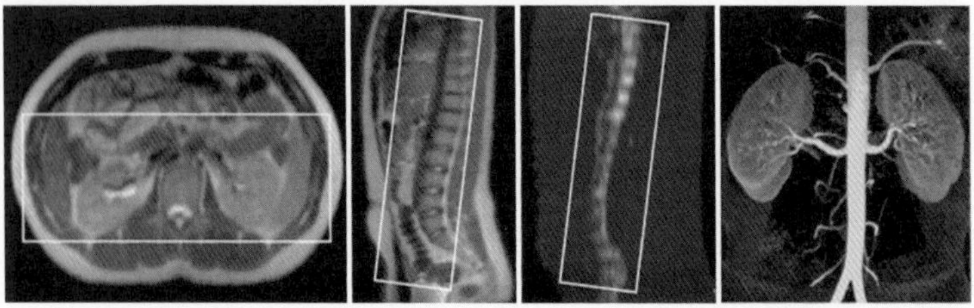

Figure 10.22 Coronal 3D CE Renal MRA planning from axial, sagittal, and scout 2D TOF MIP images is shown.

Graphical Prescription

See Figs. 10.21 and 10.22.

Peripheral Angiography (Three or Four Stations)

Peripheral MR angiography is used to image the peripheral vasculature including iliac division. With the introduction of multislice CT, peripheral angiography exams are frequently referred to CT scans. However, the fast and efficient contrast enhanced peripheral MRA and the recently developed non-contrast MRA techniques make peripheral MRA very attractive once again.

Peripheral MRA exams typically require multiple angiography exams of the peripheral vascular runoffs. Therefore, the MR scanner should be able to scan multiple locations or stations with an automatic table movement for a successful MRA exam. For CE-MRA, a precontrast, arterial, and even venous phase image can be acquired and created individually. For Non Contrast Enhanced MRA, the type of images will be dependent on the type of sequence you are using. The recent fresh blood imaging (FBI) type of acquisition can successfully acquire the arterial MRA but may not be very suitable to venous MRA due to slow flow in veins. However there are various researches going on for NCE-MRV for the time being. In any case, the acquired images are reconstructed as 3D MIP MRA images from each station and then can be pasted together to create an image of peripheral vascular tree.

Almost all the vendors today have MR scanner and whole body coil systems, which can make peripheral MRA patient positioning much simpler. However, if you have an MR scanner without the embedded whole body coil systems, you can use the magnet body coil in the bore and/or place additional coils for the region of interest.

For CE-MRA studies of peripheral MRA, the first station is almost identical to renal MRA planning. Second and third stations and critical contrast injection speed will be covered below in the patient preparation section.

Patient preparation: The patient consent form should be given to the patient with a detailed explanation on the content. The form should be carefully read, all questions must be answered with clear answers such as "YES" or "NO," and additional clarifications should be written. It must be signed by the patient or legal guardians and confirmed by MR personnel. If there are any surgical implants, radiologist on duty has to make a decision based on implant type and MR compatibility. *If there is any suspicion or lack of information on the implant, do not take any risk with the patient safety and do not scan the patient.* If the form is complete with all the information, the patient should change to MR gown and remove any clothing with any metal. It is always a good practice to remove the jewelry as well. As the last line of patient safety, it is also a good practice to scan patient with a handheld metal detector before taking the patient to MR room.

Patient positioning (three stations): If you are going to use body coil for peripheral MRA and place an additional coil for a selected region of interest, you need to first decide where you will be placing the high density coil for better image quality as shown in Figs. 10.23, 10.24 or 10.25. The coil placement might depend on patient history and symptoms. However, if you do not have

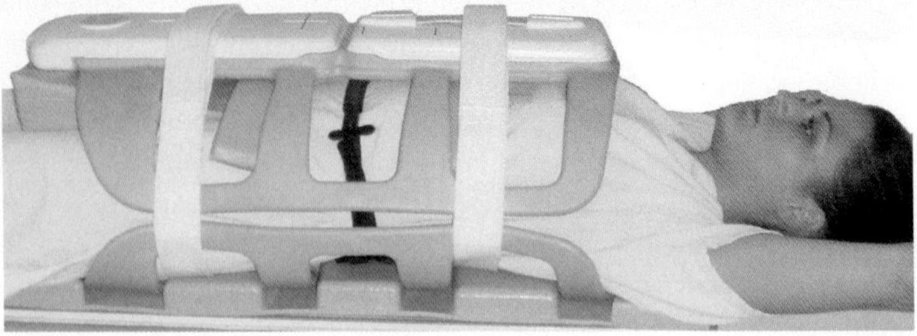

Figure 10.23 Multichannel coil can be positioned at first station if you plan to use body coil for other stations.

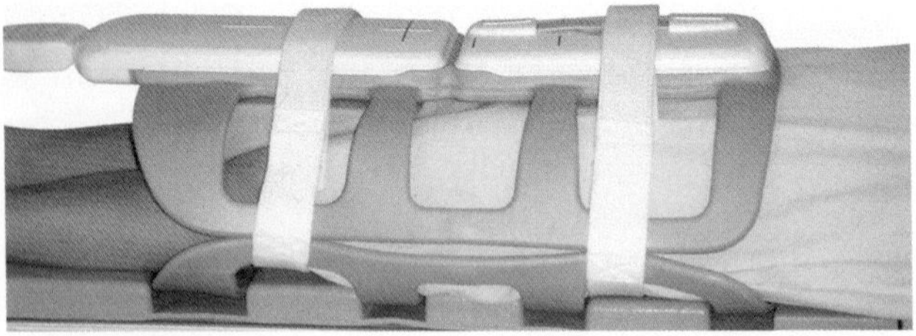

Figure 10.24 Multichannel coil can be positioned at second station if you plan to use body coil for other stations.

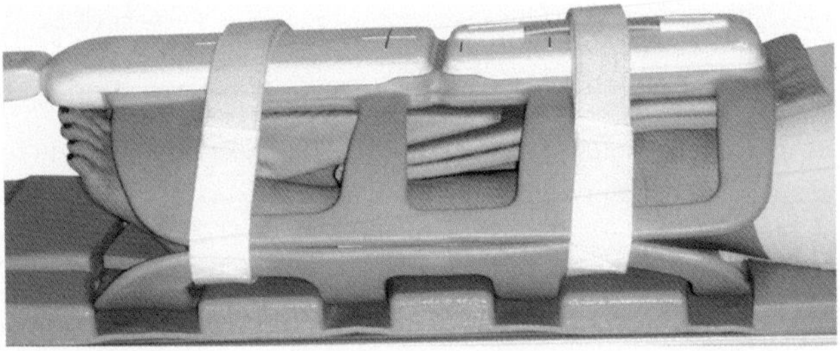

Figure 10.25 Multichannel coil can be positioned at third station if you plan to use body coil for other stations.

any preference, third station or lower legs would be the preferred location for multichannel coil as shown in Fig. 10.25. The patient body should be as straight as possible on the horizontal place for an efficient image pasting. To make the body straight, you place additional pads under the patient legs and raise them slightly. You can also place respiratory bellows simply to make sure that patient follows the breath hold instructions.

For peripheral MRA, remember that the table will move automatically according to the protocol you set up. Hence, you need to make sure the table moves to the right location and still creates an overlapped coverage with the previous station. The overlap between stations can be quite small. However, 10–20% overlap makes the image pasting more efficient. Therefore, if you choose an FOV of 48 cm, the table should move around 40 cm or less for the next station. To ensure a good overlap and accurate positioning, you can mark the center of lower stations and landmark 80 cm superior as your first station center. This way, you will know that the table will move to second station for upper legs and third station for lower legs.

When you are ready, you give the alarm/buzzer to patient's hand and test it before sending in. After landmarking the center of coil using laser lights or touch sensors, you can send the patient in and start the exam. It is always recommended to let the patient know how long the scan is going to take and also keep communicating frequently to make them as comfortable as possible in the MR bore.

Contrast injection: Double dose contrast injection can create high-quality MRA images of peripheral tree. After checking the patient renal function, you may inject about 0.3–0.4 cc/kg for 0.5 M contrast agents. Half of the total contrast agent can be injected at a rate of 1.5 cc/s and the rest can be injected at 1 cc/sec followed by 20 cc saline at the same injection rate. Higher injection rates would create venous contamination especially in lower legs. A power injector should be used for injection if available (Table 10.17).

Sample Imaging Parameters for 1.5T

Figs. 10.24–10.25.

Tips and Tricks

- The axial 2D TOF acquisition for body MRA and peripheral MRA shows major arterial vessel structures. For high resolution contrast enhanced 3D MRA, use 2D TOF MIPS in sagittal plane to make sure that you do not exclude sections of the vessel.
- For further background suppression, precontrast (MASK) 3D images are subtracted from CE MRA images.

Table 10.17 A sample Contrast Enhanced three station peripheral MRA is shown.

Sequences	Comments	Slice order
3 Plane localizer 1	Acquire 9–11 breath hold slices in each plane. Table position will be at center	
3 Plane localizer 2	Acquire 9–11 slices in each plane. Table position will be at inferior 400 mm	
3 Plane localizer 3	Acquire 9–11 slices in each plane. Table position will be at inferior 800 mm	
Axial fast TOF 1	Prescribe axial slices to cover entire region as a localizer. Use MIPs for coronal planning	S–I
Axial fast TOF 2	Prescribe axial slices to cover entire region as a localizer. Use MIPs for coronal planning	S–I
Axial fast TOF 3	Prescribe axial slices to cover entire region as a localizer. Use MIPs for coronal planning	S–I
3D FSPGR CE-1	Prescribe coronal slices to cover aorta and use localizer 2D TOF MIPS for planning	A–P
3D FSPGR CE-2	Prescribe coronal slices and use localizer 2D TOF MIPS for planning	A–P
3D FSPGR CE-3	Prescribe coronal slices and use localizer 2D TOF MIPS for planning	A–P

- For multistation angiography pasting more than 20% overlap between stations is recommended.
- Automated table movement setting differs for each vendor. For a proper peripheral station, follow the instructions given by the vendor for your system options, coil availability, and magnetic field.
- Higher SNR and better T1 enhancement on 3.0T make it possible to acquire high-quality peripheral MRA with less contrast amount.
- Embedded multichannel coil systems (TIM, GEM, ATLAS) can use parallel imaging in all stations and make it possible to cover more slices. With those systems, you can directly plan from 3 plane localizer images without worrying about excluding sections of vessels.

Graphical Prescription

See Figs. 10.26–10.28.

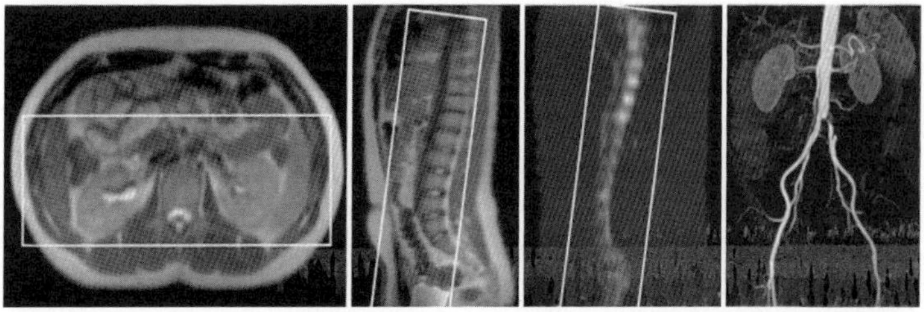

Figure 10.26 Coronal 3D peripheral MRA planning from axial, sagittal, and scout 2D TOF MIP images is shown for the first station.

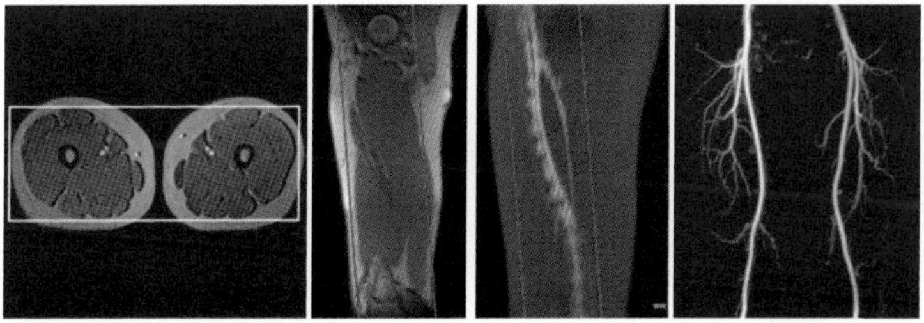

Figure 10.27 Coronal 3D peripheral MRA planning from axial, sagittal, and scout 2D TOF MIP images is shown for the second station.

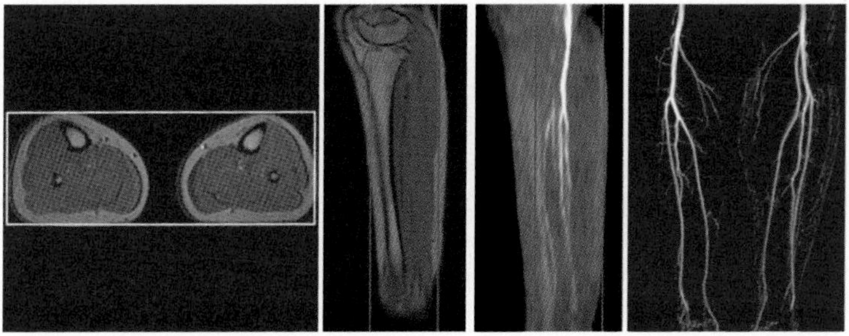

Figure 10.28 Coronal 3D peripheral MRA planning from axial, sagittal, and scout 2D TOF MIP images is shown for the third station.

Table 10.18 Three station peripheral CE-MRA imaging parameters for a multichannel coil (placed on the station) and body coil are given.

	Fast TOF localizer	3D CE first station	3D CE second station	3D CE third station
Plan	Axial	Coronal	Coronal	Coronal
Sequence	TOF	FSPGR	FSPGR	FSPGR
TE	Min	Min	Min	Min
TR	Min	Auto	Auto	Auto
BW	15.63	83.33	83.33	62.50
Slice thickness	5	2.8	2.8	2.8
Slice spacing	0	−1.4	−1.4	−1.4
FOV	40	46	46	46
Matrix	256 × 128	352 × 192	352 × 192	352 × 352
NEX/NSA	0.75	0.75	0.75	0.75
Frequent direction	R–L	S–I	S–I	S–I
Venc/number of phases		/2	/2	/2
Gating/FA	45	BH/30	BH/30	BH/30
k-space order		Centric	Elliptical centric	Elliptical centric

Contrast Enhanced MRA Considerations: Contrast Injection Dynamics and Data Acquisition Order Selection

As we discussed in earlier chapters, the MR operator can change the imaging parameters to manipulate the resulting contrast of the MR image. The inherent tissue parameters such as proton density, T1 relaxation, and T2 relaxation cannot be manipulated by the user directly. However, the contrast injection can temporarily reduce both T1 and T2 relaxations of the tissues. The T2 relaxation time reduction with contrast injection will further reduce the SNR of T2 weighted images and may not have much clinical value with the exception of brain perfusion imaging. On the other hand, the T1 relaxation time reduction with contrast injection will increase the signal from the tissue with higher amount of contrast concentration such as blood vessels, tumors, etc. Therefore; contrast injection will enhance the T1 contrast of the images. This is why we call postcontrast T1 images as contrast enhanced (CE) (Fig. 10.29).

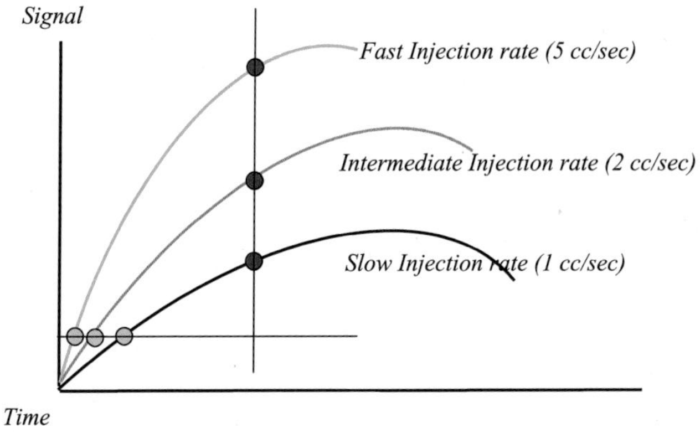

Figure 10.29 The T1 signal enhancement with different contrast injection rate is shown.

The degree of contrast enhancement will be proportional to the contrast injection rate and amount. If the same amount of contrast agent is injected, they will produce almost the same signal enhancement at the steady state. This means that if you are injection contrast agent to acquire a postcontrast T1 image for brain tumors, how fast you inject the contrast agent will have no significant effect on the resulting postcontrast images. However, this is not the case for MRA acquisitions. As shown in Fig. 10.29, the dynamic signal enhancement with contrast injection will be quite different for fast, intermediate, and slow injection rate. Let's take a look at the contrast injection rate tradeoffs.

Contrast Injection Rate Effects

Fast injection: Fast contrast injection at about 5 cc/s can be used only for brain or cardiac perfusion applications but not for MRA applications. Fast injection of 20 cc contrast agent at a 5 cc/s will create a compact contrast bolus. This bolus will create a high signal enhancement but its length will be quite short. For example, if you do a renal MRA with 5 cc/s injection, you will get an inhomogenous vessel. Depending on your timing, you will get a very bright signal in a certain section of the vessel but the rest will be fairly hypointense. In addition, the fast injection will make venous contamination more frequent in arterial MRA, especially with carotid MRA.

Intermediate injection: Intermediate injection around 2 cc/s is more commonly used for most of MRA applications. The intermediate contrast injection will create a good balance between signal enhancement and blood circulation dynamics. An intermediate injection of 20 cc contrast agent will take about 10 s to complete. After some mix up in the heart, it will pump to arterial vascular system. If we set up a typical 18-s breath hold aortic MRA protocol, we will acquire a fairly homogenous CE-MRA from the aorta. The MR acquisition times for carotid MRA can be on the order of 18 s in the older systems or 50 s on the newer systems. However, the longer carotid MRA acquisitions use specially ordered k-space acquisitions such as elliptical centric and can effectively acquire the majority of the MR signal at 5–8 s. Therefore, we can still acquire a very beautiful and uniform MRA with little or no venous contamination in carotid vessels.

Slow injection: Slow contrast injection rates between 0.5 and 1 cc/s are used in mainly peripheral vascular MRA application for the lower stations. The slow injection will create a longer duration of uniform contrast concentration in the vessels at the expense of reduced signal enhancement. A slow injection of 20 cc contrast agent will take about somewhere between 20 and 40 s to complete. After some mix up in the heart, it will be pumped to arterial vascular system. The slow injection will create a long and homogenous MR signal in the vessels. Therefore, they can be suitable only for peripheral MRA in the lower stations and sometimes 4D dynamic imaging. This is why we use two different injection rates for peripheral MRA applications. The initial intermediate injection rate for the top station will provide a beautiful MRA of the abdominal aorta and following slower injection will create peripheral runoff angiography with relatively smaller venous contaminations.

K-Space Data Acquisition Orders

In the past, MRA acquisition had been done with a standard linear data acquisition orders. However, thanks to advances in MR imaging, now, we have several different raw data acquisition orders. We are sure you will also agree with us that the new data acquisition orders make things much more complicated contrary to what we had. However, as an MR operator, you can be aware of these different techniques to make the best educated protocol selection.

The k-space or raw data ordering may vary from vendor to vendor and we provide few common acquisition orders here as fundamental information. We encourage you to consult with your MR manufacture's user manual for detailed information.

Linear filling: The linear k-space filling option acquires the k-space from top to bottom in phase encoding direction. For 3D acquisitions, it will also acquire k-space from the first slice to last in sequential order. Therefore, if your scan time is about 18 s, the center of k-space would be acquired around 9–10 s (half the time). Most of the older MRA techniques used linear k-space filling. However, it requires lower resolution and/or higher acceleration to reduce the total scan time.

Centric filling: The centric k-space filling option acquires the center of k-space first as the name indicates. Afterward, it starts filling the rest of k-space for complete information. Therefore, if your scan time is about 18 s, the center of k-space would be acquired around 6 s (a third of total time). This technique suits well for the MRA application in which capturing the arterial phase is very important. Most of the aorta and renal MRA acquisition use centric k-space ordering by default.

Elliptical centric: The elliptical centric k-space filling option acquires the center of k-space first in an elliptical fashion as the name indicates. Afterward, it starts filling the rest of k-space for complete information. Therefore, if your scan time is about 18 s, the center of k-space would be acquired around the first 2–3 s (a sixth or ninth of total time). This technique suits well for the carotid and peripheral runoff MRA application in which capturing the peak arterial phase very fast is very important. Most of the carotid and runoff MRA acquisition use elliptical centric k-space ordering.

Reverse centric: The reverse centric k-space filling option is almost an exact opposite of centric k-space filling and acquires the center of k-space last as the name indicates. Afterward, it starts filling the rest of k-space for complete information. Therefore, if your scan time is about 18 s, the center of k-space would be acquired around the last 6 s (a third of total time). This technique can be potentially used for manual control of injection timing by the user rather than automated injection contrast triggering methods.

Reverse elliptical centric: The reverse elliptical centric k-space filling option is almost an exact opposite of elliptical centric k-space filling and acquires the center of k-space last as the name indicates. It starts filling the outer parts of k-space first and leaves the center of k-space for end. Therefore, if your scan time is about 18 s, the center of k-space would acquired to be around the last 2–3 s. This technique can be potentially used for manual control of injection timing by the user rather than automated injection contrast triggering methods.

Contrast Injection Study Examples

If you were hoping that MR is getting easier, we have to tell you that it is getting more complicated with the development of new imaging techniques and k-space manipulations. The k-space or raw data manipulations are invisible to us and difficult to imagine what they can do. Therefore, it is becoming more important to follow the guidelines of your vendor for specific MRA protocol.

In the last couple of pages of the book, we will give a contrast injection scenario hoping to shed some light into the decision making process of a routine clinical day.

Practical scenario 1: Let's assume that we want to acquire an 18 s long pulmonary MRA on a 75 kg patient. What would be the delay time for elliptical centric MRA acquisition? (Consider 0.4 cc/kg).

Practical planning 1: Assuming a single dose injection with a half molar contrast agent such as omniscan, magnevist, dotarem, etc. you inject 0.4 cc/kg (30 cc total). The approximate contrast arrival to pulmonary vessels would be around 7.5 s with an injection rate of 4 cc/s. If you use an automatic triggering with a tracker placed at pulmonary aorta, the system will detect the contrast agent when the vascular signal increases 15 or 20% of the precontrast level (which will be increased only with 4.5 cc). Remaining contrast amount 25.5 cc with injection of 4 cc/sec will create a contrast bolus around 6.5 s (25.5 cc/4 cc). It is essential to collect the center of k-space during peak time. The peak time of bolus within the vessels is generally around half of the injection time, which will be 3.5 s in this example. This means we should start to fill the center of k-space with a certain delay. However, we already need some delay time to give the breath hold instruction. Therefore, we expect you to spend 4–5 s for instruction, and the acquisition has to start exactly at the time contrast detection using 18 s of elliptical k-space ordered MRA acquisition to get uniform enhancement.

As you can imagine, in clinical environment, executing a successful pulmonary MRA requires a good contrast timing planning and also a perfect patient collaboration. However, even if the patient can hold the breath easily for 18 s, it is not easy to synchronize the starting point of patient breath hold with the contrast detection time. Therefore, 4D dynamic CE MRA techniques such as TRICKS, TWIST, or CENTRA may provide much better to such demanding applications and make contrast detection timing almost absolute. In addition to reasonable CE-MRA, 4D sequences provide quite useful dynamic contrast filling information.

Practical scenario 2: Let's assume that we want to acquire an 18 s long renal MRA on a 75 kg patient. What would be the delay time for centric MRA acquisition?

Practical planning 2: Assuming a double dose injection with a half molar contrast agent such as omniscan, magnevist, dotarem, etc., you inject 0.4 cc/kg (30 cc total). The approximate contrast arrival to pulmonary vessels would be around 15–16 s with an injection rate of 3 cc/s. If you use an automatic triggering with a tracker placed at descending aorta, the system will detect the contrast agent when the vascular signal increases 15 or 20% of the precontrast level. A total of 30 cc contrast injection at 3 cc/s will create a contrast bolus around 10 s (30 cc/3s). This means if we should acquire the center of k-space 6–7 s after the arrival of contrast agent to get a uniform arterial peak. Therefore, the breath hold acquisition should 5–6 s after the contrast detection. Five to six seconds would be enough to give breath hold instructions to patients.

The contrast injection timing requires a certain degree of experience from the user not only for the timing purposes but also for interacting with the patients with a broad range of physical conditions. Even though the contrast injection can be very fast for MRA applications, its use is still off-label for MRA applications. It also requires a somewhat intervention to place the IV line. Therefore, the new NCE-MRA techniques should be used with your radiologist's approval as long as they do not interfere with a good diagnosis on the resulting images.

Chapter 11

Breast Imaging: MRI Protocols, Imaging Parameters, and Graphical Prescriptions

Traditionally, X-ray and ultrasound have been the main diagnostic tools for breast imaging due to their world-wide availability, ease of use, adequate sensitivity, and short acquisition times. The new developments of 3D like mammography imaging, state-of-art software, and hardware still make them a very powerful diagnostic tool. However, with the development of new software and hardware, modern MRI emerged as a key diagnostic tool with the highest sensitivity and specificity. Multiple imaging contrast, better soft tissue differentiation, higher resolution, and safer nature of MR imaging make breast MR imaging as one of the fastest growing imaging procedure, especially for high-risk patients.

Breast MR imaging should be done using multichannel or multielement coils for better SNR. Whenever possible, breast coils designed specifically for the anatomy of breast should be used for consistent image quality. The multiple contrast imaging of mass or non–mass-like breast lesions are very important. However, the dynamic contrast enhanced breast MRI can provide a great deal of information about the lesion type and characteristics. Signal enhancement slope and/or signal enhancement graphs can be used in combination with breast MR imaging in different lesions and patient follow-up.

A routine breast MR imaging protocol can include the following sequences:

- Fat saturated axial or sagittal FSE T2.
- Axial or sagittal FSE T1.
- Dynamic 3D gradient echo T1 during the contrast injection. The acqusition should cover at least 6–8 min post injection.

M. Elmaoğlu and A. Çelik, *MRI Handbook: MR Physics, Patient Positioning, and Protocols*, DOI 10.1007/978-1-4614-1096-6_11,

- Breast imaging with either silicone or saline implants should have either an IR sequence (STIR) or water-fat seperation sequences (IDEAL, Dixon) to better differentiate the implants from the breast tissue.
- Additional sequences such as DWI and breast spectro can be included in the routine breast protocol as well.

Patient preparation: The patient consent form should be given to the patient with a detailed explanation on the content. The form should be filled and signed by the patient with the help of MR personnel. If there are any surgical implants, radiologist on duty has to make a decision based on implant type and MR compatibility. *If there is any suspicion or lack of information on the implant, do not take any risk with the patient safety and do not scan the patient.* If the form is complete with all the information, the patient should change to MR gown and remove any clothing with any metal. The medical gown should have an opening on the chest to place to position the breasts in the breast coil. It is always a good practice to remove the jewellery as well. As the last line of patient safety, it is also a good practice to scan patient with a handheld metal detectors before taking the patient to MR room.

Patient positioning: Place the coil straight at the center of the MR table. Then you position the patient prone on the coil while the arms are extended forward and folded comfortably. The coil center should align with the center of breast mass for females and nipple for male patients.

Please make sure that you give the patient alarm/buzzer to patient's hand and test it. After landmarking the center of coil using laser lights or touch sensors, you can send the patient in and start the exam. It is always recommended to let the patient know how long the scan is going to take and also keep communicating frequently to make them as comfortable as possible in the MR bore (Fig. 11.1).

Sample imaging protocols: A sample imaging protocol for a patient referred to the MRI for breast examination is given below (Table 11.1).

Sample imaging parameters for 1.5T: Table 11.2.

Tips and tricks:

- A single oblique saturation band can be placed on axial or sagittal images to reduce the respiratory and cardiac artifacts at the expense of minimal SAR exposure increase.
- A single NEX (NSA) and higher matrix can provide beautiful T1 weighted images with higher resolution and shorter scan times.

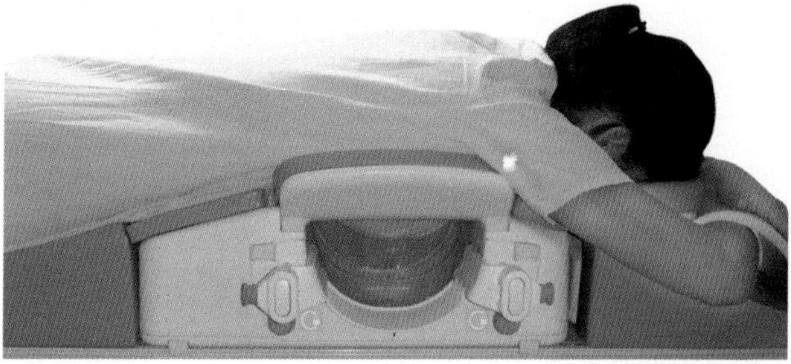

Figure 11.1 A sample feet first and prone patient breast positioning for a multichannel breast coil is shown.

Table 11.1 A sample routine breast protocol (1.5T and 3.0T).

Sequences	Protocol comments	Slice order
3 Plane or scout	Acquire ten slices in each plane	
Axial STIR or IDEAL/Dixon	Prescribe straight 3-mm axial slices to cover the breasts. This type of sequence can provide a robust fat suppression	S–I
Axial T1 FSE	Same as above	S–I
Sagittal T2 Fat saturation	Prescribe sagittal slices separately for each breast instead of a single block to cover them at once. Separate acquisition for each breast can provide much more robust fat saturation	R–L
Axial 3D dynamic multiphase (7–8 min)	Prescribe axial VIBRANT, VIBE, or similar 3D T1 weighted sequences with spectral inversion recovery for a better fat saturation	S–I
Axial delayed 3D Fat Sat T1 isotropic	This sequence can be modified from dynamic sequence for higher resolution or isotropic acquisition	S–I
Axial DWI	The *b* value should be selected 500 or larger	S–I
Spectroscopy	It should be planned on the sequence that lesion is clearly identified	S–I

- A minimum TE should be selected with 3D T1 acquisitions for shorter TR and faster acquisitions.
- The selected FOV on sagittal fat saturation images should be large enough to cover only the breast for efficient fat saturation.
- Depending on the school of thought you are following, you can choose 1-min dynamic acquisition with adequate resolution or 2-min dynamic acquisition with higher resolution.

Table 11.2 A sample routine breast protocol is shown for a multichannel dedicated breast coil.

	STIR	T1	Fat saturation T2	Dynamic VIBRANT/VIBE	3D isotropic	DWI	IDEAL/Dixon
Plane	Axial	Axial	Sagittal	Axial	Axial	Axial	Axial
Sequence type	FSE-IR	FSE	FRFSE/RESTORE	VIBRANT/VIBE	VIBRANT/VIBE	EPI	FSE
TE	45	MinFull	85	Min	Min	Min	85
TR	5275	520	4300	Auto	Auto	2500	4400
ETL	10	3	18	–	–	–	14
BW	35.71	41.67	20.83	62.50	62.50	Auto	62
Slice thickness	3	3	4	2	1	3	3
Slice spacing	0.3	0.3	0.4	–	0	0.3	0.3
FOV	35	35	18	35	35	35	35
Matrix	416 × 256	512 × 320	256 × 256	350 × 350	350 × 350	192 × 192	416 × 224
NEX/NSA	1	1	2	1	1	12	1
Frequency direction	R–L	R–L	S–I	R–L	R–L	R–L	R–L
SAT band	–	–	Auto	TI: Auto/FA: 10	Auto/10	600	–
Parallel imaging	On	On	Off	On	On	On	On

- The frequency direction for axial DWI can be chosen as R/L to reduce geometric distortions.
- DWI imaging can be performed only in one diffusion encoding direction (slice direction is preferred) with higher NEX to create high-quality DWI images.

Graphical prescription: Figs. 11.2 and 11.3.

Image processing:

The dynamic breast imaging can provide a great deal of information, especially for mass-like lesions. The dynamic imaging series includes at least one precontrast image and several postcontrast images acquired during the contrast injection. The lesions signal enhancement within the first 2 min, and the following signal enhancement pattern can be used to classify the contrast enhancement to different types. A form of image processing software can be used to display the contrast enhancement curves since visual dynamic contrast enhancement

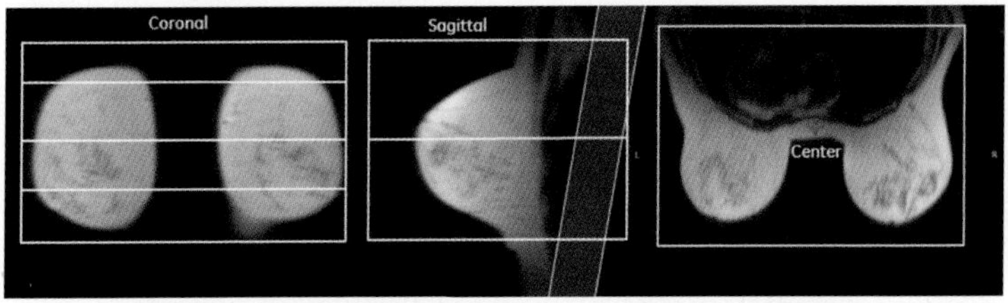

Figure 11.2 Axial planning from scout sagittal and coronal images is shown.

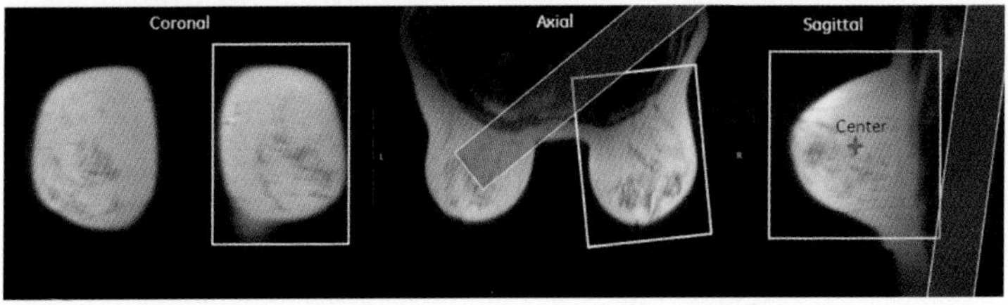

Figure 11.3 Sagittal planning from coronal and axial images is shown.

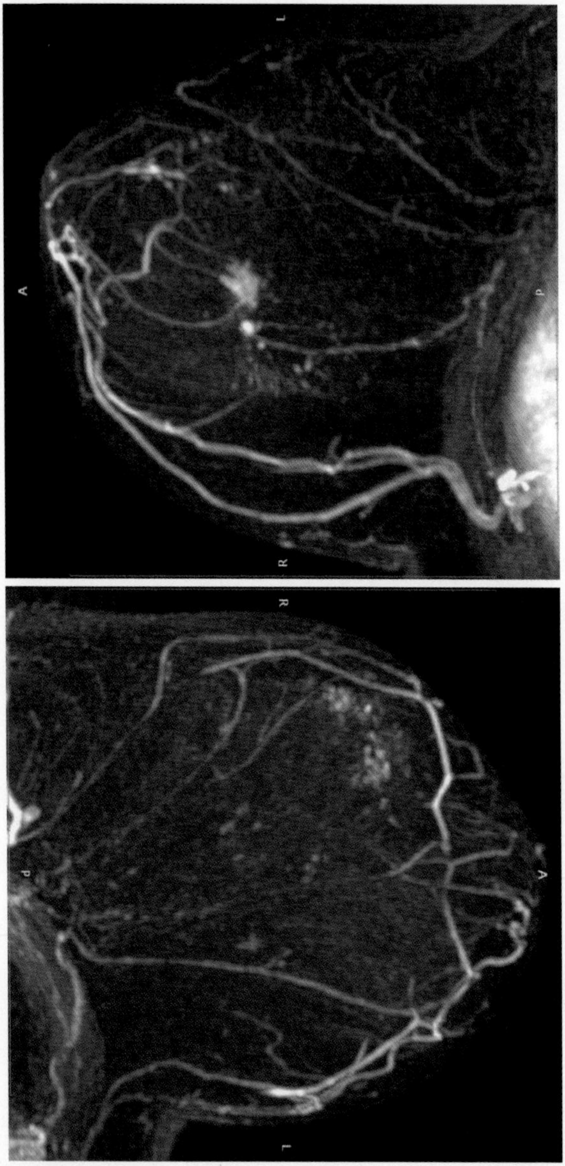

Figure 11.4 Sagittal bilateral MIP images from third phase of dynamic imaging are shown.

inspection is quite difficult. In literature, the signal enhancement patters for mass-like lesions are used to classify lesion enhancement to Type Ia, Ib, II, and III. Combination of breast MR images with image processing softwares can make the lesion detection and quantification much more efficient.

A number of different postprocessing softwares can be used to display signal enhancement graphs in absolute or percentage and wash-in and wash-out signal changes with or without patient motion correction algorithms. The recent computer aided diagnosis (CAD) tools can also show the color-coded images of lesions based on contrast enhancement percentage and wash-out characteristics of a number of lesions. The simple tools such as maximum intensity projections (MIP) over large volume or smaller volumes (subvolume MIPS) can also provide significant visual support to detect lesions easier compared to original images.

We strongly recommend our readers to keep up with the fast pace of image processing software and CAD softwares for a wide range of MRI applications (Fig. 11.4).

Further Reading

MA Brown, RC Semelka, MRI Basic Principles and Applications, Wiley-Liss, 1995.

Edelstein WA, Glover GH, Hardy CJ, Redington RW. The intrinsic signal-to-noise ratio in NMR imaging. *Magn Reson Med* 1986; 3:604–618

Elster AE, Burdette JH. *Questions and answers in magnetic resonance imaging*, 2nd ed. St. Louis: Mosby, 2001:6, 128

Baird AE, Warach S. Magnetic resonance imaging of acute stroke. J Cereb Blood Flow Metab 1998;18:583–609.

Kidwell CS, Wintermark M. Imaging of intracranial haemorrhage. Lancet Neurol 2008;7:256–267.

Suzuki M, Kishi H, Aso Y, Yashiro N, Iio M. Measurements of magnetic relaxation times of normal tissue and renal cell carcinoma. Radiat Med. 1988 Nov-Dec;6(6):263-6

P.C. Lauterbur, D.N. Levin, R.B. Marr; "Theory and Simulation of NMR Spectroscopic Imaging and Field Plotting by Projection Reconstruction Involving an Intrinsic Frequency Dimension." *J. Magn. Reson.* 59: 536-541 (1984).

Buxton RB, Frank LR & Prasad PV. (1996). Principles of diffusion and perfusion MRI. (In)*Clinical Magnetic Resonance Imaging* (vol)1 (ed 2 (Edelman RR, Hesselink JR, Zlatkin MB, eds)) Philadelphia, Saunders (pp): 233-270.

MR Technology Information Portal. http://www.mr-tip.com

J. Hornak. Basics of MRI. http://www.cis.rit.edu/htbooks/mri/

http://www.e-mri.org/

M. Elmaoğlu and A. Çelik, *MRI Handbook: MR Physics, Patient Positioning, and Protocols*, DOI 10.1007/978-1-4614-1096-6,

Norris DG. Principles of magnetic resonance assessment of brain function. J Magn Reson Imaging 2006;23:794–807.

de Bazelaire CM, Duhamel GD, Rofsky NM, Alsop DC. MR imaging relaxation times of abdominal and pelvic tissues measured in vivo at 3.0 T: preliminary results. *Radiology* 2004;230: 652-659

DW McRobbie, E Moore, MJ Graves, M Prince. MRI from picture to proton. Cambridge, UK, 2003.

C Westbrook. Handbook of MRI technique. Wiley-Blackwell, 1999.

Pretorius ES, Wickstrom ML, Siegelman ES. MR imaging of renal neoplasms. Magn Reson Imaging Clin N Am. 2000 Nov;8(4):813-36.

Bernstein MA, Huston J 3rd, Ward HA. Imaging artifacts at 3.0T. J Magn Reson Imaging 2006;24:735–46.

Le Bihan D, Poupon C, Amadon A, Lethimonnier F. Artifacts and pitfalls in diffusion MRI. J Magn Reson Imaging 2006;24:478–88.

Roberts TP, Mikulis D. Neuro MR: principles. J Magn Reson Imaging 2007; 26:823–37.

M R Prince, T M Grist, J F Debatin, 3D Contrast MR Angiography, Springer, 2003

http://www.mri-physics.com/

D D Stark, W G Bradley. Magnetic Resonance Imaging, Mosby, St. Louis, 1999

J. Gong and J.P. Hornak, "A Fast T_1 Algorithm." *Magn. Reson. Imaging* 10:623-626 (1992).

X. Li and J.P. Hornak, "T_2 Calculations in MRI: Linear versus Nonlinear Methods." *J. Imag. Sci. & Technol.* 38:154-157 (1994).

Lutsep HL, Albers GW, DeCrespigny A, Kamat GN, Marks MP & Moseley ME. (1997). Clinical utility of diffusion-weighted magnetic resonance imaging in the assessment of ischemic stroke. *Ann Neurol* 41: 574-580.

E M Haacke, R W Brown, M R Thompson, R Venkatesan. Magnetic Resonance Imaging: Physical Principles and Sequence Design. Wiley-Liss, 1999.

R R Edelman, M B Zlatkin and J Hesselink. Clinical Magnetic Resonance Imaging. WB Saunders Company, 1995.

A Celik, Validation of MR CBV Measurements, Doktora Tezi, Washington University, St. Louis, Missouri, ABD, 2000.

Bottomley PA, Foster TH, Argersinger RE and Pfeifer LM (1984). A review of normal tissue hydrogen NMR relaxation times and relaxation mechanisms from 1–100 MHz: dependence on tissue type, NMR frequency, temperature, species, excision, and age. *Med Phys* 11: 425–448

Steinhoff S, Zaitsev M, Zilles K and Shah NJ (2001). Fast T_1 mapping with volume coverage. *Magn Reson Med* 46: 131–140

Schenk JF (1995). Brain iron by magnetic resonance: T_2 at different field strengths. *J Neurol sci* 134: 10–18

Goldberg MA, Hahn PF, Saini S, Cohen MS, Reimer P, Brady TJ, Mueller PR. Value of T1 and T2 relaxation times from echoplanar MR imaging in the characterization of focal hepatic lesions. AJR Am J Roentgenol. 1993 May; 160(5):1011-7.

Rakow-Penner R, Daniel B, Yu H, Sawyer-Glover A, Glover GH. Relaxation times of breast tissue at 1.5T and 3T measured using IDEAL. J Magn Reson Imaging. 2006 Jan;23(1):87-91.

Ohtomo K, Itai Y, Furui S, Yashiro N, Yoshikawa K, Iio M. Hepatic tumors: Differentiation by transverse relaxation time (T2) of magnetic resonance imaging. *Radiology*, 155: 421–423, 1985.

Tomiha S, Iita N, Okada F, Handa S, Kose K. Relaxation time measurements of bone marrow protons in the calcaneus using a compact MRI system at 0.2 Tesla field strength. Magn Reson Med. 2008 Aug;60(2):485-8

M A Bernstein, K F King, X J Zhou, Handbook of MRI Pulse Sequences, Elsevier Academic Press 2004.

N Salibi, M A Brown, Clinical MR Spectroscopy, Wiley-Liss, 1998.

Stanisz GJ, Odrobina EE, Pun J, Escaravage M, Graham SJ, Bronskill MJ, Henkelman RM T1, T2 relaxation and magnetization transfer in tissue at 3T. Magn Reson Med. 2005 Sep;54(3):507-12.

Jones RA, Ries M, Moonen CT, Grenier N. Imaging the changes in renal T1 induced by the inhalation of pure oxygen: a feasibility study. Magn Reson Med. 2002 Apr;47(4):728-35.

Akber SF. NMR relaxation data of water proton in normal tissues. Physiol Chem Phys Med NMR. 1996;28(4):205-38.

Chen, D. 1997. Optimization of multiple overlapping thin slab acquisition (MOTSA) MRA. Med. Phys. 24, 1648 (1997).

Reimer, P., Parizel P.M. & Stichnoth, A-F., 2006. Clinical MR Imaging 2nd Ed. Germany: Springer.

Baert, A.L. & Sartor, K., Dynamic Contrast-Enhanced Magnetic Resonance Imaging in Oncology. Germany: Springer.

Brown, MA. & Semelka, RC., 2010. MRI Basic Principles and Applications. 3rd Ed. New Jersey: Wiley-Liss.

Pingitore, et al., 2006. Myocardial Viability. In: MRI of the Heart. Italy: Springer.

Paelinck, BP & Lamb, HJ, 2008. Assessment of diastolic Function by Cardiac MRI. In: Cardiovascular Magnetic Resonance Imaging. New Jersey: Humana Press Inc.

Hodler, J., Schulthess, G.K. & Zollikofer, C.L., 2007. Disease of the Heart, Chest & Breast. Davos: Springer.

Runge, V.M., Nitz W.R. & Schmeets, S.H., 2009. 2nd Ed. The Physics of Clinical MRI: Taught Trough Images. Thieme, New York.

McRobbie, W.D., Moore, E.A., Graves, J.M., Prince, M.R., 2004. MRI Picture to Proton. UK: Cambridge University Press.

Hussain, S. M., 2007. Liver MRI: Correlation with Other Imaging Modalities and Histopathology. NY: Springer.

Westbrook, et al., 2008. MRI in Practice, 3rd Ed. UK: Blackwell Publishing.

www.mrisafety.com

www.acr.org

www.fda.gov/default.htm

www.imrser.org/Default.asp

Index